MANUAL
of
ARTICULATION
and
PHONOLOGICAL
DISORDERS

Infancy through Adulthood

SECOND EDITION

Clinical Competence Series

Series Editor
Robert T. Wertz, Ph.D.
Lee Ann C. Golper, Ph.D.

MANUAL
of
ARTICULATION
and
PHONOLOGICAL
DISORDERS

Infancy through Adulthood

SECOND EDITION

Ken M. Bleile, Ph.D.

THOMSON

DELMAR LEARNING™

Australia   Canada   Mexico   Singapore   Spain   United Kingdom   United States

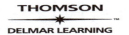

Manual of Articulation and Phonological Disorders:
Infancy through Adulthood, Second Edition
Ken M. Bleile

**Executive Director,
Health Care Business Unit:**
William Brottmiller

Editorial Editor:
Cathy L. Esperti

Acquisitions Editor:
Kalen Conerly

Developmental Editor:
Juliet Byington

Executive Marketing Manager:
Jennifer McAvey

Channel Manager:
Lisa Osgood

Marketing Coordinator:
Kim Lourinia

Editorial Assistant:
Olivia Mars

Production Coordinator:
John Mickelbank

Art and Design Coordinator:
Connie Lundberg-Watkins

Project Editor:
Daniel Branagh

Library of Congress
Cataloging-in-Publication Data

Bleile, Ken Mitchell.
    Manual of articulation and phonological disorders: infancy through adulthood / Ken M. Bleile.—2nd ed.
        p. ; cm.—(Clinical competence series)
    Includes bibliographical references and index.
        ISBN 0-7693-0256-4
    1. Articulation disorders. 2. Voice disorders.
    [DNLM: 1. Articulation Disorders—diagnosis—Handbooks.
    2. Articulation Disorders—therapy—Handbooks. WM 34 B646m 2004]
    I. Title.   II. Series.
    RC424.7.B45 2004
    616.85'5—dc22
                                    2003024193

NOTICE TO THE READER

CONTENTS

LIST OF APPENDICES

FOREWORD

com•pe•tence (kom´pə təns) n. The state or quality
of being properly or well qualified; capable.

Clinicians crave competence. They pursue it through education and experience,
through emulation and innovation. Some are more successful than others in attain-
ing what they seek. Fortunately, we have colleagues who assist us. Dr. Ken
M. Bleile is one of those. His effort, *Manual of Articulation and Phonological
Disorders: Infancy Through Adulthood,* is one of several books in the Singular
Clinical Competence Series. It is designed to move each of us further along the
path that leads to clinical competence. Dr. Bleile introduces us to the terminology,
tells us how to screen and appraise, leads us through the analysis of screening and
appraisal data, presents treatment principles, and lists facilitative techniques
designed to achieve the desired results. He is a skilled investigator and a competent clinician, and his book conveys what makes him that way. Dr. Bleile reaches
across generations—from old timers who grew up when there were only articulation disorders to recent graduates whose academic preparation emphasized phonological disorders. He creates order out of material that can be confusing, and he
demonstrates how what is known can be put into productive practice. Indeed, we
are fortunate to have colleagues like Ken Bleile who have "been there, done that,
and do it very well." Your attention to what he provides indicates your competence
and your effort to improve it, because competent clinicians seek competence as
much for what it demands as for what it promises.

Robert T. Wertz, Ph.D.
Series Editor

PREFACE

A person with an articulation and phonological disorder may be an infant, a toddler or preschooler, a school-age child, or an adult. Sometimes someone with an articulation and phonological disorder has speech as her or his only disability; more often, however, a person's difficulty in speech is embedded in other developmental and medical problems. Settings of care for a person with articulation and phonological disorder may be an early intervention program, preschool, school, hospital, or the home.

The second edition of this book, like the first, is a clinical resource for the care of persons with articulation and phonological disorders of all ages and levels of severity. This edition remains a compendium of materials and practical ideas for clinicians who wish to consider a range of clinical options, selecting those that seem good and discarding those that appear less appropriate. In addition to the chapters and appendixes included in the first edition, new and revised sections and appendixes include:

- Establishing clinical foundations of care
- Identifying milestones and individual differences in typical speech development
- Distinguishing dialect from disorder: varieties of American English
- Screening for phonological awareness
- Compiling a case history
- Finding "best bet" phonetic environments
- Selecting short-term goals and treatment targets

The first edition enjoyed wide use in the classroom as well as the clinic. Based on feedback from readers, two new chapters have been added. *Chapter 1: Foundations of Care* describes the social, linguistic, and biological foundations that underlie clinical care as described in this book. *Chapter 3: Speech Development* contains extensive discussion and clinically useful tables showing developmental milestones in speech perception and production, the connection between speech perception and production, and speech for purposes of communication.

ORGANIZATION OF THE TEXT

Key features of the text include a chapter overview of topics covered in each chapter to help direct the user to information quickly and easily. The text follows an outline format, giving clinicians the information they want without becoming lost in narrative. Throughout the text boxes highlight clinically relevant information and put clinical work in a real-life context. Chapter appendixes are an excellent resource for additional data and forms that can be used when working with clients. The text also provides a comprehensive reference list for individuals wanting to do further research on issues in articulation and phonology, as well as an index to make the text as accessible as possible.

The manual begins with a new chapter entitled *Foundations of Care*. This chapter describes the social, linguistic, and biological foundations on which clinical care is based. The types of questions addressed in this chapter include:

- Why do societies consider certain types of speech to be disordered?
- Why do speech disorders often affect language development?
- How is speech produced and perceived?
- What is the relationship between speech disorders, evolution, and brain development?
- What commonly held beliefs about speech disorders actually are speech myths?

Chapter 2: Articulation and Phonological Disorders is a practical overview of such basic topics as causes and definitions of speech disorders, the legal basis of care, medical precautions, notational conventions, transcription symbols, specialized technical terminology, and distinguishing dialect from disorder. Chapter 2 has information on African American English, Spanish-influenced English, and Asian-influenced English from Brian Goldstein; Hindi-influenced English from Jayanti Ray; Russian-influenced English from Anastasia Shilovskaya; Singapore-influenced English from Cherine Graham, Emilie Lam, Ashley Lee, Susan Loader, Isabel Tan, and Teresa To; and Turkish-influenced English from Seyhun Topbas.

The second new chapter, *Chapter 3: Speech Development*, describes developmental milestones and individual differences in speech development. Discussion and clinically useful tables are provided on speech perception, speech production, the link between speech perception and production, and speech for purposes of communication. Selected questions addressed in the chapter include:

- Why does a newborn have better speech perception than an adult?
- Why does a child babble?
- What does it mean to "learn the tune before the words"?
- How do speech demands change as a child progresses through school?

Chapter 4: Screening and Assessment describes options in nonstandardized and standardized screenings and complete assessments. The chapter concludes with appendixes of forms designed for use in clinical settings. New appendixes present case history questions and a screening test for phonological awareness contributed by Clifford Highnam.

Chapter 5: Analysis presents the most widely accepted options in articulation and phonological analysis. Major topics include measures to assess severity and intelligibility; age norms to assess prespeech vocalizations, phonetic inventories, error patterns, and consonants and consonant clusters; better methods by which to assess stimulability, key environments, key words, and responsiveness to phonetic placement and shaping techniques; and related analyses to determine adjusted and developmental age, the influence of dialect, and acquisition strategies. The chapter concludes with appendixes designed to assist clinicians in performing the major analyses described in the chapter.

Chapter 6: Treatment Principles and *Chapter 7: Facilitative Techniques* describe treatment principles and procedures, respectively. The major topics discussed in Chapter 6 include the purposes of treatment at four stages in articulation and phonological development; selection of long- and short-term goals, treatment targets, number of treatment targets, criteria for changing treatment targets, linguistic level and phonetic environments in which to introduce treatment targets; summaries of published treatment programs; and assessing treatment progress. A new appendix contributed by A. Lynn Williams compares approaches to phonological oppositions. Chapter 7 describes techniques designed to facilitate articulation and phonological development, including bombardment, metaphors, descriptions and demonstrations, touch cues, contrast therapy, building syllables and words, facilitative talk, and direct instruction. Chapter 7 concludes with extensive appendixes focusing on descriptions and demonstrations, word pairs, and phonetic placement and shaping techniques.

The book concludes with *Chapter 8: Options in Assessment and Treatment*, which summarizes the major care options for clients with articulation and phonological disorders. For convenience, the information in Chapter 8 is organized by stage of development. To illustrate, all assessment, analysis, and treatment options for a client in Stage 1 appear in the same section. This allows the reader focusing on a client in a specific developmental stage to readily consider all available care options.

My hope in writing a second edition is that the book will better meet the needs of clinicians, teachers, and students. I also hope that the new material conveys my enthusiasm for the study of that most human of topics, speech and its disorders.

Ken Bleile
September 2003

ACKNOWLEDGMENTS

I wish to thank the persons I have had the pleasure to treat during my long and ongoing apprenticeship in the study of articulation and phonological disorders. Much of the second edition of this book was written while I was an Erskine Fellow at the University of Canterbury, New Zealand. I wish to thank University of Northern Iowa's Graduate College and Department of Communicative Disorders for the sabbatical, and the Department of Speech and Language Therapy, University of Canterbury, for being such excellent hosts during my fellowship. Versions of new chapters were tried out on unsuspecting students and conference attendees, and I wish to thank the students in Foundations of Language (Fall semester 2002), my colleagues in the Republic of Singapore, and the Idaho Speech-Language-Hearing Association for their suggestions and comments. My special thanks also go to those who provided comments on earlier drafts of the manuscript, including Ann Smit and two other reviewers (anonymous) at Delmar Thomson Learning, and Elizabeth Abbott, Angie Burda, Terry Helinski, Cliff Highnam, and Joe Smaldino. Finally, I wish to thank Terry, Judy, and Zoe for making home the place I'd rather be.

For Terry, Judy, and Zoe

And for five giants in the field of articulation and phonological disorders:

Nick Bankson, John Bernthal, Barbara Hodson, Larry Shriberg, and Carol Stoel-Gammon

ABOUT THE AUTHOR

Ken Bleile is a professor in the Department of Communicative Disorders, University of Northern Iowa. During the last several years he has also served as a visiting scholar in the Ministry of Health, Singapore; in Hertzen University, Saint Petersburg, Russia; and in the University of Canterbury, New Zealand. Dr. Bleile was Speech-Language Pathology Chair of the 2003 ASHA conference, and is a recent Associate Editor for the *American Journal of Speech-Language Pathology.* Dr. Bleile is Editor of Delmar's *Clinical Resource Series* and publishes widely on speech development, pediatric head injury, and communication disorders in children with medical and developmental needs.

CHAPTER

1

Foundations of Care

The following topics are discussed in this chapter:

I. OVERVIEW

The purpose of this chapter is to describe the social, linguistic, and biological foundations on which the care of speech disorders is built. Types of questions a reader might have answered in this chapter include: Why do societies consider certain types of speech to be disordered? Why do speech disorders often affect language development? How is speech produced and perceived? What is the relationship between speech disorders, evolution, and brain development? What commonly held beliefs about speech disorders actually are speech myths?

To address these and other questions, speech and its disorders are considered from five perspectives, which are described in Section II. The role of speech in society is the topic of Section III. Speech and language are considered in Section IV, and speech production and perception is the topic of Section V. Current scientific thinking about the evolution of the human brain is the topic of Section VI, and the neurological basis of learning speech is addressed in Section VII. A summary of five perspectives on speech are presented in Section VIII, and speech myths are considered in light of ideas presented in the chapter in Section IX. A summary of clinical principles that form the foundation of care in this book are presented in Section X.

II. FIVE PERSPECTIVES ON SPEECH AND ITS DISORDERS

In Sections III through VII speech and its disorders are considered from five perspectives (Table 1–1).

Table 1–1. Five perspectives on speech and its disorders.

Perspective	Focus
Speech and Society	Social dimensions of speech
Speech and Language	Speech as a part of language
Speech Production and Perception	Speech as a channel of communication
Speech and Brain Evolution	Evolution of brain capacity for speech
Speech and Brain Development	Brain development that underlies speech learning

- **Speech and society:** Speech plays a critical role in human society. The social dimension of speech is discussed under the heading of *Speech and Society* (Section III). Included in this topic is a discussion of why societies tend to disvalue a person with a speech disorder.

- **Speech and language:** Speech is part of language. The role of speech in human language is discussed under the heading of *Speech and Language* (Section IV). The language aspect of speech is called phonology, and the word *phonological* is included in *articulation and phonological disorders* because speech disorders can arise in the speech aspect of language.

- **Speech production and perception:** In addition to being a part of language, speech also is a channel of communication. The nature of this channel is discussed under the heading of *Speech Production and Perception* (Section V). In the term *articulation and phonological disorders, articulation* refers to a type of speech problem involving the channel of communication.

- **Speech and brain evolution:** Modern human speech depends on possession of a brain sufficiently large and powerful to learn from the environment in which a child lives. The rapid evolution of human brain size over the past 2.5 million years is discussed under the heading *Speech and Brain Evolution* (Section VI). An understanding of speech disorders requires knowledge of the brain's role in speech.

- **Speech and brain development:** Speech learning and brain development are closely interconnected. The nature of brain development during childhood is discussed under the heading of *Speech and Brain Development* (Section VII). Included in this topic are discussions of how the brain and the environment interact during speech learning, how brain cells learn to connect, and the neurological basis of speech disorders.

III. SPEECH AND SOCIETY

Speech plays a critical role in human society, making possible at least four types of communication: between persons (talk), with oneself (thought), within and between groups (group identity), and across generations (cultural transmission). The roles of speech are depicted in Figure 1–1.

A. Talk

For at least the past 70,000 years, and likely much longer, humans have used speech to communicate with each other. Today, approximately

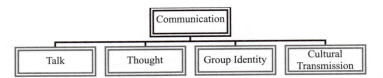

Figure 1–1. Four aspects of communication: talk, thought, group identity, and cultural transmission.

7,000 different languages exist in the world (Ethnologue, 2002). In each, the primary means of communication is the exchange of sound. Many languages have written systems in addition to spoken ones, allowing speech to be translated into graphic mediums. Modern inventions such as the telephone, DVD, and television have extended the realm of speech to transmission through electrical mediums.

B. Thought

Speech turned inward is an important vehicle of thought. Internal speech and images allow humans to regulate their own behavior, make plans, and reason. To illustrate, if you plan to ask an acquaintance to borrow a large sum of money, you might verbally rehearse what you will say, as well as reason with yourself whether this represents a good course of action. Inward speech is notoriously difficult to suppress. If you reflect a moment, inward speech often feels like a soft whisper in your mind. If you try, you can quiet this whisper, but typically only while you concentrate. When you stop concentrating, the whisper returns. A goal of many who meditate is to view the world without internal speech.

C. Group Identity

For both good and ill, speech is an important mechanism for group identity. That is, *my* group is the one that speaks *this* way, and *your* group is the one that speaks *that* way. Teenagers are particularly adept at using speech as a temporary social dialect to create group membership.

As a positive force, differences in speech celebrate human diversity and assert geographical and cultural identity. As a negative force, speech differences are used to denigrate and otherwise dehumanize groups of people. Greeks of antiquity divided the world into two groups: speakers of Greek and those unfortunate souls who spoke other languages. The Greek view was that the latter, lacking ability to think and speak Greek, were inherently inferior and largely incapable of rational thought. The speech of foreigners was considered mere noise, a kind of "bar bar bar bar," giving us the root of the word *barbarian*, or someone who speaks "bar bar" (Kitto, 1951). Of all the ways humans use to achieve group membership, speech is especially powerful for inclusion and exclusion, because in most situations a person cannot speak a community's language unless born and raised in the culture.

D. Cultural Transmission

Speech and its written equivalents are the primary means through which human beings transmit what is needful to survive from one generation to the next. Through speech and its written forms a society passes on knowledge and experiences to its children. In important and profound respects, speech serves the same function in the human species as instinct plays in others. The information a shark needs to survive, for example, is largely written in its genes. Little instruction from the environment is required. The situation for humans is different. Rather than having a survival manual as a genetic endowment, the human strategy uses speech as a mechanism through which an experienced person conveys information to a less experienced one.

E. Summary

Speech plays a central role in human society, and is the species' preeminent tool for communication. Though talking is its most obvious communicative function, speech is also critical for thought, plays a large role in determining group identity, and is essential to the transmission of culture from one generation to the next. Because speech has such a large social dimension, a speech disorder has social implications. As most parents of children with speech disorders readily attest, often the most worrisome aspect of a speech problem is not the child's pronunciation difficulty, but the possible consequences of the negative reaction of the child's peers—the child's sense of not fitting in, the resulting social isolation. Such parental concerns are real and the feared social consequences of a speech disorder sometimes occur, especially if a speech disorder persists into the later school years and adulthood. Because a speech disorder has a social dimension, a clinician's role includes understanding possible effects of the speech disorder on a person's life.

Speech Disorders in Society

Societies often denigrate a person with a speech problem. Tweety Bird is funny in part because she can't say [r], and *Four Weddings and a Funeral* and *'Tis* feature humorous clerics with similar speech problems. Sylvester the Cat lisps, as does a python-headed Egyptian god in a recent *New Yorker* cartoon who asks the god Anubis, who is sniggering, "Anubith? You find thomething humorouth?" (Shanahan, 2002). Society's message to a person with a speech problem is clear: you are comical, and someone not quite taken seriously. Or, as a lisping Ground Hog, too foolish to be aware of his own [s] problem, tells Pooh, "You've got to do something about that speech impediment, sonny!"

Though it is clear that society tends to demean persons with speech disorders, what may be less clear is that society's attention to speech disorders is out of proportion to effects such problems pose for communication, especially for those with milder disabilities. Though their speech is different from that of others, both Tweety Bird and Sylvester are perfectly understandable. Nor is it the case that certain sounds of speech are intrinsically good or bad. As the famous example of the king of Castile demonstrates, whether speech is considered disordered often has as much to do with who is speaking as it does with how words are said. As students sometimes are taught in Spanish classes, Castilian Spanish did not have a dental [s] until Castile had a king who lisped. Members of the court adopted the lisp, hoping to curry royal favor, and were followed in turn by the middle class, hoping to curry favor from the courtiers.

Why the fuss about what are, in essence, meaningless sounds, none of which are inherently better or worse than other sounds? For good and ill, societies often treat speech differences harshly because speech is a primary means through which peoples organize into groups (Section II). To varying extents societies hold the belief that "my group is the one that speaks *this* way, and your group is the one that speaks *that* way." Holding this concept, a society assigns positive attributes such as intelligence and cultivation to persons within their cultural group and may assign negative characteristics such as limited intelligence, bad manners, and vulgarity to those outside. In common with persons with foreign accents or with regional dialects, a person with a communication impairment signals not being a full-fledged member of the culture.

IV. SPEECH AND LANGUAGE

Speech has a dual nature: it is both a part of language and a channel (modality) of communication (Folkins & Bleile, 1990). As will be discussed in Chapter 2, the dual nature of speech is the basis of the conceptual distinction between phonological disorders (language disorders) and articulation disorders (disorders arising in the channel of communication). The focus of this section is the role of phonology (the language aspect of speech) in communication. The channel of communication through which language is realized is discussed in the following section (*Speech Production and Perception*).

A. Language

Language is critical to being human. No community of humans has been discovered that does not possess a language system with which to communicate. Indeed, so central is the view of humans as language users, were such a community to be discovered, they might well be considered nonhuman for the very reason that they lacked language. How can they be human if they do not possess language for communicating with each other, thinking abstractly, planning, organizing society, and transmitting culture from one generation to the next? A dark reflection of the central role of language in human affairs is that foreigners, speakers of less prestigious dialects, and persons with language disorders, because they are unable to use language in the same manner as others in their communities, may be shunned, excluded, and placed at significant social and economic disadvantage.

B. The Role of Speech

Speech is the cornerstone on which human language is built. Ironically, the most meaningful characteristic of this foundation is that it means nothing. To illustrate, the three sounds [s], [i], and [t] are meaningless, but make the word *seat* to refer to objects on which to sit. Elements such as distinctive features, syllables, and stress patterns also lack meaning (see Chapter 2 for discussion of terms). Thus, the words *below* and *ignite* share the same stress pattern (first syllable unstressed, followed by a stressed one), but mean different things.

Human speech differs from vocalizations of other species. Vocal tracts of both chimpanzees and bottlenose dolphins are capable of producing approximately 60 to 70 different sounds, each of which carries a different meaning. For example, a cry may have one meaning, a gurgle another, and lip smacking yet another. Because each sound is meaningful, the bottlenose dolphin and the chimpanzee are limited to the same number of meanings as the number of different sounds they can produce—that is, each can "talk" about 60 or 70 different things. Because human language has speech sounds without meaning, we enjoy the capacity to express a nearly infinite number of different meanings. To illustrate, because [s] lacks meaning in itself, it can be recruited to make words with such diverse meanings as *see*, *surf*, *bliss*, *sun*, and *sleet*. In no small measure, human adaptability depends on possessing a language system that allows the expression of an almost infinite number of meanings with a small set of sounds. This allows humans to enter a new environment and create vocabulary to describe the place in which they find themselves. This has allowed humans to spread out across the world and, in the future, may provide the means to explore and colonize such an unfamiliar environment as space.

C. Speech and Humanness

Humans have variously been defined as "the species that uses tools" or as "the species that tells lies." It turns out, though, that chimpanzees also use tools (Mercader, Panger, & Boesch, 2002); they sometimes dip a stick into an ant nest, and take it out covered with ants to enjoy an ant lollipop. And it turns out that the world is full of liars, from a chimpanzee that makes a cry that means, "Run! A leopard approaches!" to frighten away another chimpanzee trying to steal his food, to insects that look like leaves, to nonpoisonous spiders with the coloration of poisonous ones.

Speech has also been posited to be a unique feature of the human species (Hockett, 1960). Nearly 500 years before the modern study of linguistics, Francis Bacon, the great Renaissance poet and philosopher, defined humans according to three capacities, declaring, "We think according to nature. We speak according to rules. We act according to custom" (Wallace, 1967, p. 53). Research still must determine if the capacity for speech with meaningless elements is unique in the animal kingdom or just extremely rare (Marler, 1998; Hauser, 1996). Nonetheless, because speech is critical both to language and to being human, along with defining humans as being tool users and liars we might adopt the following definition: *humanity is the species whose cornerstone of communication means nothing*—the species whose foundation of communication is speech.

D. Summary

Speech has a dual nature, being both an aspect of language and a channel of communication. The language aspect of speech is called phonology. Speech is the foundation on which human language is built, allowing us to use finite means (a relatively small number of sounds) to create a nearly infinite number of words and sentences. So central is this ability to humanness that we might define humanity as the species whose cornerstone of communication means nothing.

Several clinical implications arise from consideration of speech and language. First, because speech is an aspect of language, a speech disorder may arise in the language domain. This is called a phonological disorder, and the idea of a language-based speech disorder is contained in the term *articulation and phonological disorder*. Second, because speech is a foundation of language, a speech disorder may produce a ripple effect across the language system. This effect occurs because speech difficulties may limit a person's ability to communicate using words, sentences, and other language elements.

V. SPEECH PRODUCTION AND PERCEPTION

Speech production and perception is the second aspect of speech's dual nature. This aspect of speech exists because of a problem that the human brain shares with those of all creatures with central nervous systems, from the small-brained shrew to the large-brained elephant. A central nervous system only understands and communicates in the language of electricity and chemicals. A brain cannot feel the wind or the touch of another person, unless those sensations are first translated into electrochemical language. Stated more broadly, a brain is unable to interact with the outside world directly, and requires translation systems to hear, smell, feel touch, see, and communicate.

How one human brain communicates with another is a fascinating speech domain. In overview, to produce and perceive speech requires the brain of the speaker to create an electrochemical message that is then converted successively into mechanical, acoustic, and hydraulic energy, before being converted back into electrochemical energy by the brain of the listener. The stages through which this energy is converted are depicted in Figure 1–2 and discussed below.

Electrochemical Energy

Broca's Area → Motor Strip → Motor Tracts

⇨

Mechanical Energy

Oral and Nasal Tracts

⇨

Acoustic Energy

Ambient Air

⇨

Mechanical Energy

Middle Ear, Round Window

⇨

Hydraulic Energy

Fluid in Cochlea

⇨

Mechanical Energy

Membrane and Hair Cells

⇨

Electrochemical Energy

Acoustic nerve → Wernicke's Area

Figure 1–2. Speech production and perception.

A. Electrochemical Energy (Broca's Area → Motor Strip → Motor Tracts)

Speech begins as electricity. Imagine that someone wants to say, "Good morning, everyone." The first step requires the brain to find electrical representations for the concepts of *good, morning,* and *everyone.* Words do not exist in a "word box" in the brain. Instead of an entire word in a single location, how a word sounds may be stored in one locale, a sight associated with a word may be stored in another, memories associated with a word means may be stored in another, how a word is pronounced may be stored in yet another, and so on. The totality of networks between brain cells is the word's meaning. A word, then, is the result of the brain coordinating an assembly operation on cell networks.

After a person selects words to be communicated, the electrochemical signal is transmitted to Broca's area, which lies in the inferior third frontal gyrus in the hemisphere that is dominant for language. In approximately 95% of the population, this hemisphere is the one on the left (Brookshire, 1997). In Broca's area, words are assembled into an electrochemical program, which is transmitted to the primary motor area (also called the motor strip), which controls voluntary movements of skeletal muscles. This lies immediately anterior to the central sulcus.

Cells on the primary motor area form an electrochemical map, called a homunculus, of the body's nerve endings. Body areas with many nerve endings appear large on the map and those with fewer nerve endings appear smaller. For example, the mouth and hands are represented by large map areas, while the back, though larger in actual size but having fewer nerve endings than the hands and mouth, is represented by a smaller map area.

From the primary motor area and several other nearby locations in the left hemisphere, the electrochemical message is sent out to the speech mechanism via the motor tracts (pyramidal and extrapyramidal tracts). The pyramidal tract carries signals to direct voluntary motor movement, and the extrapyramidal tract carries signals to direct autonomic motor impulses to voluntary muscles, including those involved in speech.

A Simple Game

Word retrieval depends in part on speech—that is, a person finds the right word guided by how a word sounds. For example, a person trying to remember the name *Tom* may search through "T" names, saying "What's his name again? Ted? Terry? No, it's Tom— that's his name." The following simple game illustrates the role of speech in word retrieval. First, ask someone to spell aloud the word *shop*. Immediately after he or she spells *shop*, ask, "What do you do when you come to a green light?" Most often a person responds, "Stop," even though, of course, traffic rules dictate that green means *go* and red means *stop*. People often confuse *stop* and *go* in this game because of *shop*, which sounds enough like *stop* to cause the retrieval of *stop*.

B. Mechanical Energy (Oral and Nasal Tracts)

At the muscles electrical energy from the brain is converted into mechanical energy (muscle movement). Muscles from the stomach upward are involved. The major muscle groups include those in the vocal tract, which consists of the nasal tract (the air space within the nose) and the oral tract (the mouth and throat).

C. Acoustic Energy (Movement of Air)

Muscle movement causes air to move up the vocal tract to be shaped by the larynx and the articulators. Movement of air molecules is acoustic energy. Similar to a rock dropped into a still lake, air ripples from the speaker's mouth to the listener's ear via the processes of condensation and rarefaction. During condensation, air molecules are closer together than normal and during rarefaction they are farther apart. Intensity of pushing of air molecules corresponds to the perception of loudness (usually measured in decibels), while the frequency at which the pushing of air molecules occurs corresponds to the perception of pitch (usually measured in Hertz). Stated differently, when air vibrates more intensely a person will likely perceive a sound as louder, and when air vibrates more frequently per second a person will likely to perceive a sound as having a higher pitch.

D. Mechanical Energy → Hydraulic Energy → Mechanical Energy (Ear)

The function of the ear is to translate vibrating air into electricity. The ear consists of three parts: the outer ear, the middle ear, and the inner ear. Air is funneled down the ear canal (outer ear). At the end of the ear canal separating the outer and middle ears lies the tympanic membrane (ear drum). At the ear drum, vibration of air (acoustic energy) is changed into mechanical energy. The ear drum vibrates, causing three small bones in the middle ear—the malleus, the incus, and the stapes—to vibrate. Mechanical energy travels across the bones. Also in the middle ear is the Eustachian tube, which connects the middle ear to the throat. If the Eustachian tube becomes closed (which sometimes happens during a cold), air to the middle ear can be reduced and the malleus, incus, and stapes do not vibrate as well. Sound is thus harder to hear.

The stapes is attached to a membrane separating the middle and inner ears, called the oval window. Movement of the stapes sets the oval window in vibration. Behind the oval window is the fluid-filled inner ear. The vibrating oval window sets fluid in motion, changing the energy from mechanical to hydraulic (liquid). Inside the inner ear is the cochlea, a small bony structure shaped like a snail's shell. Movement of fluid (hydraulic energy) presses on a membrane, changing hydraulic energy back into mechanical energy. The membrane pushes down many thousands of small hair cells lining the cochlea.

E. Electrochemical Energy (Auditory Nerve → Wernicke's Area)

Hair cells lining the cochlea are attached to nerves. As the hair cells are pressed, an electrical discharge is triggered, converting mechanical energy into electricity. The electrical message travels through the eighth cranial nerve (auditory nerve) up the brain stem, and then crosses over, so that most of the message from each ear goes to both left and right hemispheres. The electrical message is then sent to an electrical depiction of the cochlea in the temporal lobe of the cortex, close to Wernicke's area, an important region for language comprehension. The electrical message is decoded at the depiction of the cochlea and sent to Wernicke's area, where its meaning is interpreted based on information from the cochlear depiction as well as more general knowledge about context, discourse, and pragmatics.

F. Summary

For approximately 95% of the population, the cortical representation of speech is found in the frontal area of the left hemisphere. Broca's area plays a prominent role in assembling the components of speech, and the motor and premotor areas are crucially involved in preparing the speech signal for execution by the motor tracts. Through these tracts the electrical signal to speak is conveyed to muscle cells that have evolved to contract. As a result of this astonishingly complex process, muscles across nearly half the body contract in coordination, air is forced from the lungs up through the vocal tract, is shaped by the articulators, ripples through the atmosphere, is captured by the ear where it is eventually transformed back into electrical energy, and is then conveyed up the auditory tract to the temporal lobe and other cortical centers of the listener's brain, where the electrical signal is made into speech.

Several clinical implications arise from consideration of speech production and perception. First, a speech disorder may be related to the channel of communication. One type of speech disorder involves articulation of speech elements and is called an articulation disorder, giving the basis for the term *articulation* in *articulation and phonological disorder*. Second, though speaking may appear simple, it might more accurately be described as automatic rather than simple. The seeming ease with which most people speak masks great underlying complexity. The high frequency of speech disorders results in no small part because the act of speaking requires precise and coordinated activities across nearly half the body. Third, speaking involves much more than the mouth. In the speech production and perception system, the mouth is where articulators shape the air, converting mechanical energy into acoustic energy. The vast majority of persons with articulation and phonological disorders do not have mouths with a too small tongue, muscular weakness, or other malformation. Most often, the speech problem arises in the brain's control of the mouth rather than from a difficulty in the mouth itself.

A Question of Zen

A Zen riddle goes: if a tree falls in a forest and no one is there, does it make a sound? The question, intended to be unanswerable, actually has an answer: the falling tree does not make a sound. That is because sound does not exist without a listener. Movement of air made by a falling tree (or movement of air produced by a speaker, for that matter) ripples silently like water after a stone is thrown

(continued)

into a lake. Depending on the tree and how it falls, the air ripples with greater or lesser amplitude and frequency. The ripples are soundless; sound is the interpretation made by a listener in response to rippling air.

VI. SPEECH AND BRAIN EVOLUTION

Modern human speech depends on possession of a brain sufficiently large and powerful enough to learn from the environment in which a child lives. The discussion in this section presents current thinking about the evolution of human brain size.

A. Brain Size

The brain of modern humans is amazingly complex and compact (Ojemann, 1991). Approximately the size of a football, it weighs a scant 2% to 3% of total body weight, but requires almost 20% of the body's energy. This football-shaped mass contains approximately 100 billion neurons floating in a chemical bath of neurotransmitters. The brain areas that control understanding and produce speech are located in a meager 4 millimeters (1/4 inch) of the cortex at the top of the brain. The cells in the cortex are organized into folds (gyri and sulci) to maximize their numbers.

Speech and the Cortex

Building blocks of speech were laid down long ago in human beings' evolutionary past. The human auditory system is ancient and similar to that of other mammals, including the chinchilla. Human motor tracts are close equivalents to those of many other primates. A non-human primate vocal tract, though less flexible than a human one, is capable of sound production, and by all reports chimpanzees and other primates are quite vocal. But when in the long stretch of history did humans begin to use speech as they do today to talk, think, belong to groups, and transmit culture? The answer depends in large part on brain evolution, since modern human speech depends on possession of a large cortex (also called the neocortex, the prefix *neo* indicating that the cortex evolved recently in human history). Knowing when the human cortex evolved, we have at least a broad time frame during which speech likely originated.

Table 1–2. Evolution of brain size in hominid ancestors.

Hominid	Years Ago (in millions)	Body Weight (kg)	Brain Weight (g)
Chimpanzee	now	36.4	410
Australopithecus	3.9–2.8	50.6	415
Homo rudolfensis	1.9	—	700–900
Homo erectus	1.8–.2	58.6	826
Neanderthal	.3–30,000		1450
Homo sapiens	.2–now	44	1250

The human brain was not as large in the past as it is today. A list of direct and closely related hominid (humanlike) ancestors is contained in Table 1–2. A more complete map of relationships between postulated ancestors is presented in Appendix 1A (Lieberman, 1999). Table 1–2 shows named ancestors, approximately how many years ago each species lived, average body size in kilograms, and average brain weight in grams (de Waal, 2001; Mayr, 2001; Tetterall & Schwarz, 2000). Body size was determined through fossil evidence and brain size was determined through creation of a plastic or latex casts (called endocasts) made of the inner surface of fossil skulls. In considering the information in Table 1–2, ratio of body size to brain size is more important than absolute size. To illustrate, a Blue Whale and an elephant both possess large brains, but they also have large body weights; while a finch's brain weighs little, so does its body. Considering brain size relative to body weight allows comparison across species.

B. Australopithecus

Approximately 3.5 million years ago humanity's first named ancestor, Australopithecus, appeared. The most famous member of this species (or related species) is named Lucy. Lucy walked upright, and she and her kind lived on edges of rain forests. By freeing the arms and hands from locomotion, she could collect fruit and nuts, and then return to the trees to eat in relative safety. Bipedal locomotion also freed the arms to carry a young child, an ability that would be crucial later in history. Was Lucy an ape who walked on her hind legs or a primitive human? Evidence suggests she was closer to the former. Her brain size (415 grams) compared to body size is more similar to modern chimpanzees than humans. Modern primates vocalize, and there seems no reason to suppose that Lucy did not do so as well. No evidence exists, however, that Australopithecus spoke.

Early Experiments on Speech Origins

The first recorded scientific study of language origins appears in Herodotus, who reported that the Pharaoh Psammetichus (7th century B.C.) ordered two children to be raised by she-goats to determine the children's "natural" language (Godolphin, 1942; Hewes, 1992). The pharaoh claimed the children spoke Phrygian. Much later, the emperor Frederick II, the Mogul emperor Akbar, and King James IV of Scotland all subjected children to language deprivation experiments to determine their original "natural" language (Hewes, 1992). The Mogul emperor reported the children spoke no language at all, while King James IV claimed they spoke Hebrew.

C. *Homo rudolfensis*

Approximately 2.5 million years ago Earth experienced an ice age, and the climate in Africa underwent a drying and cooling period, resulting in vast areas being transformed into bush country. Hominids, no longer having the trees as a place of safety, competed with much faster and stronger plains predators such as lions, cheetahs, hyenas, and dogs. The first of human beings' big-brained ancestors, *Homo rudolfensis,* appeared nearly 1.8 million years ago. *Homo rudolfensis* had a cranial capacity of approximately 750 grams, roughly one-third larger than Australopithecus and half that of modern humans. The shift toward a larger brain must have wrought enormous changes in the social life of *Homo rudolfensis*. A brain has large nutritional requirements. Animal flesh contains the fats and proteins required by a large brain, and tool making and the regular consumption of meat seem likely to have begun in this period.

Little evidence supports the conception of a speaking *Homo rudolfensis*. However, Tobias (1987) contends that endocasts of *Homo habilus,* a near-contemporary of *Homo rudolfensis,* show size increases in Wernicke's and Broca's areas. The endocast evidence is extremely controversial, as Tobias acknowledges (Tobias, 1987). Further, such growth, even if it were occurring, could reflect other uses than speaking and listening, including skilled rock throwing or even gestural language (Corballis, 2002).

D. *Homo erectus*

Approximately 2.0 to 1.0 million years ago *Homo erectus* appeared. Built for life on the plains, taller, and having a larger brain than his predecessors, he may have controlled fire, and was the first hominid who expanded out of Africa to Europe, the Middle East, and eastern Asia. *Homo erectus* had an average cranial capacity of 826 grams, approximately two-thirds that of modern humans. Dunbar (1999) hypothesizes that increase in brain size occurred because living in the bush required larger groups for protection. Under this new condition, a larger brain offered an advantage within complex social networks.

Bickerton (1990) hypothesizes that the combination of *Homo erectus*'s brain size, range expansion, and hypothesized complex social network suggests he spoke a type of protolanguage similar to a modern human language, but without complex linguistic rules. To support this hypothesis, Bickerton (1990) observes that people often speak without knowing all the rules of a language, as with young children and persons of different language backgrounds who develop a "pidgin language" to communicate basic wants and needs.

E. Neanderthal

Approximately 300,000 years ago descendents of *Homo erectus,* archaic Neanderthal, arose in Europe and the Near East. Neanderthal, broad and heavily muscled, was adapted to cold weather. Neanderthal went extinct approximately 30,000 years ago, perhaps due to climate changes, or through either genocide or intermarrying with *Homo sapiens.* The brain size of Neanderthal averaged 1,450 grams.

Did Neanderthal use speech? Lieberman (1984) claimed not, based on evidence that Neanderthal's larynx rested high in the throat, limiting his sound-making capacities. More recently, however, researchers have challenged the anatomical evidence on which this claim rests (National Geographic, 1989). The hypothesis that Neanderthal was a speaker remains unproven.

F. *Homo sapiens*

Approximately 200,000 years ago *Homo sapiens* arose in southern Africa. Genetic evidence suggests all modern humans arose from this population, which has been dubbed "Mitochondrial Eve." The average brain weight of early modern humans was approximately 1,250 grams, the same as modern humans. The brain weight of early *Homo sapiens* was approximately three times what would be expected of a primate of similar size (Killackey, 1995; Passingham, 1982).

Researchers have yet to determine if early *Homo sapiens* used speech as we do today. The difficulty in making this determination is that speech is a behavior that leaves no direct trace in the anatomical record. That is, while brain size and larynx height may infer a capacity for speech, anatomical capacity does not mean that speech behavior actually occurred. Instead, researchers infer the presence of speech based on accomplishments that appear to require speech or similar cognitive capacities. The explosion of culture 30,000 to 40,000 years ago that gave rise to cave paintings and ceremonial burial requires symbolic representations, as does language, and so most researchers are convinced that speech must have existed by that period. More recently, Coupe and Hombert (2002) have argued that the arduous ocean crossing from Asia to Australia that occurred around 70,000 years ago would not have been possible without planning that required sophisticated language skills.

G. Summary

Possession of a large brain is essential for modern speech. During the past 2.5 million years the weight of the human brain increased threefold. Sometime during this period speech arose. No evidence suggests that Australopithecus spoke, and only scant evidence supports the idea of a speaking *Homo rudolfensis. Homo erectus* may have spoken a type of protolanguage lacking the complexities of modern languages. Possibly, the protolanguage was signed rather than spoken. Evidence for a speaking Neanderthal is uncertain, with basic questions about Neanderthal speech anatomy still unresolved. Researchers hypothesize that modern speech was established in early *Homo sapiens* at least 70,000 years ago.

Several clinical implications arise from consideration of speech and brain evolution. First, as emphasized in *Speech Production and Perception* (Section V), the cause of an articulation and phonological disorder most often lies in the brain's control of the mouth rather than in the mouth itself. Thus, it is extremely difficult to understand such disorders without considering how the brain, including how it evolved to its present-day size, functions. Second, while some children experience learning difficulty only in the speech domain, others experience other learning difficulties, and still others experience speech difficulties secondary to more general cognitive limitations or brain damage. For all such children with speech disorders, an understanding of the brain's contribution to speech is critical to provision of clinical care.

Growing Up Together

In a sense, speech and a larger brain "grew up together," speech arising as the size of cortical areas increased. The relationship between speech and brain growth is unclear. Possibly, as Chomsky (1980) has suggested, speech arose as a consequence of increased brain size—that is, speech and language is what occurs when 100 billion brain cells are packed together. Alternately—and far more likely—speech and brain growth interacted, with speech use encouraging the growth of cortical areas and increased size of cortical areas permitting greater use of speech. Within such a view, speech offered sufficient survival advantages to communities of speakers that they eventually outbred communities of hominids with less speech and smaller brains (Bickerton, 1990; Pinker, 1995).

VII. SPEECH AND BRAIN DEVELOPMENT

Most often, a person thinks of something to say, opens his or her mouth, and sounds come out, one after another. The ease of speech hides the fact that even the slowest speech requires knowledge of rules far more complex than those that underlie chess as well as motor and perceptual skills far beyond those needed to hit a home run, play a piano, or dance a ballet. Yet, while those activities require years of conscious, determined effort to master, speech is acquired early by most children and is produced almost without effort or conscious control. The fact that a child learns speech years before learning chess, swinging a bat, playing the piano, or dancing ballet is as strange as if a child learned calculus before learning to add, subtract, multiply, and divide.

This section describes the neurological foundations on which speech development depends. Five topics are considered:

- Childhood
- Cell connections
- Cell connections in speech domains
- Reflections of brain development
- A neurological basis of speech disorders

A. Childhood

Evolution has provided the human species with a brain with the capacity to learn speech, and a lengthy childhood during which learning can occur. Evolution of brain size was discussed in the previous section. The focus of this section is how the interaction between brain size and length of childhood creates the human pattern of speech learning. These ideas are summarized in Appendix 1B.

1. Development of Childhood. Human childhood, measured from birth to puberty, lasts approximately 12 years. By comparison, childhood of humankind's closest primate relative, a chimpanzee, lasts approximately three years, or roughly one-fourth as long. In human history an extended childhood grew in conjunction with a larger brain. The childhood of early hominids such as Australopithecus and *Homo rudolfensis* was similar in length to that of a chimpanzee, the length of childhood of early *Homo erectus* was intermediate between that of chimpanzees and modern humans, and that of late *Homo erectus* and Neanderthal more similar to that of modern humans (Tetterall & Schwarz, 2000).

With an extended childhood came greater need for protection, since the young were unable to fend for themselves. An important consequence of having a large brain is that early humans needed to adapt a social pattern to better protect and educate children. This entailed the creation of stable communities for group protection and strengthening bonds between parent and child, giving rise to the modern human pattern of a lengthy childhood during which the child is protected from danger while being educated about the environment. Such a system of protection and tutelage seems natural, but is only one of many possibilities. To illustrate, the childhoods of sharks and sea turtles do not include tutelage from an elder. Instead, both species are born in great numbers and disperse.

The Pelvis Isn't the Problem

Sometimes the claim is made (half-jokingly) that extensive brain growth after birth is a clever human adaptation to the female pelvis. Most mothers agree that the hardest part of giving birth involves the child's head, because it is the largest body part. Apparently, the female pelvis has reached evolutionary
(continued)

limits as regards how large it can grow. If the pelvis were any larger, women would experience difficulty walking and running. Needing a large brain to learn from the environment, but having physical limitations on how large the head can be at birth, the human adaptation is said to have most brain development occur after the child is born (Trevathan, 1987; Ellison, 2001). However, recent research has noted that the relative immaturity of the human brain at birth is only about average for higher-order mammals, being about 25% of its mature size. A kitten's brain, for example, is also about 25% of the size of an adult cat's (Gibson, 1990). If brain growth after birth is an adaptation to a too-small pelvis, it is one shared by many species.

2. **Brain Growth During Childhood.** A legacy of humankind's evolutionary past is that extensive brain development occurs as a child is acquiring speech during childhood. The human brain at birth is about 25% of its adult weight, grows maximally to 80% of its adult weight during the first few years of life, and reaches its mature size at adulthood (Gibson, 1990; Kretschmann, Kammradt, Krauthausen, Sauer, & Wingert, 1986). Brain development during childhood allows the brain to be shaped by the environment in which a child lives. Rather than possessing a genetic inheritance that includes a specialized body and mind fitted to a specific environmental niche, a human brain grows while exposed to the environment into which a baby is born. Brain development and the environment interact (Figure 1–3). A child brings an ability to grasp complex patterns and a brain that grows through interacting with the environment. The environment shapes a child's brain, narrowing the potential to learn from a wide number of possible environments to fit the actual one in which a child lives.

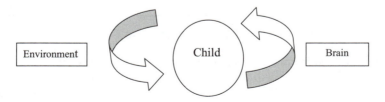

Figure 1–3. Interactions between genetic potential and the environment.

B. Cell Connections

Learning speech means making connections between brain cells. In a mature brain, it is estimated that each cell connects to approximately 10,000 other cells. Two processes underlie how brain cells establish such interconnections:

• Selective elimination

• Growth and elaboration

1. **Selective Elimination.** A brain begins with "extra" cells, approximately one-third of which are lost between birth and adulthood. Cell connections that are used are strengthened and retained, while those that are unused are eliminated. The number of cell connections remains stable throughout much of adulthood.

The process of cell selection and elimination is sometimes called neural Darwinism, arborization, or pruning—the latter two terms an analogy to how an overgrown bush is trimmed (arborized or pruned) into a specific shape (Geschwind & Galaburda, 1987). In essence, "extra" cells represent learning potential. Not knowing in advance which cells will be needed, humans (and other species as well) have the potential to learn from a wide range of environments. Loss of cell connections through arborization or pruning reflects learning. That is, cell connections are strengthened as a skill is acquired, and those not needed are eliminated. Stated more broadly, in selective elimination, additional cell connections indicate potential to learn, and elimination of cell connections indicates skill acquisition.

2. **Growth and Elaboration.** In addition to the brain possessing "extra" cells that permit learning from a range of possible environments, the environment itself stimulates growth and elaboration of cell connections. Research indicates that for many species an enriched environment promotes increased numbers of synapses per neuron in both children and adults (Quartz & Sejnowski, 1997; Chang et al., 1991; Chang & Greenough, 1984; Turner & Greenough, 1985; Bailey & Chen, 1988; Black et al., 1990). To illustrate, Black et al. (1990) increased the number of synapses per neuron in the rat cerebellum by 25% using a motor learning task. In humans, numbers of cell connections increase in old age, indicating a capacity for life-long learning and, perhaps, compensating for neuronal deaths that occur during middle and old age (Buell & Coleman, 1979).

C. Cell Connections in Speech Domains

Brain areas achieve a mature number of cell connections at different rates. Those areas responsible for sensory information mature early, while those that direct more complex functions mature later in life. Major changes in areas that affect speech include myelination on axons that transmit electrical signals between cells, maturation of the primary cortical areas for language comprehension (Wernicke's area) and production (Broca's area), and maturation of cortical areas (prefrontal cortex) responsible for executive functions that underlie speech learning, including memory, judgment, and attention (Krasnegor, Reid Lyon, & Goldman-Rakic, 1997).

1. **Myelin Sheaths.** Myelin is a white fatty substance on axons that acts as an insulator and speeds electrical transmission of signals between cells. Myelin is critical for gross and fine motor movements, including speech. The effect is evidenced by multiple sclerosis (MS), a demyelinating disease that may result in profound speech difficulties and other motor problems. Myelination of the brain begins near six months in utero, achieves its peak growth between birth and the end of the first year, and continues to grow until adulthood (Evans & Hutchins, 2002).

2. **Wernicke's and Broca's Areas.** Visual and auditory areas (including Wernicke's area) peak in number of cell connections during the first half of the first year and achieve the mature number of cell connections during the second half of the first year (Pascallis, de Hann, & Nelson, 2002). Density of cell connections in Broca's area, the functional region in the left frontal hemisphere that controls speech, does not peak until age 15 months, and does not reach a mature number of connections until ages six to eight (Simonds & Scheibel, 1989; Scheibel, 1993; Schade & van Groenigen, 1961).

Education and gender have significant effects on number of cell connections in speech and language areas. On average, persons with a university education have more dendritic connections in Wernicke's area than do those with a high school diploma, who in turn have more than those with less than a high school education (Jacobs, Schall, & Scheibel, 1993). The same study found that girls as young as age nine have more dendritic connections in Wernicke's area than do males, and that women also have brain metabolic rates approximately 15% higher than those of males (Jacobs, Schall, & Scheibel, 1993).

> ### Education and Gender
>
> In studies of education and gender the relative roles of genetics and the environment are notoriously difficult to untangle. Does a person achieve a university education because of greater potential to make connections among cells in Wernicke's area, or does a university education increase cell connections in Wernicke's area? Similarly, do women have greater genetic potential to make cell connections in Wernicke's area, or does socialization foster greater use of language in girls than boys, leading to more cell connections?

3. **Prefrontal Lobes.** The prefrontal lobes are critically important to many cognitive activities that underlie speech, including reasoning, planning, judgment, and attention. Disorders in this region are implicated in attention deficit disorder. Cell connections in the prefrontal lobes develop slowly throughout childhood and do not reach maturity until after adolescence (Sowell, Dells, Stiles, & Jernigan, 2001; Casey, Gledd, & Thomas, 2000). Teenagers are famous for lack of planning and judgment, and this has been attributed to lack of maturity of cell connections in the prefrontal lobes.

4. **Hippocampus.** The hippocampus is important to working memory, and is deeply involved in such important speech activities as memory retention and retrieval (Benes, 1997). The hippocampus, like other memory systems, develops after the child is born, especially during the second year of life (Liston & Kagan, 2002).

D. Reflections of Brain Development

Both cell connection processes (selective elimination, growth and elaboration) are implicated in speech learning. Three of many possible illustrations reflecting effects of brain development on speech acquisition include:

- Play
- Perception of tone
- Speech rate

1. **Play.** A child's brain grows rapidly during the first few years of life. A child's play reflects this growth. An infant's play with toys typically involves banging, throwing, mouthing, and shaking. Near age 12 months primitive play begins to emerge, with, perhaps, a child speaking into a pretend telephone. Full representational play begins around age 18 to 20 months and is well established by age 22 to 24 months (Hedrick, Prather, & Tobin, 1984). In representational play, a child lets one object stand for or symbolize another. To illustrate, a child may introduce absent objects into play by pretending to feed a doll without having a spoon. Such play is significant because it resembles language, in which words and sentences represent or symbolize events and objects in the real world. It is perhaps not surprising that the neurological development that permits representational play also makes possible representational language as well.

2. **Perception of Tone.** Neurological maturation of speech perception areas occurs early in life. A child typically is born with perceptual ability to acquire any of the world's languages. This must be so, because an infant has no choice regarding which language his or her parents speak. Many languages use pitch to distinguish between word meanings (called tone languages), and so a child must perceive differences between pitches. Newborns around the world notice pitch differences that in languages such as Mandarin Chinese and Vietnamese are used to signal differences between words (Pascallis, de Haan, & Nelson, 2002). Children born to English-speaking families lose this ability by the end of their first year, while those born to Chinese-speaking families retain it. A "use it or lose it" principle appears operative: children everywhere are born with the same ability to perceive pitch, but those who grow up speaking languages such as Chinese establish and retain these brain cell connections, while those who speak a non-tone language such as English lose those potential cell connections.

3. **Speech Rate.** Neurological maturation of speech production areas occurs more slowly than in speech perception areas. A child speaks more slowly than an adult and, consequently, duration of a child's phrases and sentences is longer (Kent & Forner, 1980). Relative slowness of a child's speech and increased duration of phrases and sentences may reflect that a child is less experienced than an adult in planning and executing speech. As described by Kent and Forner (1980), an adult typically speaks approximately 3 words per second, while a child 4 to 5 years old may speak 2.5 words per second, and a

2-year-old may speak 1.6 words per second. Duration of phrases and sentences of a 12-year-old are 8% longer than an adult's. Durations of phrases and sentences of a 4- to 6-year-old are 16% and 33% longer, respectively.

E. A Neurological Basis for Speech Disorders

The neurological basis for learning speech is making connections between cells. As discussed in this section, three reasons exist why a child might experience difficulty in forming cell connections for speech (see also *Causes of Articulation and Phonological Disorders* in Chapter 2 for a clinical discussion):

• Normal variation

• Environmental deficits

• Physical damage

1. **Normal Variation.** People vary in ability to form new cell connections, some accomplishing this task with seeming ease and others requiring more labor. Within a single individual, ability typically varies by subject matter. To illustrate, one person may easily learn speech and music, but struggle with math and chemistry. Another may show the opposite propensities: math and chemistry are learned easily, but speech and music require concentrated study. Ability and interests often co-occur, reinforcing each other. Alternately, a child with less initial ability in a given area may either work harder to find success or may shift interest and attention to areas in which success occurs more readily. When a person's ability in forming new cell connections in speech areas is sufficiently different from that of the community, he or she may be identified as having a speech disorder.

2. **Environmental Deficits.** Decreased environmental stimulation may result in fewer synaptic connections. For example, several studies have shown that suturing the eyes of kittens shut (thus denying input to the visual cortex) results in permanent blindness arising from a 30% to 32% reduction of number of synapses in the visual cortex (Craig, 1975; Winfield, 1981). Lifelong speech and cognitive problems of children such as Genie, who spent her early life largely reared in a closet, may reflect powerful and enduring effects of lack of environmental stimulation (Curtiss, 1977).

3. Physical Damage. Connections between cells may be affected by brain damage resulting from either organic impairment or trauma.

   a. Organic Impairment. Limitations in ability to make cell connections occur in many medical and developmental conditions associated with mental impairment, negatively affecting speech acquisition and other types of learning. To illustrate, in a rare genetic disorder called lissencephaly, a child's brain lacks gyri and sulci, vastly reducing numbers of cells available to make connections in the most recently evolved brain area, the neocortex. Speech problems and severe mental retardation are associated with this disorder.

   Children with Down syndrome often experience extreme difficulty learning speech. Decreased numbers of dendritic connections per neuron have been observed in children with Down syndrome, trisomy 18, and other forms of mental retardation (Jay, Chan, & Becker, 1990; Becker, Armstrong, & Chan, 1986). Huttenlocher (1991) indicates that the dendritic spines in cells of children with Down syndrome are narrower than in typically developing children, and that this increases difficulty in electrical current communicating between cells.

Stress and Learning

Sexual and physical abuse during childhood may result in post-traumatic stress syndrome (PTSS). As a result of abuse, the brain may release stress-related hormones that, in large quantities, damage brain functions that support speech learning, including memory, learning, and attention (De Bellis, Keshavan, Clark, Casey, Giedd, Boring, Frustaci, & Ryan, 1999; Teicher, 2002). Importantly, a speech and language disorder may also be a risk factor for physical and sexual abuse (Knutson & Sullivan, 1983). A child's communication difficulty makes her or him vulnerable to sexual predators, since the child may be a less able reporter. Within the family, physical abuse associated with communication difficulties may also occur.

---

b. Trauma. Brain trauma may affect ability of cells to connect by either reducing cell numbers or disrupting connections between cells. Speech learning may be negatively affected if trauma occurs either in speech areas or in areas that support speech learning. Trauma results from many causes and can occur anytime during childhood. The following are examples of extremely common types of brain trauma that may affect speech and other types of learning (Batshaw, 1997):

- Maternal substance abuse

- Low birth weight and prematurity

- Lead poisoning

- Closed head injury

Maternal Substance Abuse. An unborn child's fragile brain may be compromised through trauma arising from maternal substance abuse. Approximately 36% to 41% of women in the United States abuse illicit drugs, alcohol, or nicotine sometime during pregnancy (Bleile & Burda, 2003; Center on Addiction and Substance Abuse, 1996). Illicit drugs account for 11% of substance abuse, and heavy use of alcohol or nicotine the other 25% to 30%. Approximately three-quarters of pregnant women who abuse one substance also abuse other substances (Center on Addiction and Substance Abuse, 1996). To illustrate, a pregnant woman who abuses cocaine might also drink heavily.

Low Birth Weight and Prematurity. In the United States approximately 8.5% of infants are born underweight (Bleile & Burda, 2003; Guyer, Strobino, & Ventura, 1995). Many low birth weight children are born prematurely. Co-occurrence of low birth weight and prematurity varies by country; in the United States, 70% of low birth weight babies are also born prematurely. A child's likelihood of experiencing brain trauma is best predicted by birth weight, with a child weighing less being more likely to experience such damage. Many agents give rise to brain trauma in a low birth weight or premature child, including brain hemorrhages, strokes, and episodes of anoxia (Bernbaum & Hoffman-Williamson, 1991).

Lead Poisoning. In the 19th century, Bismarck of Germany recognized the injurious effect of lead on the brain and ordered that houses be built with paints lacking a lead base. As a result, present-day Germany experiences few problems from lead poisoning resulting from house paints. English-speaking countries did not follow Bismarck's excellent example, and until the mid-20th century use of lead-based paints was commonplace. Not until 1976 was unleaded gasoline well-accepted in the United States. Since removal of lead in gasoline, airborne lead poisoning has decreased dramatically.

Lead poisoning through ingestion remains a significant concern, however, especially among younger children and those with developmental disabilities who live in older neighborhoods. The Center for Disease Control estimates that 38 million homes built before 1950 still have lead-based paints on their walls. Lead may also enter a child's body through eating dirt and other nonfood items that contain flakes of lead paint. Presently, in the United States approximately 1 in 50 children ages 1 to 5 years old experience lead poisoning (defined as concentrations of 10 or more micrograms per deciliter), resulting in an average intelligence decline of 7.4 points compared to children with lead concentrations of 1 microgram per deciliter. Further, 1 in 10 children in the United States has lead concentrations of 5 micrograms per deciliter—well within the dangerous range (*New England Journal of Medicine,* 2003). Even low levels of exposure to lead may result in lowered intelligence, speech and language disorders, and behavior problems (*New England Journal of Medicine,* 2003).

Closed Head Injury. A common type of childhood brain trauma is closed head injury resulting from child abuse, falls, car accidents, and other often preventable causes. The brain floats in cerebral spinal fluid, which acts as a shock absorber, protecting the brain from impacts with the skull within which it is housed. During the event resulting in closed head injury, forward and backward movement of the brain (called *coup* and *contra coup*) causes the brain to impact the inner skull surface, and spinning motions causes the brain to spin on its axis. As a result, arteries break, blood is released into the brain, neurotransmitters may be secreted in toxic quantity, and connections between brain cells are torn and sheared. As a consequence, the brain swells, much as a shoulder does after a sports injury.

If injury is sufficiently severe, a brain may no longer support consciousness, and a person enters a coma lasting from an hour to weeks or months. If the brain is extremely damaged, the coma may be lifelong. As the brain recovers and swelling subsides, it regains function (again, somewhat like an injured shoulder regains function as swelling decreases) and a person passes through stages of consciousness. Cells that were killed are gone, but injured cells may recover and old cell connections may become operative and functional again. Presumably, growth and elaboration of cell connections allows new learning to compensate for those lost through injury.

F. Summary

Evolution has provided the human species with a brain that has the capacity to learn speech, and a lengthy childhood during which learning can occur. Brain cells connect through two basic processes: selective elimination and growth and elaboration. Through the first process cell connections are strengthened as a skill is acquired, and those not needed are eliminated. Through the second process the environment stimulates growth and elaboration of cell connections. As a consequence of evolutionary history, much brain growth occurs while a child is learning speech during childhood, as reflected by changes in play, speech perception, and speech rate. The neurological basis of speech learning involves the making of connections between brain cells. Possible difficulties in making such connections arise from normal variability, environmental deficits, and physical damage.

Several clinical implications arise from consideration of speech and brain development. First, because learning speech requires interaction between a brain capable of learning and an environment devoted to teaching, a speech problem may result either because a child experiences difficulty learning from the environment or because the environment is an inadequate teacher. Second, a speech disorder may be an isolated deficit, or may be secondary to deficits in brain systems that support speech learning. Third, a person might experience difficulty in making cell connections for speech learning as the result of normal variability, environmental deficits, or physical damage.

Genes versus the Environment

Is biology going to be to the 21st century what the revolution in computers was to the 20th? Newspaper accounts of breakthroughs in medicine have become almost daily occurrences, largely as
(continued)

outgrowths of the Human Genome Project. Recent advances in biology have deeply affected our understanding of how genetic factors may adversely impact communication. Most recently, researchers have identified genetic contributions to apraxia-like speech disorders (Lai, Fisher, Hurst, Vargha-Khadem, & Monaco, 2001) and dyslexia (Shaywitz, Shaywitz, Pugh, Mencl, Fulbright, Skudlarski, Constable, Marchione, Fletcher, Lyon, & Gore, 2002). Along with advances have come ethical concerns. Stem cell research, cloning, genetically engineered plants, and social impacts of increased longevity are only a few current examples.

Gould (1992) among others fears that advances in biology may create an intellectual framework of genetic determinism, with "what is written in our genes" replacing ideas of free will, responsibility, and self-determination. If language is an innate instinct and speech disorders result from genetic problems, what role is there in shaping the environment to facilitate speech learning? Several current linguistic theories of language innateness approach this position (Chomsky, 1980).

Information on neurological foundations of speech argues against a simple dichotomy between "the genes" versus "the environment." Rather than speech acquisition following a predetermined, innately specified path of development, genetic and environmental influences interact. Human brain size provides the tool for learning, and an extended childhood provides time during which learning can occur. During childhood, the brain grows and is shaped positively and negatively by experience. Interconnections between cells are building blocks of speech learning, and such connections are eliminated, strengthened, grown, and elaborated as a child explores and learns.

VIII. SUMMARY

Five interrelated perspectives on speech were discussed in this chapter. Essential ideas within each perspective are summarized in this section and depicted in Table 1–3.

Table 1–3. Five perspectives on speech.

Perspective	Essential Idea
Language and Society	• Speech plays a crucial role in communication between people, with oneself, within and between groups, and across generations
Speech and Language	• Speech has a dual nature: it is both a part of language and a channel of communication • Speech is the cornerstone of human language
Speech Production and Perception	• Speech production and perception is the second aspect of speech's dual nature • Speech production and perception are energy translation systems through which a brain interfaces with the world
Speech and Brain Evolution	• A large brain is essential for modern speech • Cortical areas required for speech evolved over the past 2.5 million years
Speech and Brain Development	• Evolution has provided the human species with a brain with the capacity to learn and a lengthy childhood during which learning can occur • Learning speech entails making connections between brain cells • Difficulties in making cell connections may arise due to normal variability, environmental deficits, or physical damage

A. Speech and Society

Speech has a social dimension, playing a crucial role in communication between people (talk), with oneself (thought), within and between groups (group identity), and across generations (cultural transmission).

B. Speech and Language

Speech has a dual nature: it is both a part of language and a channel of communication. The language aspect of speech is the cornerstone on which all the rest of human language is built. Because speech elements lack meaning, they afford the ability to construct a nearly infinite number of words, allowing humans to enter a new environment and create vocabulary to describe the place in which they find themselves. So central is speech both to language and to being human, humans might define themselves as the species whose cornerstone of communication means nothing.

C. Speech Production and Perception

Speech production and perception is the second aspect of speech's dual nature. This aspect of speech exists because a brain only understands the language of electricity and chemicals, and thus requires systems that translate between itself and the world. Speech production and perception is one such translation system. To produce and perceive speech requires the brain of the speaker to create an electrochemical message that is then converted successively into mechanical, acoustic, and hydraulic energy, before being converted back into electrochemical energy by the brain of the listener.

D. Speech and Brain Evolution

A large brain is essential for modern speech. Cortical areas required for speech evolved over the past 2.5 million years, during which the weight of the human brain increased threefold. Researchers hypothesize that modern speech was established in early *Homo sapiens* at least 70,000 years ago.

E. Speech and Brain Development

Evolution has provided the human species with a brain with the capacity to learn and a lengthy childhood during which learning can occur. Extensive brain development occurs during childhood, allowing a child's brain to be shaped by the environment and narrowing a brain's potential to learn from a wide range of possible environments to fit the actual one in which a child lives. Learning speech means making connections between brain cells. Difficulties in making such connections may arise due to normal variability, environmental deficits, and physical damage.

IX. SPEECH MYTHS

Nearly everyone holds beliefs about speech. One common belief is that speaking is simple. How could speaking be other than simple since people learn speech while still young children and people of all ages often talk from morning to night, the sounds and syllables flowing from the mouth, virtually without effort? If a person has "trouble saying letters," presumably something is wrong with the mouth, perhaps a malformation or muscular weakness. To correct this problem, a person sees a speech therapist, who teaches people to shape their articulators to make letters.

Though the preceding paragraph reflects widely accepted beliefs about speech, the beliefs it asserts are actually speech myths: speaking is simple, speaking is the pronunciation of "letters," speech disorders result from problems in the mouth, and speech therapy entails positioning a person's articulators to make "letters." These four myths are shown in Table 1–4 and discussed here in light of ideas presented in previous sections.

A. First Speech Myth: Speaking Is Simple

The seeming ease with which a person speaks masks enormous complexity. As discussed in *Speech and Language* (Section IV) and *Speech Production and Perception* (Section V), speech is both a part of language and a channel of communication. Both parts of its nature contribute to speech complexity. To illustrate, a person who says *dog* must find the word in memory and know how to pronounce it (language tasks), and then must pronounce it by converting energies using systems across half the body, from the cortex to the diaphragm (speech production tasks). As discussed in *Speech and Brain Evolution* (Section VI) and *Speech and*

Table 1–4. Four myths about speech and its disorders.

Speech Myths
• Speaking is simple
• Speaking is the pronunciation of "letters"
• Speech disorders result from problems in the mouth
• Speech therapy entails positioning a person's articulators to make "letters"

Brain Development (Section VII), both the language and channel aspects of speech are the result of the past 2.5 million years of brain evolution. Not all people are able to coordinate such complex language and speech production/perception activities. As discussed in *Speech and Society* (Section III), those that differ from their community in this ability may be judged to have a speech disorder.

B. Second Speech Myth: Speaking Is the Pronunciation of "Letters"

"Letters" are written representations of consonants and vowels. While speech certainly entails the pronunciation of consonants and vowels, it also involves pronouncing syllables, stress patterns, and intonation contours. As discussed in *Speech Production and Perception* (Section V), speech also entails word storage, word finding, and perception. Also, as discussed in *Speech and Language* (Section IV), "letters" are far more than sounds: they are the foundation on which human communication is built, and the capacity to build a language on this foundation gives humans their most human characteristics. A clinical implication of the idea that speech is more than "letters" is that speech disorders may arise from sources other than difficulty pronouncing consonants and vowels.

C. Third Speech Myth: Speech Disorders Result from Problems in the Mouth

On first consideration, this belief seems reasonable, since speech sounds are largely formed in the mouth, a person can reflect and feel articulators move when she or he speaks, and the mouth of a speaker is easily observed by a listener. However, as discussed in *Speech Production and Perception* (Section V), the mouth is only one part of the speech production and perception system—the part where articulators shape air, transferring speech from mechanical to acoustic energy. Rather than resulting from either a mouth malformation or weakness, far more often the type of speech disorder that is the focus of this book (articulation and phonological disorders) involve language systems and speech production and perception systems. As discussed in *Speech and Brain Evolution* (Section VI) and *Speech and Brain Development* (Section VII), during speech learning both shapes and is shaped by the environment. As emphasized in *Speech and Brain Development* (Section VII), speech learning is susceptible to damage from many different types of negative influences that can affect a person's ability to make connections between brain cells.

D. Fourth Speech Myth: Speech Therapy Entails Positioning a Person's Articulators to Make "Letters"

Helping a person shape articulators to make speech sounds is well-established clinical practice, and knowing how to shape a sound a client can pronounce into one he or she cannot is a valuable therapeutic "trick of the trade." This book contains extensive descriptions of such techniques. However, though such techniques are valuable, they work best only with selected people, typically school-aged children and adults with good attention and motivation. Further, even for such clients, because speech involves more than the mouth, more than the mouth is involved in speech therapy. As discussed in *Speech and Society* (Section III), speech has social dimensions; the impact of a person's speech disorder on his or her life is an essential aspect of all speech therapy. As discussed in *Speech and Language* (Section IV), speech also has language dimensions, and a problem in speech may affect other aspects of language. Lastly, as discussed in *Speech and Brain Evolution* (Section VI) and *Speech and Brain Development* (Section VII), speech and the brain are closely connected. A clinical implication of this idea is that an understanding of speech problem must include knowledge of the brain that makes possible the sounds that come from a person's mouth.

A Question

What exactly contributes to speech complexity? Is it a result of speech being a recent evolutionary event, making it somewhat jury-rigged, a reconfiguration of combinations of old and new brain and body circuitry? Is it because speech includes both knowing and doing, the combination of which makes speech so complex that the wonder is that more children don't experience speech difficulties? Or is it that speech is so important to societies that they label speech variations as disordered more readily than other variable activities, such as, for example, differences in gait and conversational gesturing? The reason may lie in factors combining culture, evolution, neurology, and speech anatomy and physiology. This makes speech and its disorders an exciting and challenging study, and a rich and rewarding clinical activity that requires great dedication and thoughtfulness to understand and perform.

X. FOUNDATION OF CARE

Perspectives discussed in this chapter have important implications for the care of a person with a speech disorder. The clinical implications presented throughout the chapter form 10 principles that, considered in conjunction, are the foundation of care that underlies this book. The 10 principles are highlighted in this section and are summarized in Appendix 1C. The numeric order roughly follows that in which topics were discussed in the chapter. For convenience, the sections in which ideas that support the clinical implications discussed are included.

1. A person whose speech differs from that of his or her community may be identified as speech-disordered. *Speech and Society* (Section III)

2. A speech disorder should be considered within the social context of the person with the problem. *Speech and Society* (Section III)

3. A speech disorder may impact other language domains. *Speech and Language* (Section IV)

4. A speech disorder may have a language basis, a basis in production and perception, or a combination of both bases. *Speech and Language* (Section IV) and *Speech Production and Perception* (Section V)

5. A speech disorder involves more than a problem pronouncing "letters" (consonants and vowels). *Speech and Language* (Section IV).

6. Speech disorders exist because speaking is complex. All sections, but especially *Speech and Language* (Section IV) and *Speech Production and Perception* (Section V)

7. Speech disorders are more likely to result from problems with the brain's control of speech than from malformations in the mouth. *Speech Production and Perception* (Section V)

8. A speech problem results either because a child experiences difficulty learning from the environment, or because the environment is an inadequate teacher. *Speech and Brain Evolution* (Section VI) and *Speech and Brain Development* (Section VII)

9. A speech disorder may be an isolated deficit, or may be secondary to deficits in brain systems that support speech learning. *Speech and Brain Development* (Section VII)

10. A person might experience difficulty in making cell connections for speech learning as the result of normal variability, environmental deficits, or physical damage. *Speech and Brain Development* (Section VII)

APPENDIX 1A
Family Tree for *Homo sapiens*

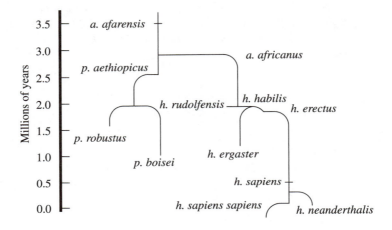

APPENDIX 1B
A Summary: Brain Development and the Environment

A legacy of humanity's evolutionary past is that extensive brain development occurs as a child is acquiring speech during childhood. Brain development during childhood allows the brain to be shaped by the environment in which a child lives. Rather than possessing a genetic inheritance that includes a specialized body and mind fitted to a specific environmental niche, a human brain grows while exposed to the environment into which it is born. A child brings an ability to grasp complex patterns and a brain that grows through interacting with the environment. The environment shapes a child's brain, narrowing the potential to learn from a wide number of possible environments to fit the actual one in which a child lives.

The following major aspects of brain development occur as the child interacts with the environment:

Brain Weight

Function: Brain size gives humans the capacity to grasp complex patterns, including those that underlie speech.

Growth: The human brain at birth is about 25% of its adult weight, grows maximally to 80% of its adult weight during the first few years of life, and reaches its mature size at adulthood.

Selective Elimination

Function: In areas of the brain responsible for speech learning as in other domains, a brain begins with "extra" cell connections. Those that are used are strengthened and retained, while those that are unused are eliminated.

Growth: Approximately one-third of cells are lost between birth and adulthood. Selective elimination occurs early in sensory areas and later in areas involved in higher cortical functions. The number of cell connections remains stable throughout much of adulthood.

Growth and Elaboration

Function: The environment stimulates growth and elaboration of cell connections, including those needed for speech learning.

Growth: An enriched environment promotes increased numbers of synapses per neuron in both children and adults, and environmental deprivation decreases numbers of cell connections. In humans, numbers of cell connections increase in old age, indicating a capacity for lifelong learning and, perhaps, compensating for neuronal deaths that occur during middle and old age.

Myelin Sheaths

Function: A white fatty substance on axons that acts as an insulator and speeds electrical transmission of signals between cells, myelin is critical for gross and fine motor movements, including speech.

Growth: Myelination of the brain begins near six months in utero, achieves its peak growth between birth and the end of the first year, and continues to grow until adulthood.

Wernicke's Area

Function: Wernicke's area is a functional region in the left temporal lobe for language comprehension.

Growth: A peak in the number of cell connections occurs during the first half of the first year; the mature number of cell connections is reached during the second half of the first year. Girls as young as nine have more dendritic connections in Wernicke's area than do males. On average, persons with a university education have more dendritic connections in Wernicke's area than do those with a high school diploma, who in turn have more than those with less than a high school education.

Broca's Area

Function: Broca's area is a functional region in the left frontal hemisphere that controls speech.

Growth: Density of cell connections in Broca's area does not peak until 15 months, and does not reach a mature number of connections until a child is six to eight years old.

Hippocampus

Function: The hippocampus is critical to working memory and such important speech activities as memory retention and word retrieval.

Growth: The hippocampus develops after the child is born, especially during the second year of life.

Prefrontal Cortex

Function: The prefrontal cortex is critically important to many cognitive activities that underlie speech, including reasoning, planning, judgment, and attention.

Growth: Cell connections in the prefrontal lobes develop slowly throughout childhood and do not reach maturity until after adolescence.

APPENDIX 1C
Foundations of Care

1. A person whose speech differs from his or her community's may be identified as speech disordered.

2. A speech disorder should be considered within the social context of the person with the problem.

3. A speech disorder may impact other language domains.

4. A speech disorder may have a language basis, a basis in production and perception, or a combination of both bases.

5. A speech disorder is more than a problem pronouncing "letters" (consonants and vowels).

6. Speech disorders exist because speaking is complex.

7. Speech disorders are more likely to result from problems with the brain's control of speech than from malformations in the mouth.

8. A speech problem results either because a child experiences difficulty learning from the environment, or because the environment is an inadequate teacher.

9. A speech disorder may be an isolated deficit, or may be secondary to deficits in brain systems that support speech learning.

10. A person might experience difficulty in making cell connections for speech learning as the result of normal variability, environmental deficits, or physical damage.

CHAPTER

2

Articulation and Phonological Disorders

The following topics are discussed in this chapter:

I. OVERVIEW

Speech is a complex activity with deep roots in human culture, evolution, language, anatomy and physiology, and brain development. As suggested in the first chapter, a person typically thinks of something to say, opens his or her mouth, and the sounds come out, one after another. The purpose of this book is to describe what to do when the typical does not happen, and the sounds do not come out, one after another. An overview of speech disorders is presented in Sections I–VI, including such essential topics as terminology, characteristics and causes, cultural components, prevalence, and legal basis of care. Phonetic symbols used in this book are described in Section VII. Special symbols and diacritics are the subjects of Section VIII, and special terminology is the topic of Section IX.

II. ARTICULATION AND PHONOLOGICAL DISORDERS

This book is concerned with speech problems called articulation and phonological disorders. The theoretical basis for the distinction between articulation and phonology was described in Chapter 1. The discussion in this section focuses on terminology and the distinction between "knowing and doing." Characteristics of articulation and phonological disorders are discussed in the following section.

A. Terminology

Terminology used in this book is similar to the usage of many authors (Bauman-Waengler, 2000; Bernthal & Bankson, 1998; Creaghead, Newman, & Secord, 1989; Lowe, 1994; Smit, 2003; Weiss, Gordon, & Lillywhite, 1987), but differs from others who prefer either articulation disorder or phonological disorder to encompass problems in speech motor control (articulation) and language (phonology) (Bernhardt & Stemberger, 1998; Fey, 1992; Hoffman, Schuckers, & Daniloff, 1989; Hodson, 1994a; Locke, 1983a; Shriberg & Kwiatkowski, 1982; Shelton & McReynolds, 1979; Williams, 2003; Winitz, 1984). Use of "articulation disorder" as the sole term is intended to emphasize that speech is a motor activity, whereas use of "phonological disorder" as the sole term is intended to emphasize that speech requires knowledge of language. Additional terminology the reader may encounter, which means approximately what is referred to here as articulation and phonological disorder, includes functional speech disorder, phonomotor disorder, speech disorder, functional articulation disorder, and—more rarely—idiopathic speech disorder. Finally, some authors, noting that persons with articulation and phonological disorders often speak similarly to younger children without speech problems, prefer to use the term delay rather than disorder (Curtiss, Katz, & Tallal, 1992; Leonard, 1985).

B. Knowing and Doing

Speech requires both language knowledge (phonology) and speech production and perception abilities (talking and listening). This is the theoretical basis for the clinical distinction between phonological and articulation disorders. Persons with phonological disorders are presumed to experience difficulty acquiring the language rules that underlie speech, while persons with articulation disorders are presumed to experience difficulty either producing or perceiving speech. To illustrate, a child with a phonological disorder might not know that [st] is a possible word initial consonant cluster (as in *stop*), whereas a child with an articulation disorder might not be able to shape his or her articulators in such a way as to pronounce [st].

In daily clinical practice, it is often impossible to distinguish between phonological and articulation causes. However, the conceptual distinction between knowing (phonology) and doing (speaking and listening) is important, because it suggests that seemingly similar difficulties may result from different causes. Possibly, a child with phonological problems also shows difficulties learning other aspects of language, including syntax and reading, while a child whose problem involves more "doing" than "knowing" has difficulties restricted to the pronunciation aspects of speech.

III. CHARACTERISTICS OF ARTICULATION AND PHONOLOGICAL DISORDERS

Not all speech problems are articulation and phonological disorders. A laryngeal anomaly, for example, may result in significant difficulties in speech motor control, but is not the type of difficulty that is amenable to the treatment principles described in this book. The types of speech problems addressed in these pages meet three criteria:

- The speech problem affects either or both phonology (language) or speaking and listening (perception and motor control).

- The speech problem arose during childhood, contains patterns similar to those found in typically developing children, and is not attributable solely to physical damage to motor or sensory systems.

- The speech problem is not the result of dialect or non-English language influences and is considered a disorder either by the client or members of the client's community.

A. First Criterion

The first criterion recognizes that speech has a dual nature, being both a part of language and a channel of communication. Virtually everyone agrees that speech disorders may arise from problems in either speech motor control (articulation disorders) or language knowledge (phonological disorders), even though research has not yet provided means to make this differential diagnosis in clinical practice.

B. Second Criterion

The second criterion distinguishes speech disorders of the types that are the focus of this book from speech problems arising directly from physical difficulties such as cranial nerve damage, unrepaired cleft palate, laryngeal anomalies, or difficulties in respiratory control. This criterion does not exclude from consideration disorders that occur in addition to problems arising from physical difficulties, nor does it exclude compensatory speech adjustments that persons with physical disabilities often develop, which are often amenable to remediation using principles described in this book.

C. Third Criterion

The third criterion distinguishes articulation and phonological disorders from dialect differences or influences of the language spoken in the client's community. The former signify difficulties in learning; the latter are part of the language system of the client's community. Selected varieties of English are depicted in Appendix 2A; although any variety of English can be affected using articulation and phonological principles, no variety of English is a type of disorder. The third criterion also recognizes that cultures and ethnic groups may differ both in what they identify as articulation and phonological disorders and in the priority they assign to remediation of various types of articulation and phonological disorders (Bleile & Wallach, 1992; Taylor & Peters-Johnson, 1986).

IV. CAUSES OF ARTICULATION AND PHONOLOGICAL DISORDERS

A child with an articulation and phonological disorder experiences difficulty learning speech from the environment. Reasons why a child might experience such a difficulty involve:

- Normal variation
- Environmental deficits
- Physical damage

A. Normal Variation

In common with many traits (including height and weight), speech development has a normal distribution, meaning that for every child who is "above average" in speech development another must be "below average." Stated more concretely, if children on the average acquire certain sounds and syllables at such or such an age, this implies that the acquisition of some children will be quicker than average and that of other children will be slower. At some point, a child who acquires speech more slowly than peers may be identified as having an articulation and phonological disorder.

B. Environmental Deficits

A second reason why a child might experience an articulation and phonological disorder is that their environment may prove an insufficient teacher. A legacy of the past two million years of human history is that the environment plays a pivotal role in shaping a child's mind. A neglected or abused child may live in an environment that does not foster speech development, resulting in slower than expected learning, or, in cases of extreme neglect, preclude virtually all speech development, as in the case of Genie, a child who lived in a closet throughout most of her early years (Curtiss, 1977). Importantly, the environment may prove an inadequate teacher of speech for reasons that benefit a child, as may occur during long-term hospitalizations. In such situations, conjunction of a child's illness and an environment focused more on medical than developmental issues may inhibit the child's ability to acquire speech.

C. Physical Damage

A third reason why a child may experience an articulation and phonological disorder is as a consequence of damage to the brain or body.

1. **Direct Damage.** Direct damage to language and to speech production and perception systems (Chapter 1) may affect speech learning, resulting in an articulation or phonological disorder. To illustrate, a child with a hearing impairment may experience an articulation and phonological disorder resulting from restricted exposure to acoustic aspects of speech. Similarly, a child with a repaired cleft palate may experience an articulation and phonological disorder as a consequence of needing to unlearn speech patterns acquired before and during repair of the cleft.

2. **Indirect Damage.** Articulation and phonological disorders also result from damage to systems that impact speech, as in the case of a child with attention deficit disorder. In attention deficit disorder, the difficulty is not specific to speech, but lies in the child's ability to concentrate sufficiently to acquire this complex aspect of communication. Intellectual impairments may also adversely affect learning. This limitation in learning includes speech, but is not specific to that domain.

3. **Single and Multiple Causes.** Causes may act alone or in conjunction with each other. A single cause does not necessarily mean a child will have a mild problem. To illustrate, severe delay relative to peers, extreme environmental neglect, or extensive physical damage may all result in significant articulation and phonological problems. However, having multiple causes of disorder often results in a more severe problem. To illustrate, a child with a severe articulation and phonological problem may experience a "ganging up effect" resulting from a combination of being slower in speech development than peers, having experienced environmental neglect, and possessing physical problems either directly or indirectly impacting speech development.

Hemispherectomy

The brain of a young child is highly flexible, showing an astonishing ability to organize and re-organize itself (Neville, 1991). A stunning illustration of this is found in children who have undergone hemispherectomy for Rasmussen encephalitis, a rare seizure disorder, in which either the right or left hemisphere is removed, depending on the locus of the seizures. Remarkably, children who undergo removal of the left hemisphere during the preschool years may not experience future speech and language difficulties (Stark, Bleile, Brandt, Freeman, & Vining, 1995; Curtiss & deBode, 1999; Curtiss, de Bode, and Mathern, 2001). I have personal knowledge of a case in which a four year old child had her left hemisphere removed and was wheeled from the surgery unit talking, joking, and singing. For this child, the seizures in the left hemisphere had caused speech to move to the remaining right. Thus, at the time of surgery the removed left hemisphere was "dead" as far as speech was concerned. Such complete recovery of speech would be surprising in children who have the surgery near adolescence or older (Vargha-Khadem, Carr, Isaacs, Brett, Adams, & Mishkin, 1997).

V. PREVALENCE

An articulation and phonological disorder is the most frequently encountered type of communication difficulty, occurring as either an isolated developmental problem or as part of a larger constellation of difficulties, including language disorders, mental retardation, respiratory problems, neurological injuries, cerebral palsy, and orofacial anomalies.

A. Prevalence of Communication Disorders

The following are prevalence statistics for communication disorders in the United States.

1. Speech and Language Disorders. An estimated 6 million children under age 18 have a speech or language disorder (Office of Scientific and Health Reports, 1988).

2. **Gender.** Two-thirds of children under age 18 with speech or language disorders are male (Office of Scientific and Health Reports, 1988).

3. **Comparison to Other Disabilities.** The most commonly diagnosed handicapping condition among persons 6 to 21 years old is learning disability (51.2%), followed by communication disorders (21.6%), mental retardation (11.5%), and emotional disturbance (8.7%) (U.S. Department of Education, 1994).

4. **Age.** Nearly 2% of persons under 18 years old have communication disorders. This number drops to below 1% of the population between 18 and 64 years old and then rises above 1% for persons 64 years and older (Schoenborn & Marano, 1989).

5. **Gender and Race.** Males younger than 45 years old are almost twice as likely to have communication disorders as females. African Americans younger than 45 years old of the same age are almost one third more likely to be diagnosed as having communication disorders as Caucasians (Schoenborn & Marano, 1989).

6. **Socioeconomic Scale.** Persons younger than 45 years old living in families making less than $10,000 annually are approximately twice as likely to be diagnosed as having communication disorders as peers living in homes making between $20,000 to $34,999 annually (Schoenborn & Marano, 1989).

7. **Educational Setting.** Nearly 85.5% of all school-age children with communication disorders receive their education in a regular classroom setting (U.S. Department of Education, 1994).

B. Prevalence of Articulation and Phonological Disorders

The following are prevalence statistics for articulation and phonological disorders.

1. **Compared to Other Communication Disorders.** Approximately 32% of all communication disorders are articulation and phonological disorders (Slater, 1992).

2. **Preschoolers.** Approximately 10–15% of preschoolers have an articulation and phonological disorders (Office of Scientific and Health Reports, 1988).

3. School-age Children. Approximately 6% of school-age children (K to 12th grade) have an articulation and phonological disorder (Office of Scientific and Health Reports, 1988).

4. Language Disorders. Approximately 75% to 85% of preschoolers with articulation and phonological disorders also experience disorders in language (Shriberg & Kwiatkowski, 1988; Paul & Shriberg, 1982).

5. Clinician Exposure. Approximately 92% of clinicians have clients with articulation and phonological disorders on their caseloads (Shewan, 1988).

VI. LEGAL BASIS OF CARE

Clinical care for articulation and phonological disorders is provided under a variety of local, state, and national laws. The following is the most pertinent legislation at the federal level (Whitmore, 2002).

A. Rehabilitation Act of 1973

This act prohibited discrimination on the basis of disability by any program or agency receiving federal funds.

B. Education for All Handicapped Children Act (P.L. 94–142 of 1975)

This act required that all children with disabilities have available a free, appropriate public education.

C. P.L. 94–142 Amendments of 1986

This amendment extended P.L. 94–142 to children birth through age 2.

D. P.L. 94–142 Reauthorized in 1990 as the Individual with Disabilities Education Act (IDEA)

This reauthorization emphasized the need for education services in the least restrictive environment, extended education services to children with autism and traumatic brain injury, and added transition services to facilitate movement from school to post-school settings.

E. Americans with Disabilities Act of 1990

This act mandated reasonable accommodations to persons with disabilities across all public and private settings.

F. Individual with Disabilities Education Act (IDEA) Amendments of 1997 (IDEA '97)

These amendments focused on improving education services for children with disabilities (Whitmore, 2002). Important mandates of this legislation for children with speech disorders include:

- Early identification of children with disabilities

- Enhanced participation of children with disabilities in the general curriculum

- Involvement of parents in their child's education

Importantly, IDEA '97 extends services to children with physical and medical conditions placing them at a high probability for future developmental delays, including those listed in Table 2–1 (Bleile & Burda, 2003; Bleile & Trenary, 2002). Safety precautions to follow when caring for children with medical needs are provided in Appendix 2B (Bleile, 1993a).

Children with Medical Needs

Speech difficulties are common among infants and toddlers with medical needs. Regardless of specific medical issues, infants and toddlers receive services similar to those given other children. The clinician's primary responsibility is to provide evaluation and intervention services appropriate to the child's developmental abilities. A difference in care provision is that the child's speech disorder is likely to occur as part of a larger picture of medical problems and developmental delay. This may make it difficult to diagnose and treat the speech disorder, especially when the child is younger and medical problems may predominate. In addition to having thorough training in typical speech and language development, speech-language clinicians working with these children should possess the following specialized training:

(continued)

- Basic knowledge of medical concepts and terminology,

- Ability to access and understand information about unfamiliar conditions and factors as the need arises,

- Knowledge of safety procedures and health precautions, and

- Ability to work well with teams that include the child's caregivers and professionals

Table 2–1. Conditions and factors present at birth or shortly thereafter with a high probability of resulting in future developmental delay.

Chromosomal abnormalities such as Down syndrome

Genetic or congenital disorders

Severe sensory impairments, including hearing and vision

Inborn errors of metabolism

Disorders reflecting disturbance of the development of the nervous system

Intracranial hemorrhage

Hyperbilirubinemia at levels exceeding need for exchange transfusion

Major congenital anomalies

Congenital infections

Disorders secondary to exposure to toxic substances, including fetal alcohol syndrome

Low birth weight

Respiratory distress

Lack of oxygen

Brain hemorrhage

Nutritional deprivation

VII. PHONETIC SYMBOLS

Extensive use of special symbols and notations is rare in clinical practice, and their use has generally been avoided in this book. Still, some special symbols, notations, and terminology are necessary; and others, although not necessary, are extremely convenient.

Symbols used to transcribe American English consonants and vowels are listed in Tables 2–2 and 2–3, respectively (International Clinical Phonetics and Linguistic Association, 1992). For convenience, American English central liquid is transcribed as [r], and the vowels [i] and [u] (which are often pronounced as diphthongs) are transcribed as [i] and [u], respectively. The consonant chart divides sounds according to place and manner, voiced/voiceless, nasal/oral, and central/lateral. The vowel chart displays sounds according to place, height, spread/unspread, and round/unround.

An American English

An effort is made throughout the book to write *American English* rather than *English*, because American English is the variety about which I know most, and varieties of English spoken in other countries are too numerous and varied to assume that what is written about one type of English necessarily pertains to another. However, rather than saying *American English*, it would be more accurate to write that the speech described in this book is *an American English*. English spoken in Hawaii, for example, is different from that spoken in Georgia or Vermont. Different ethnic and racial groups within the same geographical location add to the fascinating complexity of American speech.

VIII. SPECIAL SYMBOLS AND DIACRITICS

Special symbols and diacritics provide useful tools for describing clinically relevant aspects of speech.

A. Notations

Notations offer a convenient "shorthand" way to describe speech.

1. [ ] and / /. Square brackets indicate a phonetic transcription, and slashes indicate a phonemic transcription. Single sounds, groups of sounds, and entire words or phrases can be placed within brackets or slashes. The following examples demonstrate the use of this notation:

    a. Example: The consonant "b" as in bet.
    Notation: [b] or /b/

Table 2–2. American English consonants.

Manner of Production	Place of Production							
	Bilabial	Labiodental	Interdental	Alveolar	Postalveolar	Palatal	Velar	Glottal
Stop								
Oral	p b			t d			k g	
Nasal	m			n			ŋ	
Fricative		f v	θ ð	s z	ʃ ʒ			h
Affricate					tʃ dʒ			
Liquid								
Central				r				
Lateral				l				
Glide	w					j		

Table 2–3. American English vowels and diphtongs.

Height	Front + Sprd[a]	Central	Back – Rnd[b]	+ Rnd[c]
		Place		
Close	i			u
	ɪ		ʊ	
Close mid	eɪ			oʊ
		ə		
Open mid	ɛ		ʌ	ɔ
	æ			
Open	a			ɑ

[a] sprd = lips spread
[b] – Rnd = lips unrounded
[c] + Rnd = lips unrounded

Notes:
[ɔɪ] = tongue begins as for [ɔ] and moves toward [ɪ]
[aɪ] = tongue begins as for [a] and moves toward [ɪ]
[aʊ] = tongue begins as for [a] and moves toward [ʊ]
[ɚ] = tongue shape has both [ə]-like and [r]-like qualities

   b. **Example:** The American English voiceless stops.
   Notation: [p t k] or /p t k/

   c. **Example:** The word deep.
   Notation: [dip] or /dip/

Brackets or Slashes?

I typically transcribe a client's speech within square brackets (e.g., *bee* as [bi]). Square brackets imply nothing about the phonological status of the sounds being transcribed, whereas slashes (e.g., *bee* as /bi/) indicate that the sounds being transcribed are phonemes—that is, the sounds can distinguish between words in the client's speech, just as "p" and "b" do in adult English *pea* and *bee*. Determining which sounds are phonemes in a client's speech is a controversial procedure that is seldom performed in most clinical settings. For this reason, unless a phonemic analysis of the client's speech has been performed, I enclose a transcription in square brackets rather than slashes.

2. x → and x/y. The literal meaning of the first notation is "x becomes y"; the literal meaning of the second notation is "x for y." Both notations provide simple ways to describe speech changes. The arrow is used most often in linguistically oriented approaches, and the slash is used in more traditional approaches. The following examples demonstrate how these notations are used:

a. Example: The client says [w] for [r].
Notation: r → w w or w/r

b. Example: The client says fricatives as stops.
Notation: fricatives → stops or stops/fricatives

c. Example: The client deletes both members of consonant clusters.
Notation: CC → ø or ø/CC

3. x → y/z. This algebraic-looking notation literally means "x becomes y in the environment of z." The notation is used to describe how a phonetic or word environment affects production of speech. The "x" and "y" can be any articulation and phonological unit—features, consonants, vowels, individual sounds, syllables, or stress. The "z" typically is a distinctive feature, consonant, vowel, a syllable boundary (symbolized as "S"), or a word boundary (symbolized as "#"). The following examples demonstrate the use of this notation:

a. Example: The client says liquids as glides in the beginning of words.
Notation: liquids → glides/# _____

b. Example: The client says [s] as [z] between vowels.
Notation: s → z/V_____V

c. Example: The client says [g] as [k] at the end of syllables.
Notation: g → k/_____S

d. Example: The client deletes the first member of a consonant cluster in the beginning of words.
Notation: CC → øC/#_____

NON-ENGLISH SYMBOLS AND DIACRITICS

A. Place of Production

[ɸ] [β]**	Bilabial fricatives (two lips approximate each other)	ɸ
[̪]	Labiodental oral and nasal stops (upper teeth to lower lip)	p̪ b̪ m̪
[̪]	Dentolabial plosives and nasal (lower teeth to upper lip)	p̃ b̃ m̃
[̪]	Interdentalized (also called lisped) (tongue tip/blade between teeth)	t̪ θ̪ l̪
[̈]	Bidental (teeth approximated)	h̃ ũ
[̃]	Bidental percussive (teeth brought'percussively together)	t̃ d̃
[ɲ]	Palatal nasal (nasal stop made at palatal region)	
[x] [ɣ]	Velar fricatives (fricatives produced in the velar region)	x ɣ
[fŋ]	Velopharyngeal fricative (fricative made in velopharyngeal region)	fŋ
[ʔ]	Glottal stop (stop produced at vocal folds)	ʔ

B. Manner of Production

[↔]	Labial spreading (lips spread)	s↔ t↔
[__]	Unrounded (lips at rest, unpursed)	w̱
[ˣ]	Denasal (little air through nose)	m̽ n̽
[ˣ]	Nasal escape (air through nose)	p̽ s̽

[ˌ]	Bladed (produced with tongue blade)	s̪ z̪
[ɹ]	[w]-coloring ([r] with a [w]-like quality)	ɹ̫
[ɾ]	Flap (quick stop-like consonant as in *butter*)	ɾ
[ˡs]	Lateralized [s] and [z], respectively (air over the sides of tongue)	[ˡs] [ˡz]
[ˌˌ]	Stronger production (produced with greater force than is typical)	[f̟]
[˷]	Weaker production (produced with less force than is typical)	m
[↑]	Whistled (high pitched sound)	[s̩↑]
[ț]	Wet sound (produced with excess saliva)	ț

C. Airstream

| [↓] | Ingressive (air moves inward) | p↓ |
| [(X)] | Silent or 'mouthing' (no sound produced) | (s) |

D. Vocal Fold Activity

[ˌ] [ˌ]	Pre- and post-voicing of sounds (voicing begins or ends later than expected)	ˌb z ˌ
[(o)]	Partial devoicing (normally voiced sound is partially devoiced)	z(o)
[(v)]	Partial voicing (normally voiceless sound is partially voiced)	f(v)
[ʰ]	Pre-aspiration (sound begins with aspiration)	ʰp
[°]	Unaspirated (normally aspirated voiceless stops produced without aspiration)	p° t° k°

E. Syllables and Stress

[̩]	Syllabic (consonant standing as a syllable)	l̩
[.]	Syllable boundary (separation between syllables)	bi.twin
[']	Primary stress (syllable with main stress)	bitwín

Adapted from: "Recommended phonetic symbols: Extensions of the IPA" by the International Clinical Phonetics and Linguistics Association (1992), *Clinical Linguistics and Phonetics, 6,* 259–261. With permission.
** = Whenever two symbols are presented, the first is unvoiced and the second is voiced.

IX. SPECIALIZED TERMINOLOGY

The following terminology is commonly used to describe the speech of clients with articulation and phonological disorders. Topics are abbreviations, characteristics of speech, descriptions of errors, error patterns, influence of one sound on another, manner of production, names for sounds, phonetic and word environments, place of production, prespeech and early speech, theoretical constructs, and vowels. Definitions of terms are provided after all the topics are listed.

A. Topics

1. Abbreviations
C   CVC   V
CV   S

2. Characteristics of Speech

Aspiration	Lips spread
Blends	Light [l]
Cognates	Multisyllabic
Consonant	Nasality
Consonant cluster	Primary stress
Dark [l]	Prosody
Dentalized	Retroflex [r] and [ɝ]
Dialect	Rounding
Distinctive features	Singleton
Eggressive	Spreading

Homorganic
Homonyms
Humped [r] and [ɚ]
Ingressive
Intonation
Lip rounding

Unaspirated
Velarized [l]
Voiced
Voiceless
Voicing

3. Descriptions of Errors
Apraxia
Articulation error
Articulation disorder
Brackets
Broad transcription
Buccal (pronounced "buckle") speech
Deletion
Devoicing
Diacritics
Distortion
Dysarthria
Initial consonant deletion
Labialization
Lateral [s]
Narrow transcription
Nasalization
Omission
Pharyngeal fricative
Phonemic transcription
Phonetic transcription
Phonological error
Phonological patterns
Phonological processes
Phonological rule
Slashes
Stimulability
Stridency deletion
Substitution

4. Error Patterns
Affrication
Backing
Cluster reduction
Denasalization
Epenthesis (ePENthesis)

Lateralization
Lateral lisp
Lisping
Metathesis (MeTAthesis)
Prevocalic voicing

Final consonant deletion
Final consonant devoicing
Frontal lisp
Fronting
Gliding
Glottal replacement
Labial assimilation

Reduplication
Stopping
Syllable deletion
Velar assimilation
Vocalization
Vowel neutralization

5. Influence of One Sound on Another

Assimilation
Coalescence

Progressive assimilation
Regressive assimilation

6. Manner of Production

Affricate
Approxirnant
Fricative
Glide
Lateral
Liquid
Manner of production
Nasals
Nasal stop

Central
Continuants
Obstruent
Oral stop
Semivowels
Sibilant
Sonorants
Stop
Strident

7. Names for Sounds

Capital "E"
Caret
Digraph
Epsilon
Horseshoe

Long "s" Open "o"
Print "a"
Schwa
Theta
Thorn

8. Phonetic and Word Environments

Ambisyllabic
Arrestor
Environments
Initial sound
Intervocalic
Medial sound
Onset
Open syllable

Phonetic environments
Postvocalic
Resyllabification
Syllable initial position
Syllable final position
Word-final position
Word-initial position
Word-medial position

9. Place of Production

Alveolar
Bilabial

Labiodental
Palatal

Dental
Glottal
Interdental
Labial

Place of production
Postalveolar
Velar

10. Prespeech and Early Speech

Babble
Canonical babbling
Cooing
Jargon

Nonreduplicated babbling
Reduplicated babbling
Variegated babbling

11. Theoretical Constructs

Allophone
Coarticulation
Complementary distribution
Discrimination training
Independent analysis
Maximal pair
Metalinguistics
Minimal pair
Noncontrastive
Phone

Phoneme
Phonetics
Phonological knowledge
Phonology
Phonotactics
Perception training
Relational analysis
Rime/rhyme
Word pairs

12. Vowels

Back vowels and diphthongs
Central vowels
Close
Close-mid
Diphthong
Front vowels
High vowels

Neutral vowels
Open
Open-mid
Pure vowel
R-colored vowel
Rhotic vowel
Vowel

B. Definitions

Affricate. A consonant with a stop onset and fricative release. The American English affricates are [tʃ] and [dʒ].

Affrication. An error pattern in which stops or fricatives are pronounced as affricates; for example, *see* is pronounced as [tsi].

Allophone. A variant of a phoneme that does not affect meaning; for example, unaspirated [p°] and aspirated [pʰ] are allophones of the phoneme /p/.

Alveolar. A class of consonants produced with constriction between articulators at the alveolar ridge, which lies immediately posterior to the upper front teeth. The American English alveolar consonants are [t], [d], [s], [z], [n], [l], and [r].

Ambisyliabic. A consonant sometimes considered to belong to two syllables; for example, some investigators consider the second [m] in *mama* to be ambisyllabic.

Approximant. Liquids and glides. The American English approximants are [l], [r], [j], and [w].

Apraxia. A disorder involving voluntary, but not involuntary, speech movements. For example, a client with apraxia may not be able to respond correctly when asked to touch the lip with the tongue but when eating may lick a crumb from the lip.

Arrestor. A consonant occurring after a vowel in the same syllable; for example, "t" is the arrestor consonant in *bit*.

Articulation error. A speech error resulting from problems in speech motor control.

Articulation disorder. As defined in this book, an articulation disorder results from problems in speech motor control. Some authors use the term articulation disorder to refer to problems in both phonology and speech motor control.

Aspiration. A burst of air arising after the release of a voiceless stop in positions such as the beginning of a word; for example, in American English [t] in *tube* [tʰub].

Assimilation. The influence of one sound on another. See also **Progressive assimilation** and **Regressive assimilation.**

Babble. A prespeech vocalization in which repetitions of syllables predominate.

Backing. An error pattern in which alveolar consonants are replaced by velar consonants; for example, *tee* is pronounced as [ki].

Back vowels and diphthongs. Vowels in which the back of the tongue is the major articulator; The American English back vowels and diphthongs are [u], [ʊ], [oʊ], [ɔ], [ɔɪ], [ʌ], and [ɑ].

Bilabial. Consonants made using the two lips. The American English bilabial consonants are [p], [b], [m], and [w].

Blends. Consonant clusters.

Brackets. Transcriptions enclosed by brackets indicate that the sounds were produced; no claim is made regarding whether or not the sounds are phonemes of the language. For example, placing "b" within brackets (i.e., [b]) indicates the sound was produced, but does not indicate whether or not [b] is a phoneme. See **Phoneme.**

Broad transcription. Transcription of phonemes. Broad transcriptions are enclosed within slashes. See **Phoneme** and **Slashes.**

Buccal (pronounced "buckle") speech. Speech produced by trapping air between the cheeks; sometimes called "Donald Duck speech." Children with tracheostomies often discover they can make words and short phrases using buccal speech.

C. Consonant.

Canonical babbling. See **Reduplicated babbling.**

Capital "E" (pronounced [i]). The name for the sound transcribed [ɪ].

Caret. The name for the sound transcribed [ʌ].

Central. Sounds made with air flowing over the tongue midline. All the American English consonants are central, except [l], which is lateral.

Central vowel. Vowel in which the tongue blade is the major articulator. The American English central vowel is [ə].

Close. Vowels and diphthongs produced with the tongue raised toward the roof of the mouth. The category "close" replaces "high" in the revised International Phonetic Alphabet (International Clinical Phonetics and Linguistic Association, 1992). The American English close vowels and diphthongs are [i], [ɪ], [u], and [ʊ].

Close-mid. Vowels and diphthongs produced with the tongue in a relatively neutral position. The category "close-mid" replaces "mid" in the revised International Phonetic Alphabet (International Clinical Phonetics and Linguistic Association, 1992). The American English close-mid vowels and diphthongs are [eɪ], [oʊ], and [ə].

Cluster Reduction. An error pattern in which a consonant or consonants in a consonant cluster are deleted; for example, *speed* is pronounced as [pid] or [sid].

Coalescence. The merger of two or more sounds; for example, the pronunciation of [sp] in *spy* as [f], which appears be a coalescence of the place of production of [p] (labial) and the manner of production of [s] (fricative).

Coarticulation. The theory that sounds are blended together during speech production.

Cognates. Two sounds that differ only in voicing; for example, [p] and [b] are cognates.

Complementary distribution. Sounds that never occur in the same phonetic environment; for example, English [h] and [ŋ] are in complementary distribution.

Consonant. A sound made with marked constriction somewhere along the vocal tract.

Consonant cluster. Two or more consonants occurring within the same syllable in which the sequence of consonants is uninterrupted by vowels.

Continuants. Sounds that can be sustained for extended periods of time. The American English continuant sound classes are fricatives, nasals, liquids, glides, vowels, and diphthongs.

Cooing. A prespeech vocalization containing consonants and vowels produced at the back of the mouth.

CV. Consonant-vowel.

CVC. Consonant-vowel-consonant.

Dark [l]. [l] produced in the velar area. Also called velarized [l].

Deletion. Failure to produce a sound; for example, the pronunciation of *deep* as [di].

Denasalization. An error pattern in which nasal consonants are pronounced as oral consonants (typically oral stops); for example, *me* is pronounced *bi*.

Dental. Consonants produced with the tongue tip against the back of the upper front teeth. In American English, alveolar consonants typically are dentalized when they occur prior to an interdental consonant, as in *tenth*.

Dentalized. See **Dental.**

Devoicing. Production with partial voicing or complete lack of voicing of sounds that are typically produced with voicing.

Diacritics. Modifications made to phonetic symbols to describe phonetic details; for example, a small raised [ʰ] is a diacritic used to indicate aspiration.

Dialect. A variation of speech caused by the influence of region, social class, or ethnic or racial identification.

Digraph. The name for the sound transcribed [æ].

Diphthong. A sequence of two vowels in which only one is syllabic. The American English diphthongs are [eɪ], [aɪ], [aʊ], [ɔɪ], and [oʊ].

Discrimination training. See **Perception Training.**

Distinctive features. Attributes of sounds that distinguish one sound from another.

Distortion. An inaccurately produced sound.

Dysarthria. Motor speech disorders arising from impairments originating in the peripheral or central nervous system.

Environments. See **Phonetic environments.**

Epenthesis (ePENthesis). An error pattern in which a vowel is inserted between consonants in a consonant cluster; for example, *treat* is pronounced [tərit].

Epsilon. The name for the sound transcribed [ɛ].

Eggressive. The outward flow of air from the mouth or nose.

Final consonant deletion. An error pattern in which a consonant occurring at the end of a syllable or word is deleted; for example, *beet* is pronounced [bi].

Final consonant devoicing. An error pattern in which voiced obstruents are devoiced at the end of a syllable or word; for example, *mead* is pronounced as [mit].

Fricative. A consonant produced with a sufficiently small distance between the articulators to cause a "hissing sound." The American English fricatives are [f], [v], [θ],[ð], [s], [z], [ʃ], and [ʒ].

Front vowels and diphthongs. Vowels in which the tongue tip is the major articulator; the American English front vowels and diphthongs are [i], [ɪ], [eɪ], [ɛ], [æ], [a], [aɪ], and [aʊ].

Frontal lisp. See *Lisping.*

Fronting. An error pattern in which velar consonants (and sometimes postalveolar affricates) are pronounced as alveolar consonants; for example, *key* is pronounced [ti].

Glide. Consonants produced with relatively little constriction between articulators. The American English glides are [j] and [w].

Gliding. An error pattern in which a fluid consonant is pronounced as a glide; for example, *Lee* is pronounced [wi] or (less typically) [ji].

Glottal. Sounds produced at the vocal folds; for example, [h] is a glottal glide.

Glottal replacement. An error pattern in which a consonant is pronounced as a glottal stop; for example, *boot* is pronounced [buʔ].

High vowels. Vowels produced with the tongue raised toward the roof of the mouth. The American English high vowels are [i], [ɪ], [u], and [ʊ].

Homorganic. Sounds produced at the same place of production; for example, in American English [b], [p], [m], and [w] are homorganic.

Homonyms. Words that sound alike but have different meanings; for example, *reed* and the present tense of *read* are homonyms.

Horseshoe. The name for the sound transcribed [ʊ].

Humped [r] and [ɚ]. Production of [r] and [ɚ] with the tongue tip lowered and the bulk of the tongue raised. See **Retroflex [r] and [ɚ].**

Independent analysis. A type of analysis in which a client's speech abilities are described without reference to the language of the client's community; for example, an independent analysis might describe a client's speech as containing [p b t d], but would not indicate if these consonants are produced correctly relative to the adult language (Stoel-Gammon & Dunn, 1985). Also see **Relational analysis.**

Ingressive. Sounds made with the inward movement of air.

Initial consonant deletion. An error pattern in which the consonant beginning a word is deleted; for example, *bee* is pronounced [i].

Initial sound. A sound beginning a word or syllable.

Interdental. Consonants produced with the tongue tip protruding between the upper and lower front teeth. The American English interdental consonants are [θ] and [ð].

Intervocalic. Consonants occurring between vowels; for example, the second [b] in *baby* is intervocalic. Also see **Syllable position.**

Intonation. See **Prosody.**

Jargon. Sentence-like units in which the sounds are pronounced with little phonetic accuracy. Clients who produce jargon are sometimes said to "know the tune before the words."

Labial. Bilabial and labiodental consonants. The American English labial consonants are [p], [b], [m], [w], [f], and [v].

Labial assimilation. An error pattern in which consonants assimilate to the place of production of a labial consonant; for example, *bead* is pronounced [bib].

Labialization. Pronunciation of consonants with greater-than-expected lip rounding.

Labiodental. Consonants produced with the upper lip and lower teeth. The American English labiodental consonants are [f] and [v].

Lateral. Sounds produced with air flowing over the sides of the tongue. The American English lateral is [l].

Lateral lisp. See **Lisping.**

Lateral [s]. [s] produced with air flowing over the sides of the tongue. The symbol for lateral [s] is [ls].

Lateralization. An error pattern in which sounds typically produced with central air emission (most commonly [s] and [z]) are pronounced with lateral air emission; for example, *see* is pronounced [ls i] (see Section VIII for diacritics).

Lip rounding. See **Rounding.**

Lips spread. See **Spreading.**

Light [l]. [l] made at the alveolar place of production. Light [l] typically occurs in syllable-initial position in American English.

Liquid. A class of sounds made with a relatively large aperture between the tongue and the roof of the mouth. The American English liquids are [l] and [r].

Lisping. An error pattern in which alveolar consonants (typically fricatives) are pronounced with the tongue either on or between the front teeth; for example, *see* pronounced [s̯i]. Also called a frontal lisp. Lateral lisps are the same as lisping except the airflow comes over the sides of the tongue.

Long "s" (pronounced [ɛs]). The name for the sound transcribed [ʃ].

Manner of production. The degree of narrowing in the vocal tract and direction of air flow that occurs during the production of sounds. The American English manner of production classes are stops (oral and nasal), affricates, fricatives, liquids, glides, vowels, and diphthongs.

Maximal pair. See **Word pair.**

Medial sound. See **Word-medial position.**

Metalinguistics. The ability to reflect on language.

Metathesis (MeTAthesis). An error pattern in which the order of sounds in a word is reversed; for example, *peek* pronounced [kip].

Minimal pair. See **Word pairs.**

Multisyllabic. More than one syllable.

Narrow transcription. Transcription containing diacritics to indicate the actual speech sounds produced by a speaker. Narrow transcriptions are enclosed in brackets. See also **Brackets.**

Nasals. A class of consonants made with a lowered velum. The American English nasal stops are [m], [n], and [ŋ]. See also **Nasal stop.**

Nasal stop. A consonant made with the velum lowered and complete closure somewhere in the oral tract.

Nasality. Production of a sound with the velum lowered.

Nasalization. Non-nasal consonants (usually oral stops) are pronounced as nasal stops.

Neutral vowels. Vowels that "stand-in" for many other vowels and diphthongs in unstressed syllables; for example, [ə], [ɪ], and [ʊ] are neutral vowels for many American English speakers.

Noncontrastive. See **Complementary distribution.**

Nonreduplicated babbling. Babbling in which consonants and vowels vary within syllables; for example, *ba-di-du* or *mu-mi*. See also **Reduplicated babbling.**

Obstruent. Oral stops, affricates, and fricatives.

Omission. See **Deletion.**

Onset. A linguistic unit theorized by some researchers to occur at the beginning of syllables; for example, [sp] in *spy* and [t] in *toe* are considered onsets in some linguistic theories of syllable structure.

Open. Vowels and diphthongs produced with the tongue lying relatively flat on the floor of the mouth. "Open" replaces "low" in the revised International Phonetic Alphabet (International Clinical Phonetics and Linguistic Association, 1992). The American English open vowels and diphthongs are [a], [ɑ], [aɪ], and [aʊ].

Open-mid. Vowels and diphthongs produced with the tongue raised slightly from the floor of the mouth. The category of "open-mid" replaces "mid" in the revised International Phonetic Alphabet (International Clinical Phonetics and Linguistic Association, 1992). The American English open-mid vowels and diphthongs are [ɛ], [ʌ], [ɔɪ], and [ɔ].

Open "o" (pronounced [oʊ]). The name for the sound transcribed [ɔ].

Open syllable. Syllable ending with a vowel or diphthong; for example, *bay* and *toe* have open syllables.

Oral stop. Stop consonants that are produced with a raised velum. The American English oral stops are [p], [b], [t], [d], [k], and [g].

Palatal. Place of production at which the tongue approximates the hard palate. The American English palatal consonant is [j].

Perception training. Clinical philosophy that training helps to improve a client's ability to distinguish between different sounds, syllables, and words.

Pharyngeal fricative. A fricative produced in the pharyngeal region. Pharyngeal fricatives sometimes occur in the speech of clients with repaired cleft palates.

Phone. A sound of a language. Every consonant, vowel, and diphthong is a phone.

Phoneme. A sound that is capable of distinguishing between words; for example, [p] and [b] are American English phonemes as illustrated by the words *bee* and *pea*.

Phonetic environments. Positions in syllables in which sounds occur; for example, [t] in *beet* occurs in the syllable-final position and [d] in *buddy* occurs in the intervocalic position.

Phonemic transcription. Transcription of the phonemes of a language.

Phonetic transcription. Transcription of the sounds of a language.

Phonetics. The study of the acoustic, psychoacoustic, and production aspects of speech.

Phonological awareness. Conscious awareness of the sound structure of a language.

Phonological error. A speech error resulting from absent or limited knowledge of the phonological system of the language.

Phonological knowledge. A person's knowledge of the phonological organization of his or her language.

Phonological patterns. See **Phonological processes.**

Phonological processes. Descriptions of systematic differences between the client's speech and the speech of adults in the client's community. Phonological processes are sometimes called phonological patterns.

Phonological rule. A description of the systematic relationship between units in a phonological system.

Phonology. The study of the linguistic organization of sound.

Phonotactics. The rules for the sequential arrangement of speech sounds; for example, an English phonotactic rule is that [sp] is an acceptable word-initial consonant cluster but [ps] is not.

Place of production. The point in the vocal tract at which maximum constriction occurs during production of a sound. Place of production is sometimes called place of articulation.

Postalveolar. A place of production immediately posterior to the alveolar ridge. "Postalveolar" replaces "alveopalatal" in the revised edition of the International Phonetic Alphabet (Intemational Clinical Phonetics and Linguistic Association, 1992). The American English postalveolar consonants are [tʃ], [dʒ], [ʃ], and [ʒ].

Postvocalic. Consonants occurring after a vowel in the same syllable; for example, [t] in *eat* [it].

Prevocalic Voicing. An error pattern in which consonants are voiced when they occur before a vowel; for example, *pea* pronounced as [bi].

Primary stress. The major stress in a word; for example, the syllable *tween* carries the primary stress in *between.*

Print "a" (pronounced [eɪ]). The name for the sound transcribed [a].

Progressive assimilation. Assimilation due to the influence of an earlier occurring sound on a later occurring sound; for example, [r] is often pronounced with rounded lips in *shriek* because of the lip rounding that occurs in [ʃ]. Also see **Regressive assimilation.**

Prosody. Modifications in pitch, stress, and duration of sounds as they occur in phrases and sentences.

Pure vowel. A vowel that remains relatively unchanged throughout its production; the American English pure vowels are [i], [ɪ], [æ], [a], [ɑ], [ə], [ʌ], [ɔ], [ʊ], and [u].

R-colored vowel. See **Rhotic vowel.**

Reduplicated babbling. Babbling in which syllables are repeated; for example, *ba-ba-ba* or *da-da.* Also see **Nonreduplicated babbling.**

Reduplication. An error pattern in which a syllable is repeated; for example, the pronunciation of *water* as [wɑwɑ].

Regressive assimilation. Assimilation resulting from the effect of a later occurring sound on an earlier occurring sound; for example, [n] in *tenth* is often produced as a dental consonant because of the influence of interdental [θ]. See also **Progressive assimilation.**

Relational analysis. Analysis that compares the client's speech to the speech of the client's community (Stoel-Gammon & Dunn, 1985). An example of a relational analysis is the statement, "The client produced [k] as [t]." Also see **Independent analysis.**

Resyllabification. Movement of a sound from its original syllable; for example, [t] in the phrase *It is* often is resyllabified to *I tis* in casual speech.

Retroflex [r] and [ɚ]. [r] and [ɚ] are produced in one of two ways: humped or retroflexed. Retroflex [r] and [ɚ] are produced with the tongue body slightly retracted, the tongue tip raised, and the sides of the back of the tongue against the inside of the teeth. See also **Humped [r] and [ɚ].**

Rhotic vowel. Production of a schwa with an [r]-coloring; for example, the vowel in *merge* and the vowels in *murder.*

Rime (also called Rhyme). A linguistic unit within a syllable theorized to include the vowel and any final consonants; for example, the vowel + [nt] in *bent* is considered a rime in some linguistic theories of syllable structure.

Rounding. Lip puckering that accompanies [w] and some back vowels and diphthongs. For many speakers some lip rounding also accompanies [ʃ]. The American English back unrounded vowels are [ʊ], [ʌ], and [ɑ] and the American English back rounded vowels are [u], [oʊ], [ɔ], and [ɔɪ].

S. Syllable.

Schwa. The name for the sound transcribed as [ə].

Semivowels. A consonant that can "stand-in" for a vowel. The American English semivowels are [j] and [w].

Sibilant. Alveolar and postalveolar fricatives and the fricative portion of alveolar and postalveolar affricates.

Singleton. A sound not in a consonant cluster.

Slashes. Transcriptions enclosed by slashes indicate that the sounds are phonemes of the language; for example, /p/ is a phoneme of English. See **Phoneme.**

Sonorants. Sounds produced with relatively unobstructed airflow. The American English sonorant sound classes are nasals, liquids, glides, and vowels.

Spreading. A smile-like stretch of the lips that accompanies [s] and [z] and American English front vowels and diphthongs.

Stimulability. The ability to imitate a sound.

Stop. A class of consonants made with complete closure at some point in the vocal tract. The American English oral stops are [p], [b], [t], [d], [k], and [g] and the American English nasal stops are [m], [n], and [ŋ].

Stopping. An error pattern in which a sound (typically a fricative or affricate) is pronounced as an oral stop; for example, the pronunciation of *see* as [ti].

Stridency deletion. Deletion of strident consonants. See **Strident.**

Strident. Sounds characterized by noisiness resulting from a fast rate of air flow. The English strident consonants are fricatives and affricates in labiodental [f v], alveolar [s z], and postalveolar [tʃ dʒ ʃ ʒ] places of production.

Substitution. Replacement of one sound with another; for example, a substitution of [s] for [t] results in *see* being said as *tee.*

Syllable initial position. The beginning of a syllable; for example, [b] in *bug,* [sp] in *spy,* and [t] in *captain* occur in syllable initial position.

Syllable final position. The end of a syllable; for example, [t] in *pit,* [nt] in *mint,* and [p] in *captain* occur in syllable final position.

Syllable deletion. An error pattern in which an unstressed syllable is deleted; for example, *banana* is pronounced as [nænə].

Theta. The name for the sound transcribed [θ].

Thorn. The name for the sound transcribed [ɚ].

Unaspirated. Production of a typically aspirated oral stop without aspiration; for example, the pronunciation of *pea* [pʰi] as [pºi].

V. Vowel.

Variegated babbling. See **Nonreduplicated babbling.**

Velar. Place of production made by raising the back of the tongue toward the soft palate. The American English velar consonants are [k], [g], and [ŋ]. Vowels and diphthongs are also made in the velar position, but these are typically called back vowels and back diphthongs rather than velar vowels and velar diphthongs.

Velar assimilation. An error pattern in which consonants assimilate to the place of production of a velar consonant; for example, *teak* is pronounced [kik].

Velarized [l]. See **Dark [l].**

Vocalization. An error pattern in which a syllabic consonant is replaced by a neutral vowel; for example, beetle is pronounced [biʔu].

Voiced. Sound made with vocal fold vibration.

Voiceless. Sound made without vocal fold vibration.

Voicing. Vibration of the vocal folds.

Vowel. A sound made without marked constriction in the vocal tract.

Vowel neutralization. An error pattern in which a vowel is replaced with a neutral vowel; for example, *bat* is pronounced [bət].

Word-final position. Sounds ending a word; for example, [t] in *boat* is in word-final position. Sounds occurring in word-final position are also said to occur word finally.

Word-initial position. Sounds beginning a word; for example, [p] in *pit* is in word-initial position. Sounds occurring in word-initial position are also said to occur word initially.

Word-medial position. Sounds in the middle of a word; for example, [n] in "final" and [d] in *window* are in word-medial position. Sounds occurring in word-medial position are also said to occur word medially.

Word pairs. Words that differ by a single sound; for example, *pea* and *bee* are word pairs. Word pairs that differ by one distinctive feature in one sound are called minimal pairs (e.g., [p] and [b] in *pea* and *bee*). Word pairs that differ by more than one distinctive feature in one sound are called maximal pairs (e.g., [p] and [m] in *pea* and *me*).

APPENDIX 2A
Varieties of English

Knowledge of varieties of English is needed to distinguish disorder from possible influence of the language community. The following information illustrates eight varieties of English spoken in the United States:

- African American English (AAE)
- Spanish-influenced English
- Asian-influenced English
- Hawaiian Creole
- Russian-influenced English
- Hindi-influenced English
- Singapore Colloquial English (SCE)
- Turkish-influenced English

The descriptions of AAE, Spanish-influenced English, and Asian-influenced English are adapted with permission from the more in-depth discussion in *Cultural and Linguistic Diversity: Resource Guide for Speech-Language Pathologists* (Goldstein, 2000). The discussion of Hawaiian Island Creole is adapted from Bleile (1996). The depiction of Hindi-influenced English is adapted from Ray (in preparation), that of Russian-influenced English is adapted from Shilovskaya (2003), of Singapore-influenced English is adapted from Graham, Lam, Lee, Loader, and Ping (2003), and that of Turkish-influenced English is adapted from Topbas (1997).

Information available on forms of English described in this section varies tremendously. When sufficient information exists, patterns are shown for consonants and consonant classes, vowels, and prosody. When information is less complete, more abridged descriptions are provided. Additionally, the terminology of error patterns is suited to some English varieties, but not others. In situations where the terminology seems inadequate or misleading, a longer description of the pattern is provided.

African American English

African American English (AAE) is a variety of English spoken by many African Americans. AAE varies by region, social class, and formality of setting.

Pattern	**Word**	**Pronunciation**	**AAE**
Consonants			
Stops			
• Coarticulated glottal stop with devoiced final stop	bad	bæd	bæt?
• Devoicing of final consonants	tube	tub	tup
• Deletion of final alveolar stops	pad	pæd	pæ
Nasals			
• Absence of final nasal consonants	pan	pæn	pæ
Fricatives			
• Word initial [d] for [ð]	they	ðe	de
• Intervocalic and word final [f] for [θ] and [v] for [ð]	brother	brʌðɚ	brʌdɚ
Liquids			
• Deletion of postvocalic [r] and [l]	more	mor	mo
Consonant clusters			
• [k] for [t] in [str] clusters	street	strit	skrit
• Final consonant simplification, especially when both members of the consonant cluster are voiced or voiceless	desk	dɛsk	dɛs
• Metathesis of consonants in a cluster	ask	æsk	æks

Vowels
- The diphthongs [aɪ], [aʊ], and [ɔɪ] often neutralize to [a], [a], and [ə], respectively

Prosody

• Absence of initial unstressed syllables	about	əbaʊt	baʊt
• Stress on the first rather than the second syllable	Detroit	Detróit	Détroit
• Use of wide range of intonation contours and vowel elongations			
• Use of more level and falling final contours and rising contours			
• Replacement of absent final consonants with nasalization or lengthening of preceding vowel	cone	kon	ko: or kõ

Spanish-influenced English

Spanish contains 18 consonants and 5 vowels. Consonant clusters occur in syllable initial position and contain a stop consonant followed by either a flap or [l]. Five consonants can appear in word-final position: [l r d n s]. The following consonants exist in English, but not Spanish: [v θ ʔ h].

Pattern	Word	Pronunciation	Spanish-influenced English
• Addition	stamp	stæmp	estæmp
• Affrication	she	ʃi	tʃi
• Consonant devoicing	he's	hiz	his
• Nasal velarization	fan	fæn	fæŋ
• Stopping	vase	ves	bes
	thought	θɑt	tɑt
	though	ðo	do

Asian-influenced English

Asian-influenced English is an "umbrella" for a wide variety of languages: including Chinese, Japanese, and other variations from locations such as the Philippines, Korea, and southern and southeast Asia.

Pattern	Word	Pronunciation	Asian-influenced English
• Epenthesis	blue	blu	bəlu
	beak	bik	bik
• Final consonant deletion	gate	get	ge
• Syllable deletion	potato	potato	teto
• [l] for [r]	ray	re	le
• Stopping	vase	ves	bes
• [ʃ] for [tʃ]	cheap	tʃip	ʃip

Hawaiian Creole

Hawaiian Creole is spoken in Hawaii. Major characteristics of Hawaiian Creole include the following.

Pattern	Word	Pronunciation	Hawaiian Creole
• Stopping of [θ] and [ð]	thought	θɑt	tɑt
• Deletion of [r] after a vowel	more	mor	moə

• Deletion of final consonants	beak	bik	bi
• Backing and affrication of alveolar consonants in [r] clusters	tree	tri	tʃri

Russian-influenced English

There are 6 vowels and 36 consonant phonemes in Russian. The most common vowel is /a/. The most common consonants are /t n s/, the least common consonants are /g f/. Phonemes that appear in English and do not exist in Russian are /θ ð ŋ w r/. Phonemes that appear in Russian but do not exist in English are /i̧/ (central close unrounded), trilled /r/, velar fricative /x/, and retroflex fricative /ʂ/. In Russian, phonology stops /t d/ as well as nasals /l n/ are pronounced as either dental or postalveolar /t' d' n' l'/.

Stress and intonation in Russian language depends on the number of words in a sentence. Typically, stress falls on every word in a sentence, except for particles and conjunctions, producing an impression of "flat" intonation as compared to American English.

Pattern	Word	Pronunciation	Russian-influenced English
Consonants			
Fricatives			
• Alveolar for dental before high and mid front vowels	this	ðɪs	zɪs or dɪs
• [w] for [v]	votka	vɑtkə	wɑtkə
• [v] for [w]	we	wi	vi
• Velar for glottal	hello	helo	xɛlo
Stops			
• Postalveolar for alveolar	trendy	trɛndi	t'rɛnd'i
• Devoicing of final consonants	tube	tub	tup
Nasals			
• [n] for [ŋ]	pink	piŋk	pink
Vowels			
• [i] for [ɪ]	big	bɪg	big

Prosody
- Impression of "flat" intonation

Hindi-influenced English

Approximately 225 languages and 845 dialects are spoken in the Indian subcontinent. Hindi is the national language and is spoken by the majority of people. Hindi contains 11 different vowels and 40 different consonants.

Pattern	Word	Pronunciation	Hindi-influenced English
Consonants			
• [v] pronounced as [ß]	very	vɛri	ßɛri
• Stopping of interdental fricatives	thank	θæŋk	tæŋk
• Retroflex production of [d]	deep	dip	dip
• Deaspiration of initial stops	pen	pɛn	pᵒɛn
• Affrication	she	ʃi	tʃi
• Depalatalization	show	ʃo	so
• Addition	station	steʃƏn	isteʃƏn
• Epenthesis	blade	bled	bƏled
• Metathesis	ask	æsk	æks
Vowels			
• Lowering of tongue	roll	rol	rɔl
• Tensing of [ɪ] and [ʊ]	rim	rɪm	rim
• Use of lax vowel	gate	get	gɛt
• [ɛ] for [æ]	at	æt	ɛt

Prosody
- Substitution of one vowel for another due to change in stress placement
- Intonation contours of Hindi differ from English, decreasing intelligibility

Singapore Colloquial English

Singapore Colloquial English (SCE) is spoken in the city and Republic of Singapore. SCE shares many similarities with Chinese in terms of its syntax, and semantic and pragmatic features, which give the impression of English words embedded in Chinese sentence structures. Code switching is commonly observed in Singapore, where people frequently switch from SCE to Standard English and visa versa depending on the communication context and the parties involved in the communication. Code switching often occurs when the formality of the conversation or the communicative partner is changed, Standard English being used in formal settings, and SCE being used during informal day-to-day interaction. Interlanguage switches between English, Malay, Mandarin, or other dialects also are common, usually in informal settings. These switches can occur at phrase level, where the speaker changes languages from one phrase to the next, or they can occur within the phrase where words of another language are embedded into the phrase structure of the original language.

Pattern	Word	Pronunciation	Singapore English
Consonants			
• Initial interdental fricatives are stopped and dentalized	the	ðə	d̪ə
• Initial voiceless consonants partially voiced and unaspirated	pan	pæn	p°æn
• Deletion of initial /w/ preceding /u/	woo	wu	u
• /dz/ for /z/	zoo	zu	dzu
• Final consonants unaspirated	fat	fæt	fæt
	bad	bæd	bæd
• Final interdental fricatives are labiodental	tooth	tuθ	tuf
• Final cluster reduction	don't	dont	don
• Devoicing of final fricatives	ooze	uz	us
Vowels			
• Vowels may be shortened	bee	bi	bɪ
• Vowels may be more closed	bag	bæg	bɛg

Turkish-influenced English

Turkish is an Indo-European language, belonging to the Altaic branch of the Ural-Altay linguistic family. The language now spoken in Turkey is accepted as standard Turkish and is the descendant of Ottoman Turkish and its predecessor, the so-called Old Anatolian Turkish. Turkish contains 8 vowels and 21 consonant phonemes. Vowels are short. Turkish does not permit initial consonant clusters. Obstruents are voiceless in syllable-final position, and syllable final consonant clusters typically are sonorants + voiceless stops (examples: [rk rt nk]). Syllable final [nç st] may occur in borrowed words. Vowel and consonant harmony (assimilation) is a unique characteristic of Turkish and results in vowels and consonants within words sharing distinctive features. Turkish is a syllable-timed language in which syllables recur at regular intervals in words, phrases, and sentences.

Pattern	Word	Pronunciation	Turkish-influenced English
Consonants			
• Labiodentals as bilabials	vote	vot	βot
• Stopping of interdentals	this	ðɪs	dɪs
• Final Consonant Devoicing	tube	tub	tup
• Cluster Reduction	steep	stip	sip or tip
	beast	bist	bis or bit
• Epenthesis	blade	bled	bəled
• Palatalization of [ŋ]	king	kiŋ	kiŋ
• Partial devoicing of syllable-final nasals	mean	min	miṇ
Vowels			
• Vowel shortening	bee	bi	bɪ

Prosody

• Vowel and consonant assimilations may occur
• Errors in placement of stress may result from stress-timed alternations in words, phrases, and sentences

APPENDIX 2B

Safety Precautions for Clients with Medical Needs

Prior to providing services to any client with an articulation and phonological disorder, speech-language clinicians must be knowledgable about basic safety procedures, including cardiopulmonary resuscitation (CPR). Additionally, speech-language clinicians working with clients with medical needs must be well versed in the safety procedures for the populations with which they come into contact. Readers interested in more detailed information on medical issues affecting persons with developmental disabilities are referred to Batshaw (1997) and, for children with tracheostomies, Bleile (1993a).

A. Infection Control Guidelines

Basic infection control guidelines should be followed when providing care to all clients with medical needs.

1. Hand Washing. Many persons with medical needs have relatively weak immune systems, and diseases carried by staff are a primary source of infection. The most effective means of reducing spread of infection is through careful washing after contact with each client. Other times when hand washing should be performed are when coming on or off duty, when the hands are dirty, after toilet use, after blowing or wiping one's nose, and after handling client secretions.

To wash, wet the hands and forearms, apply soap, and wash all areas of the hands and forearms for 1 to 2 minutes, being careful to wash nail beds and between the fingers. Afterward, rinse the soap from your hands and forearms thoroughly. Use an unused paper towel to turn off the water faucet, and then discard the paper towel.

2. Toy Washing. Toys are a possible source of infection for children with medical needs, because children may place toys in their mouths, or may put their fingers in their mouths or noses after playing with an infected toy. Wear gloves to clean possibly infected toys. Wipe each toy with warm, soapy water and then rinse. Next, spray or wipe each toy with a disinfectant such as 1:10 solution of household bleach. Finally, rinse the toy well and air dry for 10 minutes.

B. Physiological Warning Signs

Clients with medical conditions sometimes experience sudden, even life-threatening, changes in their medical status. Clinicians who work with these clients must be able to recognize and respond appropriately to emergency situations if they occur. The most common physiological warning signs (or Red Flags) associated with six possibly life-threatening conditions are discussed below. If the warning signs are observed, the clinician should immediately contact the staff member (typically a physician or nurse) designated to handle medical problems.

1. **Mechanical Ventilation.** Mechanical ventilation is provided through a machine that breathes in and out for the client. The primary indicator for mechanical ventilation in children is bronchopulmonary dysplasia (Bleile, 1993b; Metz, 1993). The physiological warning signs most commonly encountered in clients receiving mechanical ventilation include changes in skin color, exaggerated breathing, coughing, alteration in heart rate or respiratory rate, and either lethargy or irritability.

2. **Tracheostomy.** Tracheostomy is a surgical opening below the larynx on the anterior neck (Handler, 1993). Persons with tracheostomy assistance breathe through a hole (stoma) placed in the anterior neck. The most common daily hazards associated with tracheostomy care involve blockages that make breathing difficult or impossible. The physiological warning signs of blockage include a blue tint around the lips or nail beds, flared nostrils, fast breathing, a rattling noise during breathing, mucous bubbles around the tracheostomy site, coughing or gagging, clammy skin, restlessness, and either lethargy or irritability.

3. **Seizures.** A seizure is a type of abnormal electrical discharge from the neurons in the cortex. Physiological warning signs associated with seizures include pallor, irritability, staring, nystagmus, changes in muscle tone, and vomiting.

4. **Shunt.** A shunt is a device that diverts cerebrospinal fluid from a brain ventricle to another part of the body where the fluid is then absorbed. Shunts are used for persons with hydrocephalus, a condition in which excess fluid causes ventricles in the brain to become enlarged. Physiological warning signs suggesting a shunt malfunction include headaches, vomiting, lethargy, and bulging fontanel (the soft spot on the heads of infants and toddlers).

5. **Gastrointestinal Conditions.** Gastrointestinal conditions involve problems in one or more of three areas: controlled movement of food through the body, digestion of food, and absorption of nutrients (Silverman McGowan, Kerwin, & Bleile, 1993). If a person cannot receive enough nourishment by mouth (per oral) to sustain life and continued growth, he or she is fed via a gastrostomy or jejunal tube placed into the stomach or small intestine, respectively. Physiological warning signs of problems with a gastrostomy or jejunal tube include the presence of formula leaking from the tube at either the clamp or skin site, in and out movement of the tube, increased irritability, and emesis.

6. **Cardiac Conditions.** Cardiac conditions are medical problems affecting the heart. They may occur as isolated medical problems or in conjunction with other disabilities. Physiological warning signs associated with cardiac conditions include changes in skin color, increased heart and/or respiratory rate, chest retractions, nasal flaring, and either lethargy or irritability.

CHAPTER

3

Speech Development

The following topics are discussed in this chapter:

I. OVERVIEW

For nearly four years I directed a speech-language pathology program in a large pediatric hospital. Children in that setting ranged in age from medically involved neonates to adolescents with recent head injuries. Included within this group were children with a wide assortment of severe developmental disabilities, including autism, feeding disorders, and self-injurious behavior. It might seem that, because it was a medical setting, preference in hiring would be given to those with the most knowledge of medically-related topics. However, an applicant with a solid foundation in typical speech and language development was valued more highly than one with greater medical knowledge and less understanding of development. The reason is that knowledge of typical development is critical for clinical reasoning, and a clinician who understands developmental topics has a more sound basis for clinical decision making than one who does not.

The purpose of this chapter is to describe the stages through which a child learns to speak, with special emphasis given to developmental information and concepts that support clinical care. Developmental stages are described in Section II. Perceptual and production building blocks are presented in Sections III and IV, respectively. The means through which a child links advanced perceptual abilities with limited means of production is the subject of Section V. Roles of speech for communication is the topic of Section VI, and a summary of speech development is presented in Section VII. Clinical implications of typical speech development are discussed in Section VIII. Readers less familiar with terminology used to describe speech may wish to read Chapter 2 either concurrent with or before reading this chapter, especially sections IV and V.

II. DEVELOPMENTAL STAGES

Speech development occurs over a number of years. For convenience, this period is divided into four stages. The time frame and major hallmarks of these stages are listed in Table 3–1.

- **Stage 1** lasts from birth to approximately 12 months. During this stage a child lays foundations for future speech development.

- **Stage 2** lasts from approximately 12 to 24 months. During this stage a child becomes a word user.

Table 3–1. Four stages in speech development and hallmarks associated with each stage.

Stages	Age Range in Typically Developing Children	Hallmark
Stage 1	birth to 12 months	Foundations
Stage 2	12–24 months	Word learning
Stage 3	24 months to 5 years	Rule learning
Stage 4	5 years through adolescence	Literacy

- **Stage 3** lasts from approximately 2 to 5 years. During this stage a child masters most major speech elements (sounds, syllables, stress patterns, prosody, and so on) within the language.

- **Stage 4** lasts from approximately 5 years through adolescence. In this stage a child masters late-acquired speech elements and lays the foundation of literacy.

III. BUILDING BLOCKS IN SPEECH PERCEPTION

To speak, a child must first discover the phonological rules that underlie the rush and garble of sound that adults produce. Making such discoveries is no small feat, since adults typically speak at rates of over nine sounds per second, and some distinctions a child must apprehend may last less than one-third of a second.

The building blocks of speech perception proceed in the following stages:

- Stage 1: A child begins life able to perceive major sound distinctions in the world's languages. By the end of Stage 1 perception is largely restricted to sounds in the language of the child's community.

- Stage 2: A child displays generally good word perception abilities, though perceptual problems arise in unfamiliar settings, when hearing rapid speech, and when distracted or uninterested.

- Stage 3: Though possessing relatively advanced speech perception abilities, difficulties in perception remain, especially during the early part of this stage.

- Stage 4: A child's speech perception abilities increasingly become adult-like.

A. Stage 1 (Birth to 12 months)

Human languages contain approximately 600 different consonants and 200 different vowels (Ladefoged, 2001). A particular language makes use of a small subset of this total number. Since the language to be learned is subject to environmental circumstances, a child must possess perceptual abilities to hear them all. A "use it or lose it" principle is followed in Stage 1 perceptual development, and advances largely consist of fine-tuning a child's abilities to fit the language of the community (Vihman, 1996; Werker & Polka, 1993).

Major perceptual developments occur in two domains: Intonation and Speech Sounds.

1. Intonation. Perception of intonation begins before birth. The fluid in which an unborn child floats, in addition to sustaining life, acts as a resonating chamber for low frequency sounds, including the mother's voice. At birth a child has had months of exposure to the mother's intonation patterns, and a newborn displays a preference for that voice above others. This preference may promote bonding between infant and mother, and first exposes a child to intonation contours of the mother's language

As described in Chapter 1, many languages use pitch (tones) to distinguish between word meanings, so a child must perceive pitch changes that potentially signal differences in meaning. Early in their first year, infants around the world appear to perceive pitch similarly. For speakers of English and other non-tone language, ability to hear pitch differences fades, while, for example, speakers of Chinese retain this skill. It may be that a child exposed to a tone language establishes and retains brain cell connections that maintain this ability, while those who speak a language such as English lose those potential connections.

2. Speech Sounds. A child must discover speech sounds buried in the rapid flow of speech—not an easy challenge to face, since sounds are seldom spoken in isolation, change in pronunciation depending on syllable position and presence of adjoining sounds, and may be spoken at rates of nine to ten per second. Finding speech sounds would probably be impossible were it not for an infant's mammalian heritage, which includes possessing a cochlea and hearing mechanism capable of categorical perception—that is, capable of dividing the speech stream into individual sounds. During the first months an infant perceives major differences between sounds found in the world's languages. This ability diminishes over the following months, and by the end of Stage 1 an infant's perception of speech sounds is largely restricted to those of the language being acquired (Vihman, 1996; Werker & Polka, 1993).

Some Flied Lice, Please

An old joke has a person from China say, "I'd like some flied lice, please" for "I'd like some fried rice, please." Most people recognize that a Chinese speaker may make speech errors affecting English [r] because that difficult sound does not occur in Chinese. What is more surprising (to an English speaker at least) is that many Chinese people also experience difficulty perceiving difference between English [l] and [r]. Similar perceptual difficulties are often experienced by speakers of other languages that do not contain these sounds. Of course, nothing is wrong with the ears of people in China, any more than ears of English speakers are disordered because they experience difficulty distinguishing pitch changes in tone languages—an aspect of languages that Chinese children perceive and produce near one year old. The problem in perception appears to result from brain maturation. During the first months of life, children around the world perceive large numbers of speech sounds. Connections between brain cells are strengthened for sounds contained in the parents' language, and are weakened for other speech sounds. As a result, a Chinese child of one year experiences difficulty perceiving the difference between [l] and [r], while an American child experiences similar difficulties with pitch changes.

B. Stage 2 (12 to 24 months)

Perceptual development in Stage 1 focused on discrimination of pitch and speech sounds. Perceptual development in Stage 2 focuses on word perception. Though a Stage 2 child possesses perceptual abilities well-adapted to the language of the community, word perception is not perfect. As with older children and adults, a Stage 2 child may experience perceptual difficulties when words refer to unfamiliar topics, are spoken quickly, or occur in longer phrases and sentences. A way in which a child in Stage 2 may differ from older children and adults is in extent of perceptual difficulties and, from an adult perspective, in willingness to assign unusual meanings to misperceived words and phrases. Evidence for such misperceptions abounds. To give just one example, during this stage a child might refer to "hair tangles" as "rectangles."

C. Stage Three (2 to 5 years)

The pattern of perceptual development observed in Stage 2 continues in Stage 3, with perception of words being good, but not perfect. To illustrate, an often heard preschool belief is that Dorothy and company went off to see "The Lizard of Oz." A more modern illustration comes from a New Zealand child, who told a visitor, "Mom has to check her Emu." (for "check her e-mail"). Such misperceptions occur more frequently in early Stage 3 than toward the end of this stage.

A relatively extreme example comes from a 26-month-old whose speech during an eight week observation period reflected the following misperceptions: "dandelion" was "dandy flower," "picnic table" was "pick me table," "clothes pin" was "pin clothes," "lawnmower" was "lawnmotor," "elbow" was "el-bone," "fire siren/noon whistle" was "fire whistle," and "butterfly" was "buzzerfly." Lastly, revealing that the child's taste buds were operative, "Tater Tot" was "little rock" (Bleile, 1987).

D. Stage Four (5 years through adolescence)

From an adult perspective, a child early in Stage 4 may make unusual interpretations of misperceived words and phrases. These may increase as the child encounters new and longer words through learning to read. A child in Stage 4 may also experience difficulties in perception of intonation when exposed to a wider range of communication styles and discourse functions. For example, in Stage 4 a child may misinterpret pitch and intonation in a phrase spoken sarcastically, such as, "Now THAT is really nice."

IV. BUILDING BLOCKS IN SPEECH PRODUCTION

Not only must children discover complex rules hidden in streams of rapidly flowing speech, they must also learn to shape the vocal tract to produce gestures that correspond to perceived sounds. The simplest of speech sounds requires muscle coordination across half the body. Astonishingly, within the first five years of life a child has largely mastered this most complex of motor activities.

The following is the developmental progression of speech production from Stage 1 through Stage 4.

- Stage 1: A child begins life producing sounds that occur while breathing and moving, and by the end of Stage 1 produces a small stock of consonants, vowels, syllables, stress patterns, and intonation contours.

- Stage 2: A child uses speech elements acquired through babbling to build a small expressive vocabulary.

- Stage 3: Early in Stage 3 a child pronounces a limited variety of sounds and syllables; by the end of Stage 3 a child has largely mastered most major speech elements of the language.

- Stage 4: A child in Stage 4 may experience difficulties pronouncing individual consonants and consonant clusters; literacy exposes a child to new vocabulary containing challenging syllabic and stress patterns.

The discussion in this section describes development of a child's speech-making abilities. Speech errors are discussed in Section V.

A. Stage 1 (Birth to 12 months)

Early in Stage 1 a child lacks cortical connections for speech, neither can an infant shape the articulators to produce consonants and vowels, syllables, pitch, and intonation.

1. Infant Vocal Tract. If, magically, a newborn could speak, it would probably sound nasally and contain a few vowels and consonants produced forward in the mouth. These characteristics result from the structure of an infant's vocal tract, which includes the following features (Kent & Murray, 1982):

- The larynx rests high in the throat, providing a protective function against choking, and descends toward the adult position during Stage 1, but does not achieve its adult position until the end of Stage 2.

- In addition to being shorter than that of an adult, an infant's vocal tract is a gradual slope rather than right-bending.

- Compared to an adult, an infant's tongue lies more forward in the mouth.

- Compared to an adult, an infant's velopharynx and epiglottis lie closer together.

2. **Prespeech Vocalizations.** Prespeech vocalizations provide "practice" for later speech development (Locke, 1983b; Locke & Pearson, 1992; Bleile, Stark, & Silverman McGowan, 1993; Vihman & Miller, 1988; Jusczyk, 1992). Development of prespeech vocalizations occurs in steps (Table 3–2).

   a. **Vegetative Sounds (Birth to 2 months).** Vocalizations made between birth and approximately two months are vegetative sounds arising as a child breathes and moves. To illustrate, if a child breathes out and the tongue is lying flat in the mouth, an [e]-like sound results, though it lacks fine motor coordination and timing of an adult-produced vowel—it is only a sound that emerges when the tongue is flat and other articulators are far apart. Similarly, consonant-like vocalizations occur as an infant expels or inhales air when articulators happen to be relatively close together.

   b. **Cooing (3 to 4 months).** Near 3 to 4 months of age vocalizations increasingly contain sounds produced near the back of the mouth (cooing). Predominance of back sounds may reflect development of myelin in homunculus areas that depict back parts of an infant's mouth (Peters & Peters, 1974).

   c. **Squealing (4 to 6 months).** Sounds produced forward in the mouth (squeals, growls, raspberries, and trills) emerge near 4 to 6 months and may reflect myelin development in homunculus areas that depict forward parts of an infant's mouth (Peters & Peters, 1974).

Table 3–2. Vocal development in Stage 1.

Age	Vocalizations
Birth to 2 months	Vegetative sounds
3 to 4 months	Cooing is well established
4 to 6 months	Vocalizations dominated by front sounds
7 to 8 months	Babbling well established

d. Babbling (7 to 8 months). Near 6 months infants begin to babble, and by 7 to 8 months 20% or more of infant vocalizations are babble. Babbling consists of a true consonant (a consonant other than [h]) and vowel in the same syllable. Consonants and vowels in syllables may either be repeated (for example, ba-ba-ba), which is called reduplicated babbling, or altered (for example, ba-da-di), which is called nonreduplicated babbling. Previously, it was hypothesized that reduplicated preceded nonreduplicated babbling in development. Research now suggests that the two forms emerge simultaneously in most children (Vihman, 1996).

Babbling is important to future speech development for three reasons: syllable development, attunement to language community, and as an origin of individual differences.

Syllable Development: Syllables are a foundation of spoken words. Through babbling a child learns to blend consonants and vowels together within the same syllable. While an infant's syllables lack the timing and motor coordination of more practiced speakers, their presence signifies a critical advance in speech development.

Attunement to Language Community: Prior to the onset of babble, infants around the world vocalize similarly. However, an infant's babble shows influence from the language to which a child is exposed, signifying an infant is becoming more attuned to the language spoken in the community (Boysson-Bardies & Vihman, 1991). To illustrate, a French baby tends to babble French consonants and vowels with French prosodic intonation contours, while an American baby babbles English consonants, vowels, and intonation contours.

Origin of Individual Differences: Importantly, babies exposed to the same language may babble differently. Selection of sounds contained in a child's babble may result partly from chance. For example, by chance an infant may have the articulators in a certain position while breathing out, resulting in a sound, which might then be babbled. Another infant, because the articulators happen to be in another position while breathing out, may build a babbling repertoire based on a different sound. To illustrate, one child may vocally stumble on labial sounds while vocalizing, and babble those, while another child may vocally stumble on [d] and babble those. Vision may also play a role in sound selection in babbling. Labial sounds, which are easily recognizable when a person speaks, seem favored by children with tracheostomies, perhaps because sounds observed on a speaker's face provide feedback lacking in their own silent vocalization (Bleile, 1998). Lastly, it is possible—though unproven—that an infant may babble sounds found in favorite objects or associated with special persons.

B. Stage 2 (12 to 24 months)

Speech development in Stage 1 provides a small stock of sounds, syllables, and intonation contours that a child uses as a scaffold to build a first vocabulary. This occurs in conjunction with brain maturation. Developments in speech allow communication of new ideas and feelings permitted by a growing cortex. More mature memory abilities facilitate acquisition of new words, while myelination and changes in the shape of the oral structure further facilitates speech production. As a result of these and other factors, a toddler talks more, and in the course of speaking stumbles on new and different sounds, syllables, and stress patterns, leading to further expansions of speech abilities.

1. Speech Domains. In Stage 2 and later stages major developments occur in the following speech domains:

- Consonants

- Vowels

- Syllables

- Stress

Consonant development is a major treatment focus and is given the most consideration. A recent review of research literature on speech production development in Stages 2 through 4, with special emphasis on Australian English, appears in McLeod (2002).

2. Consonants. Consonant development is described in terms of consonant inventories and correct productions.

Consonant Inventories = Consonant productions analyzed without regard to whether they are pronounced correctly relative to adult usage.

Correct Productions = Consonants pronounced correctly relative to adult usage.

Consonant inventories describe a child's universe of consonant-making-abilities, and analyses of correct productions describe a child's progress in consonant development relative to the language of the community. Inventory analyses predominate in Stage 2, when so many pronunciations are inaccurate relative to the adult language. As a child's consonant-making abilities develop in Stages 3 and 4, analyses of correct productions become predominant.

a. Consonant Inventories. Consonants pronounced in two or more different words are shown in Table 3–3 (Stoel-Gammon, 1985).

15 months: A child typically pronounces three different consonants word initially and none or one consonant word finally. Word-initial consonants may include [b d h].

18 months: A child typically pronounces six word initial consonants and one word final consonant. A typical word-initial consonant inventory may contain voiced oral and nasal stops and one or two glides, while a typical word-final consonant inventory may contain a voiceless stop, perhaps [t].

24 months: A child's consonant inventory may contain 9–11 consonants word initially and nearly half that number (5–6) word finally. Word initial consonant inventories may contain both voiced and voiceless stops, nasal consonants, and several glides and voiceless fricatives. Rapid expansion of the word-final consonant inventory, reflecting a child's better ability to close syllables with consonants, may contain voiceless oral stops, a nasal stop, and a fricative.

Table 3–3. Consonant inventories.

Age	Position	Number of Consonants	Typical Consonants
15 mos.	Initial	3	b d h
	Final	none	—
18 mos.	Initial	6	b d m n h w
	Final	1	t
24 mos.	Initial	11	b d g t k m n h w f s
	Final	6	p t k n r s

Individual Differences

Individual differences in speech development abound (McLeod, 2003). To illustrate, I once compared consonant inventories of children near 24 months old, all developing typically. In common with previous studies, the average number of word-initial consonants in the children's speech was 9 to 10. However, the number of different word-initial consonants among the children ranged from 5 to 14.

---

b. **Correct Productions.** In children under age 2, consonants pronounced correctly in at least two of three word positions (initial, medial, final) include [m n h w p b] (Sander, 1972). By 24 months a child may also pronounce [ŋ t k d g] correctly, and approximately 70% of a child's consonants typically are correct relative to the adult language (Stoel-Gammon, 1987).

c. **Consonant Development and Degree of Constriction.** Information on consonant development is organized by manner of production in Table 3–4 (consonant inventories) and Table 3–5 (correct consonants). For both tables, consonant classes appear on the left and are ordered, from top to bottom, according to degree of constriction between articulators. That is, oral and nasal stops are produced with the most constriction and glides with the least. To illustrate, during [d] and [n] the articulators (tongue tip and alveolar ridge) touch during production, momentarily blocking the airway, while during [w] the articulators (rounded lips and raised back of tongue) shape the airflow, but do not completely block it. Consonant inventories at 15, 18, and 24 months are displayed in

Table 3–4. Consonant inventories: relationship between development and articulator distance.

	15 mos.	*18 mos.*	*24 mos.*
Stops	b d	b d	b d g t k m n ŋ
Affricates			
Fricatives			f s
Liquids			
Glides	h	h	h w

Table 3–5. Consonants correct: relationship between development and articulator distance.

	Under 24 mos.	*24 mos.*
Stops	b p m n	b d g p t k ŋ
Affricates		
Fricatives		
Liquids		
Glides	h w	h w

Table 3–4, and correct consonants before 24 months and at 24 months are displayed in Table 3–5.

As the data in the tables suggest, early acquired consonants tend to be produced with either maximum or minimum constriction between articulators (stops and glides). Consonant classes with intermediate distance between articulators (affricates, fricatives, liquids) tend to be later acquisitions. The pattern suggested by the data is that early on a child tends to produce consonants at either end of the continuum (either with articulators touching or maximally distant from each other), and with development learns to fine-tune production to make consonants intermediate in the constriction continuum. Stated more concretely, in Stage 2 a child learns to pronounce consonants made with the articulators either touching or relatively distant from each other, and in Stage 3 a child learns to "fill in the midpoints" of the constriction continuum.

3. **Vowels.** In Stage 2, vowel development is relatively advanced compared to that of consonants (Selby, Robb, & Gilbert, 2000; Robb, Bleile, & Yee, 1999). Early acquisitions typically include "corners" of the vowel quadrangle [i u a ɑ]. Mid vowels and diphthongs often are acquired somewhat later in Stage 2 than open and closed pure vowels (Bleile, 1988).

4. **Syllables.** Open syllables (syllables ending in a vowel) predominate in Stage 2, especially during the first half of this period. Toward the end of Stage 2, a child demonstrates improved ability to close syllables with a consonant, typically a nasal or voiceless stop.

5. Stress. Words containing a single syllable predominate, though some two and even three syllable words may also occur (Kehoe, 1997). Multisyllabic words most often consist of two syllables and have primary stress on the first syllable. Pronunciation of *banana* as [nana] and *umbrella* as [belə] illustrate this.

C. Stage 3 (2 to 5 years)

During Stage 3 a child progresses from rudimentary speech-making ability to mastery of most major speech elements.

1. Intelligibility. Progress in speech development is reflected by improved intelligibility. In connected speech a child near 2 years old may be 26–50% intelligible, a child near 3 years old typically is 71–80% intelligible, and a child near 4 years old may be 100% intelligible, though pronunciation errors likely are present (Weiss, 1982).

2. Consonants. The consonant system of English is largely mastered during Stage 3.

   a. Consonant Inventories. In Stage 3 consonant inventories lose their usefulness as a measure of development, both because a child produces so many different consonant types and because a child's consonants are increasingly pronounced correctly relative to the adult language.

   b. Correct Productions. Normative information for consonants and consonant clusters in American English is presented in Tables 3–6 and 3–7. McLeod's (2002) meta-analysis and McLeod, van Doorn, and Reed (2001a, 2001b) reveal similar, though not identical, patterns in acquisition of Australian English. Tables 3–6 and 3–7 show the ages at which individual consonants and consonant clusters are acquired by 50% and 75% of children. Consonants are averaged across both initial and final word positions. Consonant clusters occur in word-initial position.

   Consonant Classes: Based on Table 3–6, individual consonants are analyzed by sound class and depicted as early, mid, and late acquisitions (Table 3–8). Based on this analysis, stops, nasals, and glides are mastered early (earlier than 3;0), affricates, liquids, and fricatives are mid acquisitions (3;0–4;0), and interdental fricatives are late acquisitions (4;6).

Table 3–6. Age of acquisition (50% to 75% correct) of American English consonants averaged across both word-initial and word-final positions.

Consonant	50%	75%	Consonant	50%	75%
m	<3;0	<3;0	f	<3;0	3;6
n	<3;0	<3;0	v	3;6	4;6
ŋ	<3;0	7;6*	θ	4;6	6;0
h	<3;0	<3;0	ð	4;6	5;6
w	<3;0	<3;0	s	3;6	5;0
j	<3;0	3;6	z	4;0	6;0
p	<3;0	<3;0	ʃ	3;6	5;0
t	<3;0	<3;0	tʃ	3;6	6;0
k	<3;0	<3;0	dʒ	3;6	4;6
b	<3;0	<3;0	r	3;6	6;0
d	<3;0	<3;0	l	3;6	6;0
g	<3;0	<3;0			

* = Transcriber difficulties may have resulted in this sound being acquired at 7;6.

Compiled from A. Smit, L. Hand, J. Frelinger, J. Bernthal, & A. Byrd, 1990. The Iowa articulation norms project and its Nebraska replication, *Journal of Speech and Hearing Disorders, 55,* 779–798.

Consonant Clusters: Consonant clusters are pronounced correctly approximately one-third of the time in connected speech by a child in the first year of Stage 3 (McLeod, van Doorn, & Reed, 2001a; McLeod, 2002). Word-final consonant clusters are more likely to be correct than consonant clusters in word-initial position. Consonant cluster acquisition is nearly complete by the end of Stage 3. Of 27 different word-initial consonant clusters presented in Table 3–7, all but six are acquired by 50% of children before 5 years of age. Of the remaining six, two are clusters in which the second consonant is [r], and four are clusters with three consonants.

3. **Vowels.** Vowel development is largely complete by 3 years of age (Selby, Robb, & Gilbert, 2000). Late acquired vowels are likely to be diphthongs, r-colored vowels, and unstressed vowels in multisyllabic words.

4. **Syllables.** At the beginning of Stage 3, a child's speech may contain syllables that are V, VC, CV, CVC, CVCV, and CVCVC.

Table 3–7. Age of acquisition (50% to 75% correct) of American English consonant clusters in word-initial positions.*

Cluster	50%	75%	Cluster	50%	75%
tw	3;0	3;6	pr	4;0	6;0
kw	3;0	3;6	br	3;6	6;0
sp	3;6	5;0	tr	5;0	5;6
st	3;6	5;0	dr	4;0	6;0
sk	3;6	5;0	kr	4;0	5;6
sm	3;6	5;0	gr	4;6	6;0
sn	3;6	5;6	fr	3;6	6;0
sw	3;6	5;6	θr	5;0	7;0
sl	4;6	7;0	skw	3;6	7;0
pl	3;6	5;6	spl	5;0	7;0
bl	3;6	5;0	spr	5;0	8;0
kl	4;0	5;6	str	5;0	8;0
gl	3;6	4;6	skr	5;0	8;0
fl	3;6	5;6			

* The Smit et al. data does not contain information for [r] consonant cluster

Complied from A. Smit, L. Hand, J. Frelinger, J. Bernthal, & A. Byrd, 1990. The Iowa articulation norms project and its Nebraska replication, *Journal of Speech and Hearing Disorders, 55,* 779–798.

Table 3–8. Early, mid, and late acquisition of sound classes in Stage 3.

Period	Sound class	Age
Early	stops, nasals, glides	Before 3 years
Mid	affricates, liquids, fricatives	3;0–4;0
Late	interdental fricatives	4;6

Based on A. Smit, L. Hand, J. Frelinger, J. Bernthal, & A. Byrd, 1990. The Iowa articulation norms project and its Nebraska replication, *Journal of Speech and Hearing Disorders, 55,* 779–798.

Reflecting the adult language, CV is likely to be the most frequently occurring syllable. As Stage 3 proceeds, syllable beginnings and endings (called onsets and rhymes) increasingly contain consonant clusters. Types of consonants within clusters diversify rapidly during the last year of Stage 3.

5. Stress. Whereas in Stage 2 a child's speech showed a preference for primary stress on the first syllable, early in Stage 3 a child can manipulate the speech mechanism to allow words beginning with unstressed syllables, as in *banana* and *umbrella* (Kehoe, 1997). As Stage 3 continues, three-syllable words with primary stress on either the first, second, or third syllable become more common.

D. Stage Four (5 years through adolescence)

By the beginning of Stage 4, a child has mastered most building blocks of speech.

1. Late Acquisitions. The following are late acquisitions in speech development:

- Individual consonants and consonant clusters

- Morphological alternations

- Syllables and stress patterns encountered through reading

2. Consonants. Most consonant classes are mastered by the beginning of Stage 4. Development continues for individual consonants and for consonant clusters.

> **a. Consonant Inventories.** Typically, analyses of consonant inventories are not performed on children in Stage 4.

> **b. Correct Productions.** A child in Stage 4 may experience difficulty learning to pronounce individual consonants and selected consonant clusters.

> *Individual Consonants:* Impressively, by 5 years of age 50% of children typically acquire the complex articulatory gestures that underlie consonants, and by 6 years of age 75% of children acquire all consonants. Consonants not acquired by 75% of children until five years or older are listed in Table 3–9. Organized into classes, these include alveolar fricatives, the post-alveolar fricative and affricates, liquids, and the voiceless interdental fricative.

> *Consonant Clusters:* Also impressively, by 5 years of age 50% of children have acquired all types of word-initial consonant

Table 3–9. Age of acquisition (50% to 75% correct) of late acquired American English consonants averaged across both word-initial and word-final positions.

Consonant	5;0	75%
s	3;6	5;0
ʃ	3;6	5;0
θ	4;6	6;0
ð	4;6	5;6
z	4;0	6;0
tʃ	3;6	6;0
r	3;6	6;0
l	3;6	6;0
	4;6	5;6

clusters, by 6 years of age the majority of consonant clusters are acquired, and by 8 years of age 75% of children have acquired the complete set. The latest acquired consonant clusters are [r] clusters and clusters with three members.

3. **Vowels.** The [r] colored schwa is acquired by 50% of children by 4;6, and is acquired by 75% of children by 5;6 (Smit, Hand, Frelinger, Bernthal, & Byrd, 1990). Other vowel development in Stage 4 consists of learning morphological alternations typically encountered in educational settings, as suggested by the following illustrative examples:

Morphological Alternations

divine/divinity
collide/collision
explain/explanation
sane/sanity
serene/serenity
obscene/obscenity

4. **Syllables.** Throughout Stage 4 a child is exposed to new vocabulary through reading, and is expected both to understand and to pronounce a wide range of complex syllable patterns, as illustrated by the following words:

Complex Syllable Patterns

electronics	(V-CVC-CCV-CVCC)
nomenclature	(CV-CVC-CCV-CV)
iambic pentameter	(V-VC-CVC, CVC-CV-CV-CV)

5. **Stress.** What is true of syllables is also true of stress. Often, with complex syllable patterns come stress patterns atypical in everyday English. This is especially true with scientific vocabulary. To illustrate, *electronics* has primary stress on the third syllable, *nomenclature* has primary stress on the first syllable, and the phrase *iambic pentameter* has primary stress on the second syllable of *iambic* and either the first or second syllable of *pentameter*, some speakers pronouncing it PENtameter and others penTAmeter.

Stress changes involving derivational morphology and compound words may challenge a Stage 4 child's speech-making abilities. To illustrate, learning to pronounce the pair *symphony* and *symphonic* entails shifting primary stress from the first syllable in *symphony* (SYMphony) to the second syllable in *symphonic* (symPHOnic). Similarly, compound words may have stress on the first syllable, while adjective + noun phrases may have stress on the second, as in the following:

Compound Word	**Adjective + Noun**
RED head	red HEAD
WHITE house	white HOUSE
GREEN house	green HOUSE
HIGH chair	high CHAIR

V. THE PERCEPTION-PRODUCTION LINK

Development of speech perception and speech production begin at opposite points but reach the same destination. Imagined as an inverted speech triangle (Figure 3–1), perceptual development begins broadly and ends narrowly. That is, a child begins life able to perceive broad perceptual distinctions needed to acquire any of the world's languages; with development, broad perceptual abilities narrow to fit perceptual distinctions encountered in the language of a child's community. Development of speech production

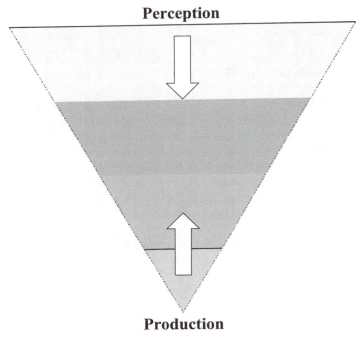

Figure 3–1. Speech development triangle.

proceeds in the opposite direction: a child begins life producing a narrow range of vegetative sounds; with development, production abilities broaden until a child can pronounce the sounds encountered in the community's language.

Though beginning at opposite points and proceeding in contrary directions, development of speech perception and production arrives at the same destination: the speech of the community. However, the two systems arrive at this point at different times, perhaps reflecting differences in arborization between the temporal and frontal lobes (see Chapter 1). The perceptual system develops early and by the end of the first year has narrowed to fit the language of the community. The production system requires a longer development time, and a child's speech abilities may not have broadened to encompass all speech elements of a language until six to eight years.

The topic of this section addresses what a child does when speech perception is more advanced than speech production, creating a mismatch between what is perceived and what can be pronounced. Evidence that speech perception abilities far exceed speech production skills is easily obtained (McLeod, van Doorn, & Reed, 2000). A simple experiment involves presenting a child with several objects that are pronounced similarly and asking the child to pick up each object after it is named. Even when an adult is extremely careful not to use eye gaze or other means to assist in object identification, a child typically experiences little difficulty in pointing to or picking up the appropriate objects. If a child's perceptual knowledge (sometimes called a representation) corresponds to the way he or she pronounces the word, selecting the right object should be impossible, since the child pronounces each similarly. The fact that most children experience little difficulty with such a task strongly suggests their perceptual knowledge is in advance of production abilities. Numerous experiments of the type just described (though much more carefully organized and executed, of course) confirm that a child perceives more than can be produced.

The following is the developmental course of linkage between speech perception and speech production:

- Stage 1: Through vocalizing a child establishes a link between the ear and mouth.

- Stage 2: A child first bridges mismatches between advanced perceptual abilities and limited pronunciation skills.

- Stage 3: A child manages mismatches between perception and production through error patterns that affect sound classes.

- Stage 4: Mismatches between perception and production decrease significantly, though they still may affect individual sounds and combinations of sounds. Such mismatches may be sufficiently slight and long-standing that a child has difficulty recognizing them.

A. Stage 1 (Birth to 12 months)

Stage 1 vocalizations establish an initial link between a child's mouth and ear. As illustrated in Figure 3–2, through vocalizing the infant learns to synchronize the velum, tongue, lips, and larynx for purposes of producing sound. A child who vocalizes also hears what is produced, linking perception to production. A child who vocalizes *mmm,* for example, learns that closing the mouth, vibrating the larynx, and emitting air through the nose creates the perception of "m." However, most often a child lacks speech-making ability to pronounce all distinctions that can be perceived.

Linking Perception and Production

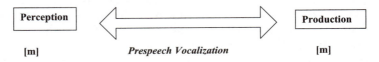

Figure 3–2. Linking perception and production.

B. Stage 2 (12 to 24 months)

Mismatches between perception and production are greatest in Stage 2. The imbalance is similar to that encountered by a student in a phonetics course exposed to languages that contain non-English consonants and vowels. After careful listening, most phonetics students perceive sounds that they cannot pronounce. Ability to perceive speech does not imply, either for phonetic students or a child in Stage 2, that the mouth can be positioned to pronounce the sound. Instead, both the phonetics student and child must discover ways to reduce mismatches between what they perceive and what their mouths are able to pronounce. A large part of speech development—and providing therapy for a person with a speech disorder—involves discovery of ways to reduce these mismatches.

1. **Linking Perception to Production.** A child handles a mismatch between perception and production through one or more of three ways: deletion, repetition, and substitution (Table 3–10). Linkages are illustrated in Figure 3–3.

Table 3–10. Three types of linkages between perception and production.

Deletions	A developmentally early linkage in which speech elements that cannot be pronounced are deleted. (Example: [but] as [bu].)
Repetitions	A developmentally early linkage in which speech elements that cannot be pronounced is replaced by repeating something that can be pronounced. (Example: *bottle* as [baba].)
Substitutions	A more developmentally advanced linkage in which speech elements that cannot be pronounced are replaced with something more pronounceable. (Example: [sut] as [tut].)

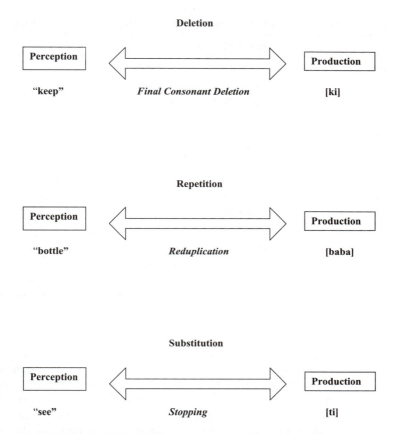

Figure 3–3. Example of linkages between perception and production involving deletion, repetition, and substitution.

2. Error Patterns. As conceptualized in this book, error patterns describe a child's linking of mismatches between perception and production. Frequently encountered Stage 2 error patterns are listed in Table 3–11, and include Prevocalic Voicing, Final Consonant Devoicing, Velar Assimilation, Labial Assimilation, Reduplication, Final Consonant Deletion, Fronting, Syllable Deletion, and Vowel Neutralization.

a. Deletions. The developmentally earliest linkage is to delete speech material that cannot be pronounced. Table 3–11 demonstrates the deletion error patterns often encountered in the speech of a child in Stage 2.

Table 3–11. Error patterns often encountered in the speech of a child in Stage 2.

Type	*Error Pattern*
Deletions:	Consonant Cluster Reduction
	Final Consonant Deletion
	Weak Syllable Deletion
Repetitions:	Labial Assimilation
	Velar Assimilation
	Reduplication
Substitutions:	Fronting
	Stopping
	Gliding
	Prevocalic Voicing
	Syllable Final Devoicing
	Vowel Neutralization

b. Repetitions. Another developmentally early linkage replaces unpronounceable speech elements by repeating something that can be pronounced. Apparently, a child finds it easier to pronounce the same sound twice than to pronounce two different sounds. This may not be unlike a hunt-and-peck typist who finds it easier to peck two identical keystrokes than to find and peck two different keys (Menn, 1976). Examples of consonant repetitions include Labial Assimilation and Velar Assimilation. This type of linkage also is employed when one syllable in a multisyllabic word is repeated several times, as in [baba] for *bottle* (Reduplication). See Table 3–11 for repetition error patterns often encountered in the speech of a child in Stage 2.

c. Substitutions. A more developmentally advanced linkage replaces unpronounceable sounds with something more pronounceable. This is similar to repetitions, except that, instead of simply repeating a previous sound, a pronounceable sound is substituted for an unpronounceable one. Table 3–11 demonstrates the substitution error patterns often encountered in the speech of a child in Stage 2.

C. Stage 3 (2 to 5 years)

Though mismatches between perception and production lessen in Stage 3, they still remain, especially during the first half of this period. Early in Stage 3 a child's error patterns may affect entire or partial classes of sounds (Table 3–12). During Stage 3 a child masters individual sounds potentially affected by an error pattern. By the end of Stage 3, errors affecting entire sound classes have largely disappeared.

1. Deletions. Deletions are increasingly less common as a child better discovers speech gestures that correspond to perceived differences between sounds. Exceptions are Final Consonant Deletion, which often is found in speech during the first half of Stage 3, and Consonant Cluster Deletion, which typically affects selected consonant clusters throughout Stage 3 (see Table 3–12).

2. Repetitions. Repetition of pronounceable speech material in place of unpronounceable material is uncommon in Stage 3.

Table 3–12. Error patterns often encountered in the speech of a child in Stage 3.

Type	*Error Pattern*	
Deletions:	Final Consonant Deletion	
	Consonant Cluster Deletion	
Repetitions:	—	
Substitutions:	Common	Prevocalic Voicing
		Final Consonant Devoicing
		Stopping
		Gliding
		Fronting
	Less Common	Denasalization
		Diphthong replacement
		Gliding of fricatives
		Frication of affricates
		Frication of liquids
		Stopping of liquids
		Backing

3. **Substitutions.** As a child's speech improves, substitutions become the dominant error pattern, affecting voice, manner, and place classes (see Table 3–12).

   a. **Voice.** Voicing can challenge a child's pronunciation abilities, especially during the early part of Stage 3. Frequently encountered error patterns that adjust voicing include Prevocalic Voicing and Final Consonant Devoicing. The former replaces a syllable-initial voiceless consonant (typically an obstruent) with its voiced cognate, and the latter replaces a syllable-final consonant (again, typically an obstruent) with its voiceless cognate. To illustrate, a child whose speech contains these patterns may pronounce *pea* [pi] as [bi] (Prevocalic Voicing) and *tub* [tʌb] as [tʌp] (Final Consonant Devoicing). Often, careful acoustic analysis reveals that a child whose speech contains Prevocalic Voicing is producing a voiceless unaspirated consonant instead of a voiced consonant. Voiceless unaspirated sounds sometimes are perceived as being between a voiceless and voiced sound. To illustrate, a voiceless unaspirated [p] may be perceived as between aspirated [p] (as occurs in *pie*) and voiced [b] (as occurs in *bye*).

   b. **Manner.** Manner classes—arranged from least to most distance between the articulators—are nasals, stops, fricatives and affricates, liquids, glides, and vowels. Often, a child stumbles on how to pronounce consonants in the classes on either end of the continuum (nasals and stops on one end of the continuum and glides and vowels on the other). Relatively uncommon error patterns affecting end-continuum sounds include Denasalization (pronunciation of a nasal consonant as an oral stop) and replacement of a diphthong with a pure vowel. Sounds on the midpoint of the continuum prove more problematic for a child's developing speech-making abilities.

   Fricatives and Affricates: A child in Stage 3 may experience great difficulty discovering how to shape the mouth to pronounce fricatives and affricates. A child unable to pronounce one or more fricatives often substitutes a stop consonant made near the same place in the mouth, thereby maintaining the sound's obstruent quality, but losing its continuous air flow (Stopping). Less commonly, a child maintains the continuous nature of the airflow, pronouncing a fricative as a glide (Gliding), which maintains the sound's continuous nature, but loses its friction quality.

Affricates may also present challenges to a child's pronunciation abilities. A frequently encountered substitution is to maintain the stop onset of the affricate, giving rise to, for example, [t] for [tʃ] (Stopping). A less common example would be when a child pronounces the fricative part of the affricate, giving rise to [z] in place of [ ].

Liquids: Often, the closest approximation to a liquid that a Stage 3 child can achieve is a glide (Gliding). Less frequently, a child pronounces liquids as fricatives, preserving the continuous nature of [l r], while replacing their non-turbulent airflow with a turbulent one. A more distant approximation of a liquid is a stop (Stopping), which preserves the consonant nature of the sounds while losing their continuous, non-turbulent airflow.

c. **Place.** Error patterns may replace one or more consonants made at a difficult to pronounce place of production with a consonant made at a place of production that a child already uses. American English consonant places of production are bilabial, labiodental, interdental, alveolar, postalveolar, palatal, velar, and glottal (see Chapter 2). Places of production most likely to challenge the speech abilities of a child in Stage 3 include interdental, postalveolar and velar. Dental consonants (tongue tip placed between upper and lower front teeth) appear both difficult to perceive and produce, and, consequently, occur in fewer than five percent of the world's languages (Ladefoged, 2001). A child may not acquire facility with this place of production until the end of Stage 3 or early in Stage 4. Postalveolar and velar consonants, especially during the early part of Stage 3, may be pronounced in the alveolar region (Fronting). Less commonly, a child may replace consonants made in the front of the mouth (typically, alveolar and postalveolar consonants) with velar ones (Backing).

D. Stage 4 (5 years through adolescence)

Mismatches between what a child can perceive and pronounce lessen as Stage 3 ends. Instead of entire sound classes, a child in Stage 4 may experience pronunciation difficulties affecting individual sounds. When such mismatches occur in late Stage 3 and throughout Stage 4, a child's regular way of talking may be so well established that "reminders" are needed to realize a mismatch between perception and production exists. The value of techniques such as discrimination training and minimal pairs lies in helping a child discover perceptual and production mismatches.

Residual errors is a useful term coined by Smit (2003) to describe individual sounds that may challenge pronunciation skills of a school-age child. Likely residual errors often are late-acquired sounds and consonant clusters. Tables 3–13 and 3–14 depict sounds and consonant clusters not acquired by 75% of children at the end of Stage 3. Sounds most likely to occur as residual errors are liquids, postalveolar affricates and fricatives, alveolar fricatives, [r] colored schwa, and interdental fricatives. Consonant clusters likely to be residual errors are, from most to least likely, three member clusters, two member Liquid clusters, and two member [s] clusters.

Table 3–13. Likely residual errors in Stage 4.

Consonant
s
ʃ
θ
ð
z
tʃ
ɚ
r
l

Table 3–14. Likely consonant cluster residual errors in Stage 4.

Consonant Clusters	*Age*
Three member clusters	7;0–8;0
Two member Liquid clusters	5;6–6;0
Two member S clusters	5;0

VI. SPEECH FOR COMMUNICATION

Speech serves human society as a vehicle for communication between individuals, between groups, and across generations (see Chapter 1). The type of communication most directly relevant to clinical practice occurs between individuals (talk). The following is the developmental progression of speech for communication between individuals from Stages 1 through 4:

- Stage 1: A child learns "my turn–your turn" structure of conversation and a small stock of word meanings.

- Stage 2: A child increasingly uses words to express thoughts, wishes, and feelings.

- Stage 3: Communication increasingly includes unfamiliar persons. A child's speech abilities are made possible and are extended by attainment in syntax, morphology, and discourse.

- Stage 4: Speech serves as a foundation of literacy. Increasingly, speech becomes a way to explore the world, and a child learns uses of speech in formal and diverse educational and social settings.

A. Stage 1 (Birth to 12 months)

A child does not begin life knowing that sound is used to communicate. Through a combination of brain growth, stimulation from the environment, fine-tuning of perceptual abilities, and vocal play, during the first year the foundations are laid for future developments in communication. Learning the "my turn–your turn" pattern of conversation and the special relationship between sound and meaning are major accomplishments in Stage 1.

1. First Conversations. A conversation typically involves back-and-forth volleys of speech. A child acquires rudiments of conversational turn taking during the first year. By 3 to 4 months an infant may coo, grunt, or squeal when spoken to, and by 7 months may vocalize on seeing a bottle. Through the first half of Stage 1 vocalizations typically are largely reflexive, occurring as a child moves, is excited, or is upset. To illustrate, during the first half of Stage 1 an infant sitting in a high chair may reach forward to obtain a bottle, grunting as a consequence of diaphragm compression. Sound making may assume a ritualized quality toward the end of Stage 1. For instance, by 10 months an infant sitting in a high chair may seek to obtain a bottle by looking at a parent and emitting a short, ritualized grunt. Such a ritualized noise lies between a reflective sound and a word.

2. **Sound and Meaning.** Human language rests on the special relationship between sound and meaning. Early in life a child grasps that sound is special in this regard. Behaviors reflecting this awareness include an infant 4 to 6 months old responding to the sound of his or her name, and an infant 6 to 7 months turning to look when a family member is named (example: "Where's Daddy?").

3. **First Words and Sign Language.** Though some infants may produce one or two words near 5 or 6 months old, most commonly—though not always—such words are spoken from a few days to several weeks and then disappear. For most children, ability to speak words emerges closer to 11 or 12 months. An interesting research finding is that an infant acquires hand signs a few months earlier than spoken words (Corballis, 2002), suggesting that an infant may find gesturing with the hands easier than gesturing with the mouth.

4. **Discovery of Meanings.** Two aspects of communication facilitate discovery of word meanings: intonation and context.

   a. **Intonation.** A caregiver's intonation is a tremendous help to infants when the meaning of words is unclear. To illustrate, near six months a child stops an activity when a parent says "no" in a commanding voice (Hedrick, Prather, & Tobin, 1984). Parents often assume a child understands *no* and, by ceasing the action, is demonstrating compliance. However, compliance is based on intonation rather than knowing what *no* means. If parents wished, they could change *no* to *yes* (or *dog* or *bus*, for that matter), maintaining a commanding voice, and a child would likely respond as if "no" were spoken.

   b. **Context.** An infant's ability to discover word meanings appears strongly influenced by context. Like adults, an infant learns words that are functionally important and are heard frequently in highly familiar and predictable contexts. For an infant, word meanings likely to fit this description refer to caregivers, favorite pets and toys, and are found in daily routines such as bathing, mealtimes, diaper changes, and bedtime.

   To better see the similarity between infant and adult learning, imagine a person in a foreign country who doesn't know a word of the language. If the visitor were in a bar and pointed to a beer glass, the bartender might pour a beer and stretch out a hand, palm up, saying "Deeb." While not knowing the exact meaning of "Deeb," a visitor would likely assume it meant something like, "pay me for the beer," since in a bar a bartender typically asks for money after pouring a drink. The visitor's knowledge of a familiar context (a bar) narrows possible meanings of words. Though not knowing if "deeb" is one word, several words, means "pay me," is the amount of money owed, or simply means "please," the visitor suspects the word or words has something to do with payment. The same visitor would have far less chance to determine the meaning of "deeb" if it were only heard once and outside a familiar context—for example, overheard while walking down a street. Similarly, an infant has little chance to understand the meaning of a word if it is seldom heard and does not occur in familiar contexts.

B. Stage 2 (12 to 24 months)

By the end of Stage 1 a child grasps that sound can signify differences in meaning, may speak a few words, and has learned the back and forth, "my turn to make sound, your turn to make sound" quality of conversation. In Stage 2 a child has developed a small expressive vocabulary, increasingly uses speech to communicate, and has strategies that reduce speech complexities.

1. Expressive Vocabulary. Near the beginning of Stage 1 a child's expressive vocabulary (words spoken by the child) may consist of two or three different words (Table 3–15). By 18 to 20 months a child may achieve an expressive vocabulary of approximately 50 different words, and by 24 months, the end of Stage 2, a child may have an expressive vocabulary of over 100 different words (Capute, Palmer, Shapiro, Wachtel, Schmidt, & Ross, 1986).

Table 3–15. Growth in size of expressive vocabulary in Stage 2.

Age	Number of Words
12 to 13 months	2 to 3 words
14 to 15 months	4 to 6 words
16 to 17 months	7 to 20 words
20 to 21 months	50 words

2. **Word Combinations.** Early in Stage 2 a child's speech may contain both single words and a few longer utterances such as "Mommy go" and "Go home now." To a child such utterances may seem like long words rather than sentences. Toward the last months of Stage 2, a child regularly places words together to form two and three word sentences, and by the end of Stage 2 a child's speech regularly contains a mix of single words and two and three word sentences.

3. **Speech for Communication.** A child's growing ability to use speech to interact with others is a pivotal accomplishment of the first two years. At first, sound is little more than an activity that accompanies interactions with caregivers, similar to eye gaze and arm waving. Gradually, however, sound replaces eye gaze and pointing as a child's primary means of communication, allowing expression of increasingly complex thoughts and needs permitted by a rapidly evolving neurological system. A toddler in the first months of the second year typically communicates using facial expressions, gestures, single words, and vocalizations. A toddler near 16 to 18 months old uses words to express wants and needs, and by 20 months uses words to relate experiences (Hedrick, Prather, & Tobin, 1984). To illustrate, a 20-month-old child might say "doggy" to her father when he comes home (as my daughter once said to me when she was that age), telling him a story about a remarkable event earlier in the day that involved meeting a neighbor's dog. (As an aside, "doggy" was the entire story. No one claims 20-month-old children tell a great story, only that they tell stories.)

Regressions Seldom are Regressions

Regressions involve loss of a previously mastered ability. They may be as small as loss in phonetic accuracy in a single word, or may be as large as loss of previously correct stress patterns, syllable shapes, and sound classes (Bleile & Tomblin, 1991; Menn, 1976). Regressions, small and large, occur commonly in speech development, especially during Stage 2, and may last from days to months. Parents sometimes notice larger, longer-lasting regressions, commenting that a child "used to say it correctly, but now doesn't." Or, "My child used to say it right, but now it sounds more like baby talk." Regressions often arise as a child generalizes and overgeneralizes "regular ways to talk." Similar to a morphological overgeneralization in which, for example, a preschooler overgeneralizes the past tense marker to

(continued)

say, "I goed home," regressions in speech represent developmental progress. Rather than proceeding in a straight line, speech development zigzags and sometimes even regresses as a child generalizes and overgeneralizes regular ways of talking. Unless a regression in speech is concomitant with changes in neurological status, its presence is not cause for concern and, indeed, may signify an important developmental advance.

4. **Communication Strategies.** A Stage 2 child may develop one or several strategies to facilitate verbal communication, including:

- Selectivity

- Word-based learning

- Favorite sounds and word recipes

- Homonym seeking and avoiding

- Gestalt learning

Strategies are not mutually exclusive. A child whose speech demonstrates a high degree of selectivity, for example, may or may not also be a word-based learner or a homonym seeker or avoider.

a. **Selectivity.** Many children follow a strategy of "picking and choosing" words to say based on their ability to pronounce them. First described by Ferguson and Farwell (1975) and first studied experimentally by Schwartz and Leonard (1982), selectivity has been shown to occur widely among both typically developing children and those with articulation and phonological disorders (Schwartz, 1988; Leonard, 1985). Twin hallmarks of selectivity are: (1) a child more readily attempts words that possess speech elements (sounds, syllables, and stress patterns) that can be pronounced, and (2) selectivity does not typically occur in a child older than 1;10.

Selectivity allows children to ignore the many sounds that cannot be pronounced, and to communicate instead with words that contain those sounds that lie within their narrow range of speech abilities. The interpretation given here is that selectivity functions as a developmental mechanism that bootstraps a child from prespeech vocalization into speech. To illustrate, suppose that both

Child A and Child B produced CV syllables during babbling, but that the babble of Child A consisted mainly of labial consonants while that of Child B consisted primarily of alveolar ones. Selectivity would draw Child A toward an early expressive vocabulary containing CV syllables and labial consonants (for example, *bee* and *boo-boo*), while Child B would be drawn to a first expressive vocabulary containing CV syllables and alveolar consonants (for example, *daddy* and *day*). Weeks and months later, suppose that Child A stumbled on [t] during the course of speaking while Child B stumbled on [k], Child A would then be drawn to attempt to pronounce words such as *toe* while Child B might be drawn toward attempting to pronounce words such as *key*. Thus, selectivity provides a late Stage 1 and early Stage 2 child a transitional stepping stone from babbling to speech, and a means to acquire a small expressive vocabulary.

b. **Word-based Learning.** Another frequently encountered strategy focuses on functional and useful words, but gives little attention to how the words are pronounced. This strategy is particularly common in the first half of Stage 2, when the challenging task of connecting what can be perceived to what can be pronounced is especially great. For a child following a word-based strategy, words are pronounced as isolated "items" rather than as part of a language system.

A child's word-based strategy is somewhat analogous to how a person in a foreign country may learn words such as *dinner*, *taxi*, and *museum* because they are functional and useful, but know little of the phonology of the language. I have been in such a situation when visiting a country with a language I did not know, and while there learning a few dozen polite greetings and useful phrases. We would not dignify what I did by saying I was learning a language; rather, I learned isolated words, and said them just well enough to be understood (sometimes). A child with a word-based strategy follows a similarly cavalier approach to pronouncing first words: they are pronounced just well enough to be understood, with little or no systematic approach to pronunciation in evidence. As a result, such a child may pronounce words that contain a word initial [m] in the adult language as [m] in some words, [p] in others, and [b] in yet others. Only later does the child come to realize that a number of different words may begin with the same sound, and, thus, may all be pronounced similarly.

c. Favorite Sounds and Word Recipes. While some children "pick and choose" (selectivity) and others pronounce haphazardly (word-based learning), still others prefer to base communication on a few favorite speech elements. To illustrate, a favorite consonant may be an [s] that is used to end all words (Ferguson & Macken, 1983). A more extreme communication strategy is called word recipes, a term intended to convey that a child, like some inexperienced cooks, may use a few recipes over and over again (Menn, 1976; Waterson, 1971). For a novice cook, all meals may end up tasting like spaghetti. For a child with a word recipe strategy, all words may end up sounding like [di] or some other narrow set of speech elements.

d. Homonym Seeking and Avoiding. Two other strategies that a child may follow involve homonyms, words that sound alike but mean different things (Ingram, 1975). A vocabulary with large numbers of homonyms can severely limit a child's ability to communicate, and may be particularly harmful during periods when a child has a large number of meanings to express and only a small stock of sounds and syllables through which to express them. In such a circumstance, children divide into two groups. Those in the first group speak in ways that seem to avoid homonyms (homonym avoiders). This strategy makes it easier for the listener to discern the message, but increases the burden on a child's limited pronunciation abilities. Those in the second group seek homonyms (homonym seekers), increasing the burden on a listener to determine a child's message, but easing the burden on a child's pronunciation abilities.

e. Gestalt Learning. Another communication strategy bypasses words in favor of phrase and sentence melody. Even in the early part of Stage 2, the speech of a child following such a strategy (called a gestalt learner) may contain phrases with good intonation and relatively poor pronunciation of individual sounds. This may be because a child is more focused on intonation than words, or because of difficulty discovering individual words in the stream of speech. In a colorful and insightful phrase, Ann Peters has said that such children "learn the tune before the word" (Peters, 1977, 1983).

C. Stage 3 (2 to 5 years)

By the beginning of Stage 3 a child typically communicates using speech and has amassed a stock of words that can be understood and pronounced. In Stage 3 a child's universe of conversational partners expands from family members and close friends to unfamiliar persons in a range of social roles. Growth in speech abilities makes important advances in syntax and morphology possible, which in turn stretches and expands a child's speech skills.

1. **Leaving the World of Familiars.** Many children in Stage 3 attend preschool or other programs and settings that include persons outside immediate family and friends. In these environments, a child's daily life may for the first time regularly include unfamiliar persons, both children and adults. The rules for when and how to talk in these settings are often different from those with which a child is familiar. Further, a child at home with family and friends shares enormous amounts of experience, permitting successful communication despite limited speech abilities. If a child says "ball," a parent may know that "ball" refers to a favorite toy that rolled under a couch earlier that day. If a child says the same thing in preschool, a teacher may wonder, "Do you want a ball? Did someone take your ball? Do you want to draw a ball? Do you want me to get you a ball?" To be understood in this new world of unfamiliar persons, a child must include more words (and, thus, more sounds) in the message, filling in those parts that shared experience provided at home. Additionally, speech must be pronounced more systematically and clearly for the meaning to be understood.

2. **Syntax and Morphology.** Speech is critical to developments in syntax and morphology.

   a. **Syntax.** As pressure to communicate grows in Stage 3, a child increasingly relies on syntactic means to convey messages, requiring sounds be combined in longer and more complex ways. At the beginning of Stage 3, a child's speech likely contains single words and short, two and three word sentences. By three years, a child's speech contains short sentences of four or more words, and by four and one-half years, near the end of Stage 3, sentences may be embedded one inside the other, such as "My mother is waiting for me."

   b. **Morphology.** In addition to stringing together words to make sentences (syntax), a child in Stage 3 also uses speech to modify word and sentence meaning (morphology). This begins shortly before two years and continues throughout Stage 3 (Brown, 1973). Examples of morphemes acquired during this period include present progressive –ing (*He is running.*), regular plural –s (*dogs and cats*), articles (*a, an, the*), and irregular past (*come/came, break/broke*). Speech development both supports and is expanded by acquisition of morphology. To illustrate, modifying meaning through morphology entails pronouncing unstressed syllables (present progressive, articles), ending syllables with sometimes challenging consonants (regular plural), and making vowel alternations (irregular past).

D. Stage 4 (5 years through adolescence)

By the beginning of Stage 4, a child has largely acquired the building blocks of speech, has experience with speech in environments outside the home, and can use speech to convey ideas and feelings through means of a large vocabulary, syntax, and morphology. Near the beginning of Stage 4, a child typically begins formal education, our society's principle method of cultural transmission. Uses of speech expand dramatically and diversify in Stage 4, reflecting and supporting a child's social and educational development. Chief among these developments, a child learns to translate speech into other mediums, especially printed representations (reading). Through reading and pronunciation of longer and more complex sound combinations, speech abilities are further expanded.

1. **Phonological Awareness.** Major aspects of modern cultures are transmitted from one generation to the next through formal education. This transmission is achieved primarily through speech and its written representation, reading. Learning how speech is represented in print entails the child having awareness of speech. Growth in phonological awareness occurs during the late preschool and early school years.

   Dodd and Gillon (2001) indicate that development of phonological awareness proceeds as shown in Table 3–16. Near the end of Stage 3 a child first demonstrates ability to divide words into syllables. By five and one-half years of age a child demonstrates awareness of rhyme and alliteration, and can isolate individual sounds in words. Between six and one-half and seven years of age a child learns to segment a word into individual sounds.

2. **Speech Demands in School.** Speech demands change and increase as a child progresses through the educational system (Highnam, 2003). Table 3–17 summarizes changing demands placed on speech.

Table 3–16. Development of phonemic awareness in late Stage 3 and early Stage 4.

Age	Description
4;6–4;11	Syllable segmentation
5;0–5;5	Rhyme awareness
	Alliteration awareness
	Phoneme isolation
6;6–6;11	Phoneme segmentation

Adapted from Dodd and Gillon (2001). Exploring the relationship between phonological awareness, speech impairment and literacy. *Advances in Speech-Language Pathology, 3(2),* 139–147.

Table 3–17. Changing school demands in Stage 4.

Grades	Changing School Demands
K	Learn outside of an immediate context
1–2	Learn to read and write
3–6	Read and write to learn
7–10	Students assume responsibility for their own learning
10–12	Students become independent learners and need to process large volumes of language information in short periods of time

a. **Kindergarten.** In the first school year a child increasingly is exposed to speech devoted to topics outside an immediate context. For example, a child may learn about continents or types of flowers, without the context of traveling to each continent or standing in a flower bed.

b. **First and Second Grade.** A child acquires foundations of literacy, including how such speech elements as consonants, consonant clusters, and vowels are realized in written forms.

c. **Third through Sixth Grade.** A child increasingly uses reading and writing to learn. Speech makes possible or facilitates such important social and educational activities as:

- Undertaking projects with peers

- Making class presentations and oral reports

- Answering questions in class

- Participating in extracurricular activities such as drama

- Discussing ideas

- Expressing feelings

d. Seventh through Ninth Grade. A child must possess sufficient proficiency in speech and reading to assume responsibility for learning.

e. Tenth through Twelfth Grade. A child stands on the threshold of adulthood and is expected to process large quantities of information in short periods of time.

Something Speech Does

A polite eighth grade boy was made quarterback of his junior high football team and shortly thereafter began acting verbally aggressive at home. A visit to the school counselor revealed he was having difficulty separating aggressiveness needed on the football field from the way he was to behave at home. The counselor and the boy talked this over and soon problems at home largely disappeared. As discussed in Chapter 1, speech has great power as a thinking tool. The example of the eighth grade quarterback illustrates how speech can direct and guide thinking during a sometimes difficult developmental period.

VII. SUMMARY: STAGES IN SPEECH DEVELOPMENT

The discussion in this chapter has focused on how a child learns to speak. The long period over which speech development occurs was divided into four stages.

A. Stage 1

Stage 1 lasts from birth to approximately 12 months. During this stage a child lays foundations for future speech development. A review of specific developments follows.

1. Perception. An infant is born able to perceive major sound distinctions in the world's languages. By the end of Stage 1 perception is largely restricted to sounds found in the language spoken in the child's community.

2. Production. A child begins life producing sounds that occur while breathing and moving, and by the end of Stage 1 produces a small stock of consonants, vowels, syllables, stress patterns, and intonation contours.

3. Perception-Production Link. Through vocalizing a child establishes a link between the ear and mouth.

4. Communication. A child learns the "my turn–your turn" structure of conversation and a small stock of word meanings.

B. Stage 2

Stage 2 lasts from approximately 12 to 24 months of age. During this stage a child becomes a word user.

1. Perception. A child displays generally good word perception abilities, though perceptual problems arise in unfamiliar settings, when hearing rapid speech, and when distracted or uninterested.

2. Production. A child uses speech elements acquired through babbling to build a small expressive vocabulary.

3. Perception-Production Link. A child first bridges mismatches between advanced perceptual abilities and limited pronunciation skills.

4. Communication. A child increasingly uses words to express thoughts, wishes, and feelings.

C. Stage 3

Stage 3 lasts approximately 2 to 5 years. During this stage a child masters most major speech elements (sounds, syllables, stress patterns, prosody, etc.) of the language.

1. **Perception.** Though possessing relatively advanced speech perception abilities, difficulties in perception remain, especially during the early part of this stage.

2. **Production.** Early in Stage 3 a child pronounces a small stock of sounds and syllables; by the end of Stage 3 a child has largely mastered most major speech elements of the language.

3. **Perception-Production Link.** A child manages mismatches between perception and production through error patterns that affect sound classes.

4. **Communication.** Communication increasingly includes unfamiliar persons. A child's speech abilities both make possible and are extended by attainment in syntax, morphology, and discourse.

D. Stage 4

Stage 4 lasts from approximately 5 years through adolescence. In this stage a child masters late-acquired speech elements and lays the foundation for literacy.

1. **Perception.** A child's speech perception abilities increasingly become adult-like.

2. **Production.** A child in Stage 4 may experience difficulties with individual consonants and consonant clusters; literacy exposes a child to new vocabulary containing challenging syllabic and stress patterns.

3. **Perception-Production Link.** Mismatches between perception and production decrease significantly, though they still may affect individual sounds and combinations of sounds. Such mismatches may be sufficiently slight and long-standing that a child has difficulty recognizing them.

4. Communication. Speech increasingly becomes a way to explore the world, and a child learns uses of speech in formal and diverse educational and social settings.

VIII. CLINICAL IMPLICATIONS

Clinically, typical speech development provides a conceptual framework, an assessment tool, and a foundation of treatment.

A. Conceptual Framework of Speech Development

The following are ten major points in the conceptual framework of speech development that underlies this book.

1. Speech plays a critical role in human society, facilitating talking, thinking, group identity, and cultural transmission.

2. Speech has a dual nature, as a part of language and a channel of communication.

3. Speech is deeply rooted in human evolution and biology.

4. Speech development requires a brain capable of learning and an environment dedicated to teaching.

5. Speech development shapes and is shaped by brain development.

6. During speech development a child learns to link together perceptual and production abilities for purposes of communication.

7. During the first year a child lays the foundations of speech development.

8. During the second year a child increasingly communicates through speech.

9. During the preschool years a child masters most major speech elements.

10. During the school years speech facilitates reading and both supports and is extended by educational and social development.

B. Assessment

Knowledge of typical speech development plays a central role in assessment and is used in conjunction with other means to determine eligibility for services, ascertain therapy progress, and make differential diagnoses (Tyler, Tolbert, Miccio, Hoffman, Norris, Hodson, Scherz, & Bleile, 2002).

1. **Eligibility.** A critical first step in therapy, and one mandated both by law and common sense, is to determine if a person is eligible for treatment. A clinician considers many factors in making this important decision, including typical speech development. To illustrate, a clinician may decide to provide speech services to a child based in part on slower than expected speech development relative to his or her peers.

2. **Therapy Progress.** Respect for a client—and, in many situations, to satisfy requirements of agencies that fund clinical services—requires therapy progress be assessed on a regular basis. Information obtained through assessment helps a clinician with such important decisions as whether to continue or end therapy, or whether to maintain or alter clinical goals. To illustrate, based in part on information about typical speech development, a clinician might end therapy because a client's progress has become comparable to peers. Alternatively, if a client has not been progressing in therapy, a clinician might consult a guide on typical speech development to help select a different therapy goal.

3. **Differential Diagnosis.** Therapy proceeds most rapidly when focused on a client's deficit area. To give a health care example, if a person visited a physician complaining of a sore throat, an attempt would be made to assess the reason for the problem. If its cause were a cold, one recommendation would result, and if its cause was cancer, another recommendation and treatment plan would follow. Differential diagnosis is equally important in therapy for a person with a communication disorder. A clinician, knowing that delay seldom affects all communication domains equally, performs a differential diagnosis to map peaks in ability and valleys of disability. For example, speech would likely be a therapy focus if, based on information about typical speech development, a clinician determined that a child demonstrated particular delay in that domain. Alternately, if a child's speech development was more advanced compared to other communication areas, a clinician might select non-speech therapy goals.

C. Treatment

Typical development provides a framework within which to organize treatment of articulation and phonological disorders. Goals of treatment change depending on a child's developmental stage.

1. Developmental Levels. Stages refer to levels that correspond to the client's articulation and phonological development—this may or may not be the same as the client's chronological age (procedures to determine the age level most closely corresponding to the client's level of articulation and phonological development are described in Chapter 5). For example, a school-age child in Stage 3 receives treatment using principles developed to treat clients whose speech contains errors affecting sound classes. Naturally, specific treatment activities are selected based on the client's interests rather than level of articulation and phonological development. An adult in Stage 4, for example, receives treatment using principles developed to treat clients with errors affecting a few late-acquired consonants, consonant clusters, and unstressed syllables in more difficult multisyllabic words with the particular activities and instructions modified to reflect adult interests.

2. Stages. Treatment goals corresponding to each stage are listed in Table 3–18.

a. Stage 1. A child in Stage 1 may be an older child with a delay in articulation and phonology or an infant with a medical or developmental disability putting him or her at risk for future delays in speech development.

Table 3–18. Treatment goals in four stages in speech development.

Stages	Age Range in Typically Developing Children	Treatment Goals
Stage 1	0–12 months	Facilitate development of vocal skills that underlie later speech development.
Stage 2	12–24 months	Facilitate development of a functional vocabulary for purposes of communication
Stage 3	24 months to 5 years	Facilitate acquisition of major speech elements
Stage 4	5 years through adolescence	Facilitate development of literacy and eliminate errors affecting late-acquired speech elements.

For a child in Stage 1 treatment focuses on laying foundations for future speech development. Possible treatment goals to facilitate articulation and phonology development include:

- Increase opportunities to vocalize

- Acquire developmentally advanced vocalizations

- Teach functional, high-frequency words in familiar contexts

- Facilitate conversational turn-taking

b. Stage 2. A child in Stage 2 may be an older child delayed in articulation and phonological development, or, in common with a Stage 1 child, someone with a medical need or developmental disability putting him or her at risk for future delay in speech development.

Treatment focuses on expressive vocabulary based on research that indicates expressive vocabulary (words actually used for communication, rather than simply words the client understands) is a primary means through which younger children acquire the rules of speech and language (Ferguson & Farwell, 1975). Articulation and phonological problems are also thought to be major factors in limiting expressive vocabulary development in such diverse populations as children with Down syndrome and otherwise typically developing children with expressive language delay (Miller, 1992; Paul, 1991).

Possible treatment goals to facilitate articulation and phonology development include:

- Stimulate expressive vocabulary development

- Encourage speech for communication

- Reduce homonyms

- Reduce variability

c. Stage 3. A child in Stage 3 typically is a preschooler or school-age child with a delay in speech development. Concurrent language disorders are extremely common (see Chapter 2). Medical and developmental problems occur among children in Stage 3, but less commonly than among children in Stage 1 or 2.

Treatment facilitates acquisition of rules underlying classes of speech elements. Possible treatment goals to facilitate articulation and phonology development include:

- Reduce or eliminate errors affecting classes of speech elements
- Facilitate speech in phrases and sentences
- Encourage use of speech in settings outside the home

d. Stage 4. A child or young adult in Stage 4 typically is either without other developmental problems or experiences mild to moderate problems in other developmental domains. In Stage 4 reading and language-related learning disabilities tend to co-occur with speech difficulties.

Treatment focuses on helping clients achive mastery of acquired speech elements and development of speech skills related to literacy. Possible treatment goals to facilitate articulation and phonology development include:

- Facilitate mastery of late-acquired consonants and consonant clusters
- Teach pronunciation of literary and scientific vocabulary
- Increase phonological awareness
- Encourage use of speech in social and educational settings

APPENDIX 3A

10-Point Conceptual Framework
of Speech Development

1. Speech plans a critical role in human society, facilitating talking, thinking, group identity, and cultural transmission.

2. Speech has a dual nature, being both a part of language and a channel of communication.

3. Speech is deeply rooted in human evolution and biology.

4. Speech development requires both a brain capable of learning and an environment dedicated to teaching.

5. Speech development both shapes and is shaped by brain development.

6. During speech development a child learns to link together perceptual and production building blocks for purposes of communication.

7. During the first year a child lays the foundations of speech development.

8. During the second year a child increasingly communicates through speech.

9. During the preschool years a child masters most major speech elements.

10. During the school years speech facilitates reading and both supports and is extended by educational and social development.

CHAPTER

4

Screening
and Assessment

The following topics are discussed in this chapter:

137

I. OVERVIEW OF SCREENING

A screening is performed to determine if the client's articulation and phonological development is appropriate for his or her chronological age or developmental age (see Chapter 5, Section VI). Screenings are most successful in
settings in which the clients do not show a high incidence of articulation and
phonological problems, including well baby clinics, preschools, and grade
schools. In settings where potential clients may have a higher incidence of
articulation and phonological disorders (e.g., early intervention programs
and Head Start centers), screenings should be undertaken with more caution,
because they impose an additional time burden on the clinical staff, who may
need to screen and perform complete assessments on large numbers of
clients. Approximately five minutes should be allotted for an articulation and
phonological screening.

II. NONSTANDARDIZED SCREENINGS

Screenings can be performed using either nonstandardized or published
screening instruments. The following is an example of a nonstandardized
clinical screening procedure for clients of different chronological ages.

The Setting

Provide screenings (and complete evaluations) in a room sufficiently
quiet to hear speech. The room should be clean and free of distractions
but not sterile. Toys and other playthings should be kept out of the sight
and reach of younger clients. If possible, have parents or professional
caregivers familiar with the client present with infants and toddlers. If
a client has physical limitations or special motoric needs, positioning
should be undertaken with guidance from occupational or physical
therapy (Bleile, in press; Bleile & Miller, 1994). If the client has a
(continued)

medical condition, a nurse or other qualified staff member knowledgable about the client's medical status should be consulted to rule out the existence of medical complications that would either interfere with the assessment or exacerbate the client's medical problems (Bleile & Miller, in press).

A. All Ages

If a caregiver is present, ask if he or she is concerned about the client's speech. Spend a moment to study the client's face, looking for signs of gross structural abnormalities. If time permits and the client is cooperative, open the client's mouth and shine a penlight at the roof of the mouth to look for repaired or submucous clefts. The latter often appear as a blue tint at midline. With infants it is often easier to insert a gloved finger in the mouth than to peer in with a penlight. Be sure to wash any powder off the glove before inserting it in the client's mouth. Note any gross abnormalities in teeth (including malocclusions) and tongue size. Ask the client's caregivers questions to determine if risk factors are present (see Section VII), which might suggest that the client should receive a full evaluation, even if a delay in articulation and phonological development does not yet exist.

B. Infants (9 to 12 months)

Ask the caregiver to help elicit vocalizations. Also ask, "Does your baby make babbling noises?" If the caregiver answers yes, probe further by asking, "What do the sounds sound like?" The purpose of these questions is to determine if the child engages in reduplicated babbling (repetition of identical consonants, such as *ba ba*) or nonreduplicated babbling (repetition of different consonants, such as *ba da*), skills that emerge between 7 and 9 months of age. Refer the infant for a speech-language evaluation if the caregiver indicates that the child does not make noise or does not engage in reduplicated or nonreduplicated babbling.

C. Toddlers (18 to 24 months)

Ask the caregiver to play with the child to elicit speech. Also ask the caregiver: "Does your child speak yet?" or "Does your child use words to communicate?" The purpose of this question is to discover if the child speaks more than three words, a skill that emerges near 13 months of age. If the caregiver answers affirmatively, ask "What words does your child say—can you give me examples?" If the caregiver answers any of these questions negatively, refer the child for a speech-language evaluation.

D. Preschoolers, School-age Children, and Adults

Ask the client, "What did you have for breakfast today?" or "What did you do today?" Also compare the client's development to age norms on consonant and consonant cluster acquisition using an instrument of the clinician's choosing or the one provided in Appendix 4A. If the client fails to produce the consonants and consonant clusters expected of persons of his or her age, a referral should be made for a complete speech-language evaluation. An instrument to screen phonological awareness in kindergarteners is provided in Appendix 4B (Highnam, 2002).

III. PUBLISHED SCREENING INSTRUMENTS

If the decision is made to use a published screening instrument, the clinician has a wide range of instruments from which to choose. The most widely used instruments are listed below.

Predictive Screening Test of Articulation (PSTA)

Authors: Van Riper, C., & Erickson, J. (1968). Predictive screening test of articulation. *Journal of Speech and Hearing Disorders, 34,* 214–219.

Comments: Developed to identify children whose speech is likely to improve without treatment; intended for use with first graders.

Preschool Language Scale 3 (PLS-3)

Authors: Zimmerman, I., Steiner, V., & Pond, R. (1992). *Preschool Language Scale 3.* Columbus, OH: Charles E. Merrill.

Comments: A language test that contains a screening subtest for speech; intended for use with children 1 through 7 years old.

Quick Screen of Phonology (Quick Screen or QSP)

Authors: Bankson, N., & Bernthal, J. (1990). *Quick Screen of Phonology.* Chicago, IL: Riverside Press.

Comments: A picture naming test developed by two highly regarded clinical investigators; intended for use with children 3 through 7 years old.

Screening Deep Test of Articulation (Screening Deep Test)

Author: McDonald, E. (1968). *Screening Deep Test of Articulation.* Pittsburgh, PA: Stanwix House.

Comments: Offers a relatively in-depth screening (90 items); intended for use with children kindergarten through 3rd grade.

Speech and Language Screening Test for Preschool Children (Fluharty)

Author: Fluharty, N. (1978). *Speech and Language Screening Test for Preschool Children.* Bingingham, MA: Teaching Resources.

Comments: Elicits speech using real objects; intended for use with children 2 through 6 years old.

Templin-Darley Screening Test

Authors: Templin, M., & Darley, F. (1969). *Templin-Darley Screening Test.* Iowa City: University of Iowa Bureau of Education Research and Service.

Comments: A well-known screening test; intended for use with children 3 through 8 years old.

Test of Minimal Articulation Competence (T-MAC)

Author: Secord, W. (1981). *Test of Minimal Articulation Competence.* San Antonio, TX: The Psychological Corporation.

Comments: A complete assessment instrument that includes a quick (3- to 5-minute) screening test.

Yopp-Singer Test of Phonemic Segmentation (Yopp-Singer)

Authors: Yopp, K. (1995). A test for assessing phonemic awareness in young children. *The Reading Teacher,* 49, 20–29.

Comments: A quick 22-item screening test with normative data for kindergarteners.

IV. OVERVIEW OF ARTICULATION AND PHONOLOGICAL ASSESSMENTS

A complete articulation and phonological assessment is performed to achieve one or more of three goals:

- To determine the client's current level of and prognosis for future articulation and phonological development,

- To determine if the client's problem is severe enough to warrant intervention, and

- To provide information useful in planning treatment, if that is found to be warranted.

A. Steps in Articulation and Phonological Assessment

Typically, a complete articulation and phonological assessment is part of a speech-language evaluation. The articulation and phonological assessment consists of three sections: initial observation, collection of the speech sample, and hypothesis testing.

1. Initial Observation. During the initial observation the clinician listens to the client's spontaneous speech, makes notes about particular speech errors, and formulates an initial impression of the client's perceived intelligibility. Depending on the client's developmental level, the spontaneous speech sample can be obtained by asking the client to describe a picture, to respond to questions such as "What did you have for breakfast?" or simply by listening to the client speak during conversation. Approximately 3 to 5 minutes are allotted for the initial observation.

2. Collection of the Speech Sample. The clinician collects a speech sample for later analysis using either nonstandardized procedures, published instruments, or a combination of both. The relative strengths and limitations of nonstandardized procedures and published instruments are listed in Tables 4–1 and 4–2, respectively. Nonstandardized assessments, as summarized in Table 4–3, are often the primary or sole form of assessment for clients in Stage 1 or Stage 2, are used in conjunction with standardized assessment instruments for clients in Stage 3, and may serve as an adjunct to standardized tests for clients in Stage 4. Whatever combination of nonstandardized and standardized assessments are performed, the clinician should allow 10 to 30 minutes for collection of the speech sample, depending on the extent of the client's articulation and phonological problems.

3. Hypothesis Testing. Hypothesis testing is undertaken to obtain additional information about the client's articulation and phonological disorder. During the collection of the speech sample, for example, a client might pronounce *key* as [ti], raising the question of whether this pronunciation results from an error pattern that turns all velar

Table 4–1. Strengths and limitations of nonstandardized assessment procedures.

Variable	Characteristics
Strengths	Flexible procedures allow the clinician to adapt the assessment to the clients learning style
	Can be used with clients who are not testable by other means
	Can be used when no published test is suitable to the client's needs or developmental level
	Often provides more in-depth analysis than typically is provided by a published assessment instrument
Limitations	Requires greater knowledge by the clinician
	Use of flexible procedures may impair reliability
	Some nonstandardized procedures require more time than is available in most clinical settings

Table 4–2. Strengths and limitations of standardized assessment instruments.

Variable	Characteristics
Strengths	Promotes reliability by use of standardized procedures and speech samples
	Provides an overview of important speech assessment topics
	Often is time-efficient
	Results are often accepted by insurance companies and other third party payers
Limitations	Not all clients have sufficient cognitive and attention skills to perform well on published tests
	Many published instruments do not analyze speech in sufficient depth to be used with clients who have severe articulation and phonological disorders

Table 4–3. Use of nonstandardized procedures and standardized instruments at four developmental levels.

Developmental Level	Assessment Strategy
Stage I	Primarily nonstandardized assessments supplemented by standardized instruments
Stage 2	Primarily nonstandardized assessments supplemented by standardized instruments
Stage 3	Combination of nonstandardized procedures and standardized instruments
Stage 4	Primarily standardized assessment instruments supplemented by nonstandardized assessment procedures

stops into alveolar stops. Alternately, the client might produce [f] correctly in one word, and the clinician may want to know if the client is able to produce [f] correctly in other words. In general, hypothesis testing requires from between a few minutes to 30 minutes, depending on the nature and complexity of the client's articulation and phonological problems. Time permitting, hypothesis testing is undertaken during the evaluation session at which the speech sample is collected. Hypothesis testing may also be undertaken over several sessions concurrent with the onset of treatment.

Hypothesis testing can be undertaken using a wide variety of procedures. The author's preference is to use word probes such as those provided in Appendixes 4B and 4C. These probes can be used either to test individual sounds (sound probes) or error patterns (error probes). Word probes also provide a time efficient means to perform pre-tests and posttests and to search for key phonetic environments and key words (see Section V in Chapter 5). Typically, word probes are not used to test all the client's errors, but focus instead on the sounds and error patterns that seem likely treatment goals. To illustrate, a client's speech might show the error patterns of Fronting, Stopping, Prevocalic Voicing, and deletion of abutting consonants word medially (e.g., the pronunciation of *window* as *widow*). In this situation, it would be appropriate to perform word probes to test hypotheses related to Fronting, Stopping, and Prevocalic Voicing, but not the error pattern affecting abutting consonants word medially. This is because, given the nature of the client's other error patterns, the error pattern affecting medial consonants is not likely to be selected as an early treatment goal.

What's in a Name?

Error patterns include all errors that affect more than one sound. This includes such traditional articulation categories as lisping and lateralization, as well as what are called phonological processes or phonological patterns. The term *error pattern* was chosen to avoid biasing the discussion to either an articulation or phonological perspective.

V. NONSTANDARDIZED ASSESSMENTS

The following are procedural guidelines for undertaking a nonstandardized assessment.

Multiple Error Patterns

Most clients in Stage 2 and Stage 3 experience difficulties with more than one aspect of articulation and phonological development. A client, for example, may experience problems with both pronouncing fricatives and producing voiceless consonants. The result may be two error patterns: Stopping and Prevocalic Voicing, both of which may occur in the same word. A client, for example, might say *see* as [di] because the combination of Stopping and Prevocalic Voicing converts [s] into [d]. Identifying the effects of multiple error patterns can be challenging. The information in Appendix 4D illustrates how commonly occurring combinations of error patterns may affect consonants and consonant clusters.

A. Sample Size

In general, a nonstandardized assessment requires a sample of between 50 to 100 utterances. Smaller samples are typically collected during initial evaluations with clients in Stage 1 and Stage 2, because these clients often vocalize and speak less. Whenever possible, two or three productions of the same words should be obtained for clients in Stage 2 and early Stage 3, because these clients are often variable in how they say words (see the discussion of short-term goals in Chapter 6).

B. Transcription System

Speech is transcribed using the International Phonetic Alphabet (IPA) or an equivalent system. As summarized in Table 4–4, the client's level of articulation and phonological development largely determines whether whole words or isolated sounds are transcribed. With clients in Stage 1, either the entire vocalization is transcribed phonetically or a checklist system is used (see Appendix 5J). Whole words are transcribed when the client is in Stage 2 or Stage 3, because the presence of a sound in one part of a word can affect the production of another sound elsewhere in the word. Typically, isolated sounds are transcribed if the client is in Stage 4.

The Reluctant Child

If a young child appears reluctant to enter the evaluation room, ask "Do you like to play?" Most children nod or say yes and then come willingly. Another technique that sometimes works is to tell the child that you have a new toy you want the child to play with, which is a very special toy that the child will be the first one to use.

Table 4–4. Transcription at four levels of development.

Developmental Level	Type of Transcription
Stage 1	Entire vocalization or checklist
Stage 2	Whole word
Stage 3	Whole word
Stage 4	Individual sounds or check mark system

C. Non-English Symbols and Diacritics

Different non-English symbols and diacritics are likely to be needed depending on the client's level of articulation and phonological development. (See Chapter 2 for the list of non-English symbols and diacritics used in this book.)

1. **Stage 1.** Stage I vocalizations are not well-described by most systems of non-English symbols and diacritics. For most clinical purposes, a checklist system bypasses the need for diacritics (Vannucci, 1994). Appendix 5J contains a sample vocalization checklist. If detailed phonetic transcriptions are needed, the reader is referred to discussions in Oller (1992), Proctor (1989), and Stark (1980).

2. **Stage 2.** The non-English symbols and diacritics most likely to be needed for transcription of the speech of clients in Stage 2 include labiodental stops (often produced for bilabial stops), bilabial fricatives (often produced for [f] and [v]), unaspirated voiceless stops (often produced in place of aspirated stops), wet sounds (wet sounding speech often occurs in clients with oral motor problems), and glottal stops. The most difficult of these sounds to hear are unaspirated, voiceless stops and glottal stops.

   a. **Labiodental Stops.** Labiodental stops often sound like bilabial stops, but can be identified by the upper teeth touching the lower lip, which may be similar or identical to the position used for [f] and [v].

Diacritics

Extensive use of diacritics is time consuming and leads to transcriptions in which the phonetic symbols become lost among all the accompanying wiggles, wavy lines, and circles. On the other hand, using too few diacritics results in missing clinically significant aspects of speech. The following general rules may prove helpful in deciding which diacritics to include in transcriptions:

- Include only those diacritics that are clinically relevant. Do not attempt the nearly impossible task of transcribing all the phonetic details of the client's speech.

(continued)

- On the top of the first page of the transcription sheet list the diacritics you are likely to need based on the client's level of articulation and phonological development, recognizing that all of them might not be needed or that other diacritics may also be needed.

- While transcribing the client's speech, if you hear the client produce a sound in a way that you cannot readily describe, transcribe the closest approximation of the sound you are able to make, and place an "X" under it. For example, if you hear something "[s]-like," but somehow different than standard [s], transcribe it as [s] with an "X" underneath. Continue placing "X" under the [s] until you are able to identify how the client is producing the sound. When this occurs, define the "X." For example, you might indicate at the bottom of the page that "X = voiceless lateral postalveolar fricative."

- Exclude diacritics that describe relatively minor, predictable aspects of speech production. For example, do not use diacritics to indicate that [s] is produced with lip rounding when preceding [w] in *sweet* or that [r] is usually produced without voicing when following voiceless consonants in such words as *pride.*

- Exclude diacritics that describe aspects of speech that the client produces in an adult manner. For example, do not use diacritics to indicate stress patterns and syllable boundaries that conform to that of the adult language. To illustrate, do not use a diacritic to indicate stress if the client says *begin* with stress on the second syllable, but do so if the client says the same word with stress on the first syllable.

b. Bilabial Fricatives. Bilabial fricatives often are perceived as sounding like a cross between a fricative and a glide and can be identified by the client's lips coming together close or identical to the position for [p] and [b].

c. Voiceless, Unaspirated Stops. Voiceless, unaspirated stops are often mistaken for voiced stops. There are several options to practice hearing these sounds.

(1) Perception. Most American English speakers who hear voiceless unaspirated stops report that the sound "jumps" between the aspirated voiceless sound and its voiced counterpart (e.g., [pʰ] and [b]). If you hear a [b] that "jumps" in perception between [pʰ] and [b], it may be a voiceless unaspirated stop.

(2) Phonetic Drills. Several phonetic drill books have tapes of voiceless, unaspirated stops (Edwards, 1986; Shriberg & Kent, 1982).

(3) Native Speaker. Ask a speaker of a language that has voiceless, unaspirated stops to produce [p], [t], or [k].

(4) Production. Sometimes, making a sound facilitates hearing it better. To do this, place your hand in front of your mouth and say [pʰ]. Feel the puff of air on your hand. Now, keep repeating [pʰ], working to reduce the puff of air on your hand. When the puff of air is gone, but the sound is not quite [b], it is probably a voiceless unaspirated [p].

d. Glottal Stops. There are several ways to train yourself to hear glottal stops:

(1) Word-initial. The word *ice,* if said forcefully, begins with a strong glottal stop. Repeat the word several times aloud, tuning your ear to the glottal stop.

(2) Word-final. A glottal stop at the end of a word sounds like the preceding vowel was cut off very suddenly. Say *bee* several times, cutting off the vowel each time.

(3) Between Vowels. Glottal stops that replace consonants in the middle of words (as in *funny*) sound like someone trying to imitate a Cockney accent. To practice, try saying *funny* several times with a Cockney accent.

3. Stage 3. The same non-English symbols and diacritics are used to transcribe the speech of clients in Stage 2 and Stage 3 (labiodental stops, unaspirated voiceless stops, wet sounds, and glottal stops). Additional diacritics likely to be needed include [w] coloring of [r], as well as lisped, lateralized, and bladed productions of [s] and [z].

a. **[w] Colored [r].** [w] coloring of [r] often is perceived as being between [w] and [r].

b. **Lisping.** During lisping [s] and [z] are produced with the client's tongue either touching the teeth or protruding slightly between the teeth as for [θ] or [ð]; however, the tongue may be either more forward or retracted than for [θ] and [ð]. Air may also be released over the sides of the tongue, in which case the sound is called a lateral lisp ([ls] and [lz]).

c. **Lateralized.** Lateralized [s] and [z] can be identified by feeling for release of air by placing the hand near the sides of the client's mouth.

d. **Bladed.** Bladed production of [s] and [z] often is perceived as an [s] or [z] with [ʃ]- or [ʒ]-like qualities, although the tongue may not be retracted as far back as it is for [ʃ] and [ʒ].

4. **Stage 4.** Transcriptions for clients in Stage 4 are likely to need the same non-English symbols and diacritics as for clients in Stage 3 ([w] coloring of [r] and lisped, lateralized, and bladed production of [s] and [z]).

D. Information Maintenance

There are no agreed-upon methods to maintain client information. The client's utterances can simply be transcribed on a piece of paper or on a sheet such as that presented in Appendix 4E. The use of a form is illustrated in Table 4–5.

Table 4–5. Example of a transcription sheet.

Word	Transcription	Environments			Other Environments		
		#___	V_V	___#	___	___	___
pea	b pi		p→b				
stoop	øtuø stup		st→øt		p→ø		

1. **Word.** The word is the presumed meaning of the word (or phrase). A question mark is used if the clinician is uncertain of the client's meaning. If a client points to a dog and says [du], for example, the word is *dog.* If the clinician is uncertain if *dog* is the presumed meaning of [du], the word is *?dog.*

2. **Transcription.** The transcription is the phonetic rendition of the word (or phrase). The transcription of *pea,* for example, is [pi]. Differences between this and the client's pronunciation of the word are indicated directly above the sounds in error. The [b] for [p] pronunciation in *pea,* for example, is indicated by transcribing [b] above the crossed-out transcription of [p]. Deletion of consonants (as occurs for [s] in *stoop*) is indicated by the null (zero) sign.

3. **Environments.** The environments indicate where the sound or sounds occurred. The most commonly used environments are beginnings of words (#____), ends of words (____#), and between vowels (V____V) (see Chapter 3 for definitions of environments). Vowels are usually indicated by "V." If the client pronounces *stoop* as [tu], for example, the first error occurs in a word-initial environment and the second error occurs in a word-final environment.

4. **Other Environments.** Other environments are environments that may be added as need arises. A clinician, for example, might add a syllable-initial environment (S____) to describe the production of [h] in words such as *behind.*

E. Recording Speech

Decisions must also be made as to whether video or audio tapes will be used for later transcription and analysis.

1. **Repetitions.** If recording the client's speech, repeat the word after the client so that you can later identify what the client said. Also say in a quiet voice any characteristics that might be difficult to identify on the tape (e.g., "Oh, I saw your tongue between your teeth").

2. **Recording Devices.** Select a high-quality recording device from among the wide variety of excellent recording equipment available commercially.

3. **Microphones.** If possible, record speech samples using a lapel microphone unless the client's movements appear likely to produce too much noise. Free standing microphones are often best to use with these clients. If possible, two microphones are used in case the client moves around.

4. **Recording Procedures.** Shriberg (1993) recommends the following recording procedures:

   a. Record the speech in a quiet environment.

   b. If the environment is noisier than optimal, reduce the mouth-to-microphone distance if the noise is constant, or have the client repeat the utterance if the noise is transient.

   c. Use high-quality recorders with an impedance-matched external microphone and high-quality cassette tapes.

   d. Place the cassette deck on a different surface from the microphone and as far away as possible to avoid noise from the tape deck interfering with the recording.

   e. Place the microphone approximately 6 to 8 inches from the client's lips.

   f. Adjust the volume control so the client's vowels cause the VU meter to peak just below the distortion range (In general, volume levels between one half to two thirds of the highest volume yield the best signal-to-noise ratios).

To Record or Not Record?

If you believe recording improves your clinical work, then by all means record, but remember that it will take just as long to listen to an audio tape or watch a video tape as it did to make the recording, and that transcribing the tape is likely to require much additional time. Because of the time it takes, extensive recording of clients' speech is probably not practical outside of university settings. For this reason, many clinicians restrict use of recordings to challenging clinical cases, for educational purposes, and—less often—to document clinical progress.

F. Types of Speech Samples

One of the most important clinical decisions involves the types of speech samples to collect. Methods for collecting speech samples are listed in Table 4–6.

1. **Spontaneous Speech.** Spontaneous speech is the preferred sampling technique because it is most representative of how the client talks (Ingram, 1994; Morrison & Shriberg, 1992; Morrison & Shriberg, 1994). The major limitation of spontaneous speech samples is the length of time it can take to transcribe them, especially if the client speaks in sentences of three or more words. Further, longer utterances usually must be tape recorded to be transcribed, which adds greatly to the time needed to complete the analysis. For this reason, many clinicians prefer to spend a few minutes early in the session listening to the client's spontaneous speech, perhaps making notes about particular speech errors and the client's level of severity and/or intelligibility. The initial impression of the client's spontaneous speech is then used to guide the subsequent analysis of the client's elicited speech.

2. **Elicited Speech.** There are four major speech elicitation techniques: naming, sentence completion, delayed imitation, and imitation.

Table 4–6. Methods used to collect a speech sample.

Elicitation Techniques	Definition
Spontaneous speech	Naturally occurring speech
Elicited speech	
Naming	Single words typically elicited through naming objects or pictures
Sentence completion	Single words typically elicited through the client finishing the clinician's sentence
Delayed imitation	Single words typically elicited through placing a short phrase between the clinician's model and the client's response
Imitation	Single words typically elicited through the clients immediate imitation of the clinician's model

a. **Naming.** Naming involves asking a client to name pictures or objects. For example, the clinician asks, "What is this?" or engages in an object identification game in which the client names objects pulled from a box.

b. **Sentence Completion.** Sentence completion involves asking the client to end a sentence begun by the clinician. For example, the clinician might pick up an object or picture and say, "Here/This is a ____." A useful variation of this procedure which tests morphological endings is to say, "Here is a ____. Here is another ____. Now I have two ____." One advantage of sentence completion tasks over naming procedures is that sentence completion elicits speech somewhat faster. More importantly, sentence completion tasks direct the client to say the words you want to elicit.

c. **Delayed Imitation.** Delayed imitation involves placing a short phrase between the clinician's request to say a word or phrase and the client's response. For example, the clinician says, "This is a dog." Now you say it./"Now you say it." The phrase provides a small amount of time during which the client must hold the word in memory, which presumably makes this task slightly more reflective of cognitive skills than immediate imitation. Delayed imitation is quick and useful when the clinician wants to elicit a large number of words from the client.

d. **Immediate Imitation.** Immediate imitation involves having the client immediately repeat something said by the clinician. For example, the clinician says, "Say these words after me," followed by the words. Immediate imitation is the least natural elicitation technique, but it has the advantage of offering a speedy way to elicit a large number of words.

H. Elicitation Activities

Activities used to collect speech samples change according to the client's chronological age and for clients who have intellectual impairments or cognitive deficits, level of cognitive development.

Leave Your Dignity at the Door

The curricula of most graduate schools does not include course work on smacking your lips, singing, tickling, and puffing out your cheeks, but these are some of the techniques that often work best with infants. The best advice for working with the youngest of clients is to leave your dignity at the door and enjoy yourself.

---

1. **Infants and Toddlers.** The optimal elicitation technique is to observe the child interacting with his or her caregivers. Begin by asking the caregiver, "'Will you play with your child a few minutes so I can get a better idea how your child sounds?" If the caregiver is not available, the clinician should interact with the child. Whether the caregiver or clinician is the elicitor, have the following objects present and introduce and remove them one at a time to avoid overwhelming the child.

   a. **Birth to 6 Months.** Infants from birth to 6 months old tend to vocalize while shaking a small rattle, listening to a music box start and stop, watching a black and white mobile, holding a hand-held or noise-making toy, and playing with a simple busy box.

The Problem May Not Be Speech

Sometimes a client's articulation and phonological disorder is the first indication of larger problems in language and cognitive development. In some cases, a client's family will say their child has a speech problem, even when they suspect that their child may have more extensive developmental problems, because a speech problem seems correctable and is easier to deal with emotionally. Other times, a client's family will say their child has a speech problem, having no inkling that their child's speech is part of a larger picture of developmental difficulties. Because language and cognitive disorders sometimes manifest first as speech problems, the clinician should perform a thorough language evaluation of all young clients who are referred for problems with speech development.

---

b. 6 to 12 Months. Infants 6 to 12 months old tend to vocalize while looking in a mirror; watching bubbles; or playing with pop-up toys or manipulable toys, such as a drum or toy cars.

c. 12 to 18 Months. Toddlers 12 to 18 months old tend to speak while riding a wagon or tricycle, looking at a simple picture book with an adult, putting together and taking apart Mr. and Mrs. Potato Head, or "talking" on a play telephone.

d. 18 to 24 Months. Toddlers 18 to 24 months old tend to speak while playing with and dressing a doll, looking at a picture book with an adult, playing with building blocks, putting together a big-piece puzzle, or "talking" on a play telephone.

2. **Preschoolers (2 to 4 Years).** The following ideas may help elicit speech either directly or through the help of a caregiver.

a. Reading. Read a picture book with the client and have the client name and describe actions in the pictures.

b. Shopping. Play "shopping" with pretend food, play money, and a cash register.

c. Tea Party. Have a tea party or make a meal using toy dishes, utensils, and cooking equipment.

d. Dress a Doll. Help the child dress a doll. The adult holds a doll, and the child names the pieces of clothing to put on the doll. Alternately, the adult wears a puppet, and the child tells the puppet how to dress the doll.

e. Puppets. The adult and the child wear finger or hand puppets and have the puppets take turns telling stories such as Little Red Riding Hood or The Three Little Pigs.

f. Broken Toy. Present the child with a broken toy that has a missing part and ask the child, "What's wrong?" or "Why won't it work?"

g. Misnaming. The adult (or a puppet) misnames common objects, saying things like, "This is a dog" while pointing to a toy cat. The hope is that the client will correct the adult by giving the appropriate name for the object.

3. Late Preschoolers and Younger Grade School Children. The following ideas help to elicit speech from late preschoolers (4 to 5 years of age) and younger grade school children (through third grade).

a. Spontaneous Speech

(1) Family Photos. If possible, ask the client's caregivers to bring in a family photo album and have the client tell you about the album photos.

(2) Picture Sequence Cards. Lay out picture sequence cards and have the client use the pictures to tell a story.

(3) Most Favorite/Least Favorite. Ask the child to tell you what is his or her favorite/least favorite cartoon, television program, food, animal, and so on. Alternately, ask the child, "What did you have for breakfast?" or "Where's your favorite place to go in the entire world?"

(4) Broken Toy. Present the child with a broken toy and ask him or her to tell you what is wrong and how to fix it.

(5) Tell a Story. Give the child a picture book and ask him or her to tell a story. Alternately, wear finger or hand puppets and either have the child tell a story to the puppet or have the puppet tell the story.

(6) Play Acting. Play act with the child using favorite activities and characters, for example, playing house, going grocery shopping, or pretending to be Bugs Bunny, or the Power Rangers.

(7) Explain a Game. Have the child explain a game to you or a puppet, for example, jacks, Cootie, Old Maid, or hide-and-seek.

(8) Funny Clothes. Enter the room wearing something funny (perhaps upside-down toy glasses), hoping the child will notice and discuss it.

(9) Treasure Hunt. Play treasure hunt in which the clinician visually impairs a stuffed animal with sunglasses, so that the child has to describe where the treasure is hidden in the room.

(10) Bizarre Questions. Ask the child bizarre questions, for example, "Are you married?" or "I like your shoes. Can I have them?"

b. Single Words

(1) Turn Over the Cards. Play a game in which the child is allowed to turn over and remove picture cards from a table after naming what is on the card.

(2) Bingo. Play Bingo, allowing the child to pick a picture from a bag, name the picture, and match it to a sheet in front of him or her.

(3) Tossing Games. Play ball or bean bag toss, instructing the child to toss a ball or a bean bag to a board with pictures on it and to name the pictures he or she hits.

(4) Steps. Place picture cards on steps and have the client climb the steps, naming the picture cards on each step.

(5) Toy Car. Place cards on a table or the floor and let the client drive a toy car over the cards, naming each card the car rolls over. Alternately, have the child roll a ball and name the card on which the ball stops.

(6) Magic Box. Show the child a "magic box" or a lunch bag. Play a game in which the child reaches into and pulls out and names objects or pictures from the box or bag. Alternately, draw a picture of a cartoon character with a big mouth on a piece of paper, for example, Cookie Monster or a lion. Place the picture over the opening of a cardboard box and instruct the client to reach in and tell you what is in Cookie Monster's (or the lion's) mouth.

(7) Lights Off. Place objects around the treatment room before the client arrives. When the client arrives, turn off the light and have the client shine a flashlight around the room, naming objects as they are found.

(8) Play Teacher. Let the child play teacher by wearing glasses and using a pointer to name objects placed around the room.

4. Older Grade School Children and Adolescents. Ask the client one or more of the following questions.

a. Blame. Have you ever been blamed for something you didn't do?

b. Dump Truck. What would you do if someone dropped a dump truck of popcorn in your living room?

c. Ball on a Roof. Can you tell me how to get a ball off a roof?

d. Christmas Tree. How do you decorate a Christmas tree?

e. Sandwich. Can you tell me how you make a peanut butter and jelly sandwich?

5. Adults. Ask the client one or more of the following questions.

a. Today. What were you doing before you came here today?

b. Store. Would you describe the route from your home to the nearest grocery store?

c. Kitchen. Would you describe your kitchen for me?

VI. PUBLISHED ASSESSMENT INSTRUMENTS

The following published instruments offer a wide range of approaches to assess articulation and phonological disorders. Specific procedural guidelines for the tests are included with the individual assessment instruments. When applicable, I indicate whether the test instrument is oriented primarily to analyzing error patterns (typically, phonological processes) or individual sounds (typically, consonants and consonant clusters). Unless otherwise noted, each test requires approximately 30 minutes to complete.

Arizona Articulation Proficiency Scale (Arizona or AAPS)

Authors: Fudala, B., & Reynolds, W. (1986). *Arizona Articulation Proficiency Scale.* Los Angeles, CA: Western Psychological Services.

Comments: A traditional test of individual sounds.

Assessment Link Between Phonology and Articulation (ALPHA)

Author: Lowe, R. (1986). *Assessment Link Between Phonology and Articulation.* East Moline, IL: LinguiSystems.

Comments: A carefully designed assessment instrument for children 3 years and older.

The Assessment of Phonological Processes—Revised (APP-R)

Author: Hodson, B. (1986). *The Assessment of Phonological Processes—Revised.* Danville, IL: Interstate Publishers and Printers.

Comments: One of the most popular tests of error patterns, it is intended for children with multiple error patterns and takes about 50 minutes to complete. Also comes in a computer version.

The Assessment of Phonological Processes—Spanish (APP-S)

Author: Hodson, B. (1986). *The Assessment of Phonological Processes—Spanish.* San Diego, CA: Los Amigos Association.

Comments: The Spanish version of the popular APP-R.

Austin Spanish Articulation Test (ASAT)

Author: Carrow, E. (1974). *Austin Spanish Articulation Test.* Austin, TX: Teaching Resources Corporation.

Comments: A traditional test of individual sounds; one of the few tests available to assess Spanish speakers.

Bankson-Bernthal Test of Phonology (Bankson-Bernthal)

Authors: Bankson, N., & Bernthal, J. (1990). *Bankson-Bernthal Test of Phonology.* Chicago, IL: Riverside Press.

Comments: A carefully designed error pattern assessment instrument developed for children 3;0–7;11 by two highly respected clinical investigators.

Children's Speech Intelligibility Test (CSIT)

Authors: Kent, R., Miolo, G., & Bloedel, S. (1994). Children's speech intelligibility test. *American Journal of Speech-Language Pathology, 3,* 81–95.

Comments: A word-recognition test of intelligibility for children with limited speech abilities; this test is in the developmental stage, and the authors do not necessarily recommend it for use in intelligibility assessment.

Clinical Probes of Articulation Consistency (C-PAC)

Author: Secord, W. (1981). *Clinical Probes of Articulation Consistency.* San Antonio, TX: The Psychological Corporation.

Comments: A collection of probes for individual consonants and vowels; requires approximately 5 minutes per consonant probe and 10 minutes per vowel probe.

Compton-Hutton Phonological Assessment (Compton-Hutton)

Authors: Compton, A., & Hutton, S. (1978). *Compton-Hutton Phonological Assessment.* San Francisco, CA: Carousel House.

Comments: A test of error patterns that contains a good selection of multi-syllabic words; intended for children with multiple error patterns.

Computer Analysis of Phonological Processes: Version 1.O. [Apple II series computer programs]

Author: Hodson, B. (1985). *Computer Analysis of Phonological Processes Version 1.* Danville, IL: Interstate Printers and Publishers.

Comment: Computer version of the popular APP-R.

Computerized Profiling

Authors: Long, S., & Fey, M. (1994). *Computerized Profiling.* Austin, TX: Psychological Corporation.

Comments: A new computer analysis for the Macintosh computer program and MS-DOS systems.

A Deep Test of Articulation (McDonald Deep Test)

Author: McDonald, E. (1964). *A Deep Test of Articulation.* Pittsburgh, PA: Stanwix House.

Comments: A test of individual sounds that provides detailed information on phonetic environments; comes in picture and sentence forms; requires approximately 1 hour to complete,

The Edinburgh Articulation Test (Edinburgh)

Authors: Anthony, A., Bogle, D., Ingram, T., & Mclsaac, M. (1971). *The Edinburgh Articulation Test.* Edinburgh, UK: E & S Livingston.

Comments: A traditional test of individual sounds and consonant clusters developed for children between 2 and a half to 6 years old.

Fisher-Logemann Test of Articulation Competence (Fisher-Logemann)

Authors: Fisher, H., & Logemann, J. (1971). *Fisher-Logemann Test of Articulation Competence.* Boston, MA: Houghton Mifflin.

Comments: A traditional test of individual sounds.

Goldman-Fristoe Test of Articulation (Goldman-Fristoe or GFTA)

Authors: Goldman, R., & Fristoe, M. (1986). *Goldman-Fristoe Test of Articulation.* Circle Pines, MN: American Guidance Service.

Comments: A well-respected test of individual sounds for late preschoolers and school-age children.

The Khan-Lewis Phonological Analysis (Khan-Lewis or KLPA)

Authors: Khan, L., & Lewis, N. (1986). *The Khan-Lewis Phonological Analysis.* Circle Pines, MN: American Guidance Service.

Comments: A well-designed test that uses pictures from the GFTA to identify error patterns.

Lindamood Phoneme Sequencing Program for Reading, Spelling, and Speech (LIPS)

Authors: Lindamood, P., & Lindamood, P. (1998). *Lindamood Phoneme Sequencing Program for Reading, Spelling, and Speech.* Austin, TX: Pro-Ed.

Comments: A popular test of phonological awareness.

Logical International Phonetic Programs (LIPP)

Authors: Oller, K, & Delgado, R. (1990). *Logical International Phonetic Programs.* Miami, FL: Intelligent Hearing Systems.

Comments: Offers in-depth speech analysis for Version 1.03 (MS-DOS computers).

The Macintosh Interactive System for Phonological Analysis

Authors: Masterson, J., & Pagan, F. (1994). *The Macintosh Interactive System for Phonological Analysis.* San Antonio, TX: *The Psychological Corporation.*

Comments: A new procedure to analyze speech using a Macintosh computer.

Natural Process Analysis (NPA)

Authors: Shriberg, L., & Kwiatkowski, J. (1980). *Natural Process Analysis.* New York: John Wiley.

Comments: A well-respected test of error patterns for use with children with severely delayed speech; analysis is based on spontaneous speech samples; no specific stimuli are required; requires approximately 1½ hours to administer.

Phonological Assessment of Child Speech (PACS)

Author: Grunwell, P. (1986). *Phonological Assessment of Child Speech.* Boston, MA: College-Hill Press.

Comments: An impressive comprehensive test for children with multiple error patterns.

Phonological Awareness Test

Authors: Robertson, C., & Salter, W. (1997). *The Phonological Awareness Test.* East Moline, IL: LinguiSystems.

Comments: A commonly used test of phonological awareness.

Phonological Process Analysis (PPA)

Author: Weiner, F. (1979). *Phonological Process Analysis.* Austin, TX: Pro-Ed.

Comments: Tests 16 error patterns; requires approximately 45 minutes to complete with a cooperative child.

Photo Articulation Test (PAT)

Authors: Pendergast, K., Dickey, S., Selmar, J., & Soder, A. (1969). *Photo Articulation Test.* Danville, IL: Interstate Printers and Publishers.

Comments: A long-time stand-by test of individual sounds for ages 3 through 12 years; pocket-size cards are convenient; requires approximately 15 minutes to complete.

Process Analysis: Version 2.0. [Apple II series computers]

Author: Weiner, F. (1986). *Process Analysis: Version 2.* State College, PA: Parrot Software.

Comments: Computer version of the PPA designed for Apple computers.

Programs to Examine Phonetic and Phonologic Evaluation Records: Version 4.0. [MS-DOS systems].

Author: Shriberg, L. (1986). *Programs to Examine Phonetic and Phonologic Evaluation Records: Version 4.0.* Hillsdale, NJ: Lawrence Erlbaum.

Comments: Computer version of the highly regarded NPA.

Smit-Hand Articulation and Phonology Evaluation (SHAPE)

Authors: Smit, A., and Hand, L. (1997). *Smit-Hand Articulation and Phonology Evaluation.* Los Angeles, CA: Western Psychological Services.

Comments: An excellent evaluation instrument based on strong normative data and with outstanding photograph stimulus items.

Spanish Articulation Measures (SAM)

Author: Mattes, L. (1993). *Spanish Articulation Measures.* Oceanside, CA: Academic Communication Associates.

Comments: Assesses Spanish-speaking children's acquisition of individual sounds and elimination of error patterns.

The Templin-Darley Tests of Articulation (Templin-Darley)

Authors: Templin, M., & Darley, F. (1969). *The Templin-Darley Tests of Articulation.* Iowa City: University of Iowa Bureau of Educational Research and Service.

Comments: A classic test of individual sounds for late preschoolers and school-age children.

Test of Minimal Articulation Competence (T-MAC)

Author: Secord, W. (1981). *Test of Minimal Articulation Competence.* San Antonio, TX: The Psychological Corporation.

Comments: A traditional test of individual sounds; requires approximately 10–20 minutes to complete.

Test of Phonological Awareness (TOPA)

Authors: Torgesen, J., & Bryant, B. (1994). *Test of Phonological Awareness.* Austin, TX: Pro-Ed.

Comments: A new test of a child's awareness of individual sounds in words.

Weiss Comprehensive Articulation Test (WCAT)

Author: Weiss, C. (1980). *Weiss Comprehensive Articulation Test.* Chicago, IL: Riverside.

Comments: A well-respected test for preschoolers to adults.

VII. RELATED ASSESSMENTS

Other aspects of a complete speech-language evaluation can have an important influence on the articulation and phonological assessment.

A. Language Assessment

The language assessment (especially information on language reception abilities) helps establish the client's upper potential for articulation and phonological development. In most cases, a child 10 years of age with mental retardation, whose major language reception abilities approximated a child 3 years of age, for example, would be expected to have (at best) the articulation and phonological abilities of a child 3 years of age. (See Chapter 6 for further discussion of developmental age.)

B. Hearing Screening

The hearing screening establishes whether the client has a hearing impairment that might affect his or her articulation and phonological development.

C. Case History

Several questions asked during the case history can help to determine if the client is either at-risk for an articulation and phonological disorder in the future or presently has an articulation and phonological disorder adversely affecting his or her life. Sample case history questions for a preschooler are provided in Appendix 4G.

1. At-risk Conditions. At-risk conditions include genetic, medical, and environmental factors. Positive answers to any of the following questions should alert the clinician that the client may be at-risk for problems in articulation and phonological development:

- Does anyone in the client's immediate family have a speech problem?
- Does the client have a hearing impairment?
- Does the client have any neurological or cognitive handicaps?
- Does the client have any medical difficulties or genetic factors that might interfere with present or future articulation and phonological development?
- Was the client born more than 4 weeks prematurely?
- Does the client have any structural or functional abnormalities of the face or oral motor system?
- Is the client a long-term hospital patient?
- Has the client experienced neglect?

2. **Effect on Life Situation.** The following questions may serve to determine if speech is adversely affecting the client's life situation.

- Ask caregivers of infants and toddlers, "Do you feel that your child has speech problems (problems in vocalizing for infants) that interfere with your interactions?"
- Ask caregivers of preschoolers, "Does your child get frustrated when he or she can't be understood?" or "What does your child do when he or she can't be understood?"
- Ask late preschoolers and school-age children, "Do people sometimes have trouble understanding you when you talk?" or "If you had three wishes, what would you wish for?" (If the child wishes for better speech or wishes to be understood better, the clinician should consider that a sign for concern.) Alternately, ask the client's caregiver, "Do other children tease your child about his/her speech?"
- Ask adults, "Does your speech interfere with your job?" or "How do you feel about your speech?" or "How does your speech affect your life?"

D. Oral Cavity Assessment

The oral cavity assessment helps to determine if the client has gross oral cavity abnormalities that might interfere with speech production (Mason & Wickwire, 1978). The oral cavity assessment requires gloves, a mirror, a penlight and a tongue depressor. The evaluator should wear gloves, and universal health precautions should be followed. The oral cavity assessment proceeds as described in the steps below. A sample form for the oral cavity assessment is provided in Appendix 4H.

The Oral Cavity

The speech mechanism is so flexible that persons speak well with high palates, small teeth, a small or large tongue, and many other mild to moderate structural and movement problems. Only the grossest abnormalities are capable of nullifying the human capacity to develop compensatory strategies to minimize physical limitations. If the oral cavity assessment reveals gross abnormalities of structure or movement, the client should be referred to an otolaryngologist, orthodontist, or neurologist.

---

1. **Face.** Sit at eye level across from the client and observe his or her face. Muscle weakness or spasticity might suggest cerebral palsy. Muscle weakness or drooping of one half of the face might suggest paralysis.

2. **Breathing.** Observe the client breathing. Mouth breathing might indicate blockage of the nasal airway. If a problem is suspected, ask the client to close his or her mouth and breathe onto a mirror placed under the nose. An unfogged mirror or inability to breathe through the nose would be additional evidence that the nasal airway is not open.

3. **Lips.** Observe the client's lips for drooling, which might indicate the presence of dysarthria or another oral motor deficiency. Ask the client to perform the following activities to test for movement disorders:

   a. **Spreading.** Ask the client to say [i] (to test lip spreading).

Which Consonant Remains?

When a consonant cluster is reduced, which consonant remains? Typically, but not always, the consonant that remains is the one, acquired earlier, according to age norms (see Chapter 5). For example, [st] is likely to be reduced to [t] and [br] is
(continued)

> likely to be reduced to [b]. The same principle applies to clusters with three consonants. For example, [spr] is likely to be reduced to either [p] or [sp], whereas the [r], being acquired latest in development of the three sounds, is the consonant most likely to be deleted.

b. Rounding. Ask the client to say [u] (to test lip rounding).

c. Rapid Movements. Ask the client to say [pʌpʌpʌ] (to test rapid movements of the lips).

4. Jaw. Turn the client's head to each side, and look for gross retrusions or protrusions of the maxilla or mandible.

5. Teeth. Ask the client to open his or her mouth so you can examine the teeth.

a. Missing Teeth. Look for missing teeth. Missing front teeth have the most direct effect on speech, especially on [s] and [z].

b. Bite. To observe the client's bite, instruct the client to bite down lightly on the back teeth and to open the lips. In a normal overbite the upper front teeth are about one quarter inch in front of the lower teeth and cover about one third of the top of the lower teeth.

c. Overbite. Note if the client has an excessive overbite or an open bite (i.e., the upper teeth do not cover part of the lower teeth at any point along the dental arch).

6. Tongue. Observe the client's tongue.

a. Size. Determine that the tongue is not grossly large or small. A tongue that appears shriveled either on one or both sides might indicate paralysis,

b. Reach. Ask the client to touch the alveolar ridge with his or her tongue tip. A client whose tongue tip cannot reach the alveolar ridge may have a short lingual frenum (i.e., the attachment under the tongue).

    c. Laterality. Instruct the client to move his or her tongue laterally to test its mobility.

7. Hard Palate. Instruct the client to extend his or her head back.

    a. Clefts. Observe the client's hard palate for signs of repaired or unrepaired clefts, fistulas, and fissures.

    b. Coloration. Observe the midline of the client's hard palate, using a penlight if needed. Normal coloration of the midline is pink and white. A blue tint in the midline could indicate a submucous cleft. A blue tint lateral to the midline is not a cause for alarm. If a blue line is found at the midline, gently rub the posterior portion of the hard palate, feeling for a cleft.

8. Soft palate. Instruct the client to open his or her mouth three quarters of maximum to get the best velar elevation.

    a. Clefts. Observe the soft palate for signs of repaired and unrepaired clefts, fissures, and fistulas.

    b. Coloration. Look for a normal pink and white coloration at the midline. As with the hard palate, a blue tint at midline may indicate a submucous cleft. A blue tint lateral to the midline is not a cause for concern.

    c. Nasality. Ask the client to produce a sustained "ah." A nasal sounding "ah" may indicate difficulty closing the nasal tract. Determine whether the client can elevate his or her velum to the plane of the hard palate.

9. Uvula. Ask the client to say a sustained "ah" and observe his or her uvula. A bifid uvula (it looks like two uvula) might indicate the presence of other anatomical problems.

10. Fauces. Ask the client to say a sustained "ah" and look for signs of redness, inflammation, or movement of the faucial pillars that might indicate infection.

11. Pharynx. Ask the client to say a sustained "ah" and look at the back of his or her throat. Presence of a Passavant's pad might indicate a possible velopharyngeal valving problem.

APPENDIX 4A
Sample Consonant Screening Items

A. Introduction

To screen for articulation and phonological disorders, (1) obtain a short spontaneous speech sample to help develop an initial impression of the client's level of intelligibility or severity of involvement and (2) elicit the underlined sounds shown on the following pages. The typical ages at which the underlined sounds are acquired are listed in parentheses (Smit, Hand, Frelinger, Bernthal, & Byrd, 1990). To illustrate the information gathering procedure, a spontaneous speech sample might be obtained by asking, "What did you have for breakfast?" To elicit the underlined sounds, a client aged 4;10, for example, would be asked to say the words in Category C, the closest category below the client's chronological age. Clients older than 5 years of age are compared to the age norms in Category D. A client is placed within a category based on developmental age instead of chronological age if intellectual limitations or a cognitive impairment exists. Clients with no risk factors (see Section VII) who miss more than one underlined sound should be referred for a complete articulation and phonological assessment. Clients with risk factors (see Section VII) should be referred for a complete evaluation if they miss one underlined sound.

B. Elicitation Procedures

Elicit either isolated words or sentences using the phrase, "Repeat after me: _____. Now you say it." If the client answers too quickly, say "First wait for me to finish," followed by repetition of the word or sentence.

Example

Begin the screening with an example of the procedure.

Isolated word: "Repeat after me: dog. Now you say it."

Sentence: "Repeat after me: The man walked home. Now you say it." If the client answers too quickly, say "First wait for me to finish," followed by repetition of the sample.

Sample Consonant Screening items

A. For Clients   3;6–3;1 1

<u>tw</u>in	_____	(3;0)
<u>q</u>uick	_____	(3;0)
<u>s</u>on	_____	(3;6)
<u>z</u>oo	_____	(3;6)
<u>sk</u>ip	_____	(3;6)
<u>pl</u>ay	_____	(3;6)

Or: "My <u>tw</u>in is <u>q</u>uick." (3;0)
     "My <u>s</u>on <u>pl</u>ays at the <u>z</u>oo." (3;6)

B. For Clients 4;0–4;5

<u>s</u>on	_____	(3;6)
<u>z</u>oo	_____	(3;6)
<u>sk</u>ip	_____	(3;6)
<u>pl</u>ay	_____	(3;6)
plea<u>se</u>	_____	(4;0)
<u>pr</u>ide	_____	(4;0)
<u>dr</u>y	_____	(4;0)
<u>cr</u>owd	_____	(4;0)

Or: "My <u>s</u>on <u>pl</u>ays at the <u>z</u>oo." (3;6)
     "Plea<u>se</u> don't make the baby <u>cr</u>y." (4;0)

C. For Clients 4;6–4;1 1

<u>pl</u>ease	_____	(4;0)
<u>pr</u>ide	_____	(4;0)
<u>dr</u>y	_____	(4;0)
<u>cr</u>owd	_____	(4;0)

<u>th</u>umb _____ (4;6)

<u>gr</u>ape _____ (4;6)

<u>sl</u>ip _____ (4;6)

Or: "Plea<u>se</u> don't make the baby <u>cr</u>y." (4;0)

"The boy <u>sl</u>ipped on a <u>gr</u>ape." (4;6)

D. For Clients 5 Years or Older

<u>th</u>umb _____ (4;6)

<u>gr</u>ape _____ (4;6)

<u>sl</u>ip _____ (4;6)

<u>tr</u>ee _____ (5;0)

<u>spr</u>ing _____ (5;0)

<u>str</u>ing _____ (5;0)

<u>spl</u>ash _____ (5;0)

Or: "The boy <u>sl</u>ipped on a <u>gr</u>ape." (4;6)

"The water <u>spl</u>ashed on a <u>tr</u>ee." (5;0)

APPENDIX 4B

Screening Tool for Phonological Awareness (Highnam, 2002)

A. Introduction

Among the most important things to know about phonological aware-ness screening is that this knowledge is curriculum driven. Thus, how well children perform is dictated by what they have been taught. This fact makes developing "norms" difficult since children enter school with a variety of educational experiences. Moreover, children's performance at a given grade level will vary depending upon (1) how phonological awareness is addressed in the curriculum, and (2) when, in the course of the school year, the screen is administered. Having said that, some phonological tasks appear to be simpler and more easily learned than others, and an approximate sequence of difficulty is represented in this screening tool. Item 2, Letter Names, is technically phonics and not phonological awareness. This knowledge, however, is highly predictive of reading success and kindergarten/elementary teachers are especially interested in children's performance on these items. Upper-case letters are used because they are less easily confused by kindergarteners than lower-case letters.

Children's performance may be scrutinized in two ways: total scores and area scores. If the screen is administered to an entire class of children, a spread of scores from lowest to highest may reveal a segment of children at the bottom of the spread who need further testing. In a class of 15–20 children the clinician may discover 2–5 children who clearly lag behind others in their overall phonological awareness. A second look may reveal other children who perform poorly in certain areas in relation to their peers, but their overall scores are typical. These children appear to have "holes" in their phonological awareness that should be probed further.

B. Elicitation Procedures

Children should be screened one-by-one in a quiet area without distrac-tions. These materials are not formatted for screening groups. Each administration requires approximately 10 minutes. One point is awarded for each response item with the exception of letter names. In this cate-gory children must know both letter names and sounds to earn credit, and each item is worth 1/2 point. This segment also requires that examiners prepare block upper-case letters printed on index cards to serve as stimulus items. Specific instructions for each segment are included on the protocol.

Screening Items

1. Rhyming

Direction: I'm going to say a word and I'd like you to say a word that rhymes with it.

Example: pot ————

If the child rhymes correctly, go directly to the stimulus items. If the child does not rhyme correctly, provide a rhyming word (dot). Say, "Pot—dot, they sound the same." Then proceed to the stimulus items.

Stimulus	*Response*	*+/ -*	
Cat	_____	_____	
Fog	_____	_____	
Night	_____	_____	Score _____

2. Letter Names

Direction: I'll show you a card with a letter on it. Tell me the name of the letter. Then tell me what sound you think it makes.

For letter sounds, score as correct (1) plosive + schwa, (2) continuent + schwa, and (3) continuent only. Both letter names and sounds must be correct to earn credit. Each item earns ½ point for a total of 5 possible points.

Letter	*Response*			*Letter*	*Response*	
	letter name / sound +/–				letter name / sound +/–	
B	__ __ __ (.5)			D	__ __ __ (.5)	
P	__ __ __ (.5)			T	__ __ __ (.5)	
G	__ __ __ (.5)			M	__ __ __ (.5)	

F	___ ___ ___ (.5)	S	___ ___ ___ (.5)
R	___ ___ ___ (.5)	L	___ ___ ___ (.5)

Score ___ *

* = Round total score up to nearest whole integer. For example, a score of 2.5 would be rounded up to 4.0.

3. Segmenting Words into Syllables

Direction: I'll say a word and you clap how many parts it has.

Demonstration: Examiner says "circus—cir (clap)—cus (clap)"

Pronounce these words clearly but at a normal rate

Word	*Response*	*+/–*
Tiger	_____	____
Poodle	_____	____
Elephant	_____	____
Alligator	_____	____ Score ____

4. Segmenting Words into Phonemes

Direction: I will say a word. I'd like you to say each sound that you hear in the word.

Example: The word is "CUP." Listen to the sounds. /k/ – /ʌ/ – /p/.

Score as correct only those items with three separate segments and correct phoneme productions.

Word	*Response*	*+/–*
Fan (3)	_____	____
Boat (3)	_____	____
Worm (3)	_____	____
Fur (2)	_____	____ Score ____

5. Blending

Direction: I will say the parts of a word. You see if you can tell me what word it is.

Example: birth-day (pronounced at one segment per 1/2 second). Provide correct response, if necessary.

Word	Response	+/–	
Hot-dog	_____	____	
B - oy	_____	____	
F - i - sh	_____	____	
t - o - p	_____	____	
b - l - a - ck	_____	____	Score ____

6. Isolation

Direction: I will say a word. Tell me what the *beginning* or the *first* sound is.

Example: What's the first sound in "foot"? (provide correct response, if necessary)

Word	Response	+/–
Sun	_____	____
Book	_____	____

Direction: This time, tell me the ending or last sound in the word.

Word	Response	+/–
Leaf	_____	____
Cut	_____	____

7. Deletion

Direction: I'm going to ask you to say a word and then say it again without one of its parts.

Example: Say <u>light</u>bulb
Now say it without the *light.* (provide correct answer, if necessary)

Say water<u>ski</u>
Now say it without the *ski.* (provide correct answer, if necessary)

Delete the portion of following words that is underlined.

Word	*Response*	*+/−*	
<u>Cow</u>boy	_____	_____	
<u>F</u>oot	_____	_____	
<u>D</u>og	_____	_____	
Cu<u>p</u>	_____	_____	Score _____

Total Score _____

APPENDIX 4C

Word Probes for Consonants, Consonant Clusters, and [ɚ]

A. Introduction

The following sound probes are used either during the initial elicitation or follow-up hypothesis testing to help determine whether a client in Stage 3 or Stage 4 is able to produce a sound correctly. The sound probes may also be used to test for stimulability, key phonetic environments, key words (see Section V in Chapter 5), and for pre- and post-testing (see Chapter 6). To illustrate, stimulability of [s] might be tested by asking the client to repeat the sound lists for [s]. Similarly, a pretest for [k] might be obtained by having the client say the word list for [k] at the onset of treatment, and a post-test might be obtained by having the client say the same sound list after the client is thought to have learned how to produce [k]. The sound probes that follow test consonants, consonant clusters, and [ɚ] in the most commonly tested phonetic environments: word initially, between syllables (between vowels when possible), and word finally. Most often, five words for each sound are presented, although fewer words are used for several sounds for which it was harder to find words. The clinician should create additional probes to test more words and different phonetic environments, as the need arises.

B. Procedures

Elicit the words through naming, sentence completion, delayed imitation, or imitation. Transcribe the entire word if the client is in Stage 3; transcribe isolated sounds if the client is in Stage 4. To determine the sounds for which a client is stimulable, have the client imitate a sound and place a check mark next to sounds the client imitates correctly.

Word Probes for Consonants, Consonant Clusters, and [ɚ]

Oral Stops

[p]

# ___	S ___ S	___ #
pan ___	puppy ___	mop ___
pot ___	papa ___	map ___
pony ___	diaper ___	hop ___
pie ___	muppet ___	pop ___
pin ___	sleepy ___	ape ___

[b]

# ___	S ___ S	___ #
bee ___	baby ___	crab ___
bat ___	Abby ___	bib ___
book ___	hobo ___	tub ___
boot ___	hobby ___	fib ___
bike ___	tuba ___	web ___

[t]

# ___	S ___ S	___ #
tea ___	Patty ___	ate ___
tail ___	water ___	bat ___
toe ___	waiter ___	pot ___
tie ___	twenty ___	foot ___
tag ___	Rita ___	boat ___

[d]

# ___	S ___ S	___ #
dive ___	daddy ___	kid ___
dog ___	soda ___	mud ___
doll ___	caddy ___	bed ___
dot ___	Sunday ___	sad ___
dam ___	birdie ___	head ___

(continued)

Oral Stops (*continued*)

[k]

#__	S__S	__#
key ___	bucket ___	bike ___
cat ___	lucky ___	sick ___
kite ___	broken ___	duck ___
coat ___	sneaky ___	book ___
candy ___	icky ___	peek ___

[g]

#__	S__S	__#
gum ___	buggy ___	bag ___
good ___	tiger ___	leg ___
guy ___	wiggle ___	frog ___
goat ___	piggy ___	big ___
go ___	groggy ___	dog ___

Fricatives and Affricates Fricatives

[f]

#__	S__S	__#
fun ___	sniffle ___	safe ___
feet ___	taffy ___	hoof ___
fire ___	sofa ___	knife ___
fog ___	gopher ___	cough ___
face ___	offer ___	off ___

[v]

#__	S__S	__#
vine ___	movie ___	dove ___
van ___	navy ___	live ___
vote ___	lava ___	wave ___
very ___	diver ___	brave ___
valley ___	never ___	move ___

[θ]

# ___		S ___ S		___ #	
think	___	nothing	___	teeth	___
thief	___	panther	___	with	___
thumb	___	something	___	north	___
thick	___	author	___	mouth	___
thanks	___	Kathy	___	broth	___

[ð]

# ___		S ___ S		___ #	
that	___	weather	___		___
this	___	feather	___		___
them	___	brother	___		___
then	___	either	___		___
these	___	neither	___		___

[s]

# ___		S ___ S		___ #	
sun	___	icy	___	bus	___
soap	___	messy	___	kiss	___
sit	___	castle	___	face	___
say	___	bossy	___	hiss	___
see	___	Bessie	___	horse	___

[z]

# ___		S ___ S		___ #	
zoo	___	daisy	___	keys	___
zero	___	busy	___	please	___
zoom	___	freezer	___	buzz	___
zip	___	lizard	___	news	___
zebra	___	music	___	eyes	___

[ʃ]

# ___		S ___ S		___ #	
shoe	___	wishing	___	dish	___
sheep	___	ocean	___	crash	___
shiny	___	washer	___	wash	___
shut	___	fishy	___	wish	___
shell	___	dishes	___	splash	___

[ʒ]

S ___ S		___ #	
Asia	___	garage	___
vision	___	beige	___
leisure	___	treasure	___
measure	___		
seizure	___		

(continued)

Fricatives and Affricates (continued)

Affricates

[tʃ]

#___		S___S		___#	
chair	___	itchy	___	watch	___
chew	___	teacher	___	peach	___
chain	___	matches	___	witch	___
cheese	___	nature	___	catch	___
chase	___	pitching	___	ouch	___
cheep	___	watching	___	speech	___

[dʒ]

#___		S___S		___#	
jump	___	magic	___	judge	___
jet	___	cages	___	huge	___
juice	___	edges	___	page	___
joy	___	ranger	___	cage	___
jar	___	danger	___	badge	___
joke	___	ages	___	stage	___

Liquids, Glides, and [ɚ]

Liquids

[l]

#___		S___S		___#	
light	___	pillow	___	ball	___
laugh	___	sailor	___	fall	___
left	___	valley	___	eel	___
lie	___	alley	___	doll	___
ow	___	balloon	___	yell	___

[r]

#___		S___S		___#	
rain	___	story	___	car	___
row	___	marry	___	air	___
root	___	hero	___	chair	___
run	___	very	___	bear	___
ring	___	arrow	___	boar	___

[w]

#___		S___S	
wind	___	flower	___
we	___	rowing	___
web	___	tower	___
win	___	growing	___
wet	___	shower	___

[ə˞]

C___C		C___#	
worm	___	fur	___
girl	___	her	___
bird	___	tower	___
shirt	___	over	___
burn	___	pepper	___

[j]

___#	
yes	___
yard	___
you	___
used	___
yell	___

[h]

S___S		#___	
crayon	___	home	___
million	___	he	___
onion	___	hat	___
billion	___	hi	___
Mayo	___	help	___

183

Nasal Stops

[m]

# ___		S ___ S		___ #	
moon	——	gummy	——	dam	——
me	——	comet	——	boom	——
mud	——	mummy	——	aim	——
mop	——	mama	——	swim	——
meat	——	hammer	——	game	——

[n]

# ___		S ___ S		___ #	
nice	——	running	——	spoon	——
no	——	honey	——	pan	——
knife	——	winner	——	train	——
nut	——	rainy	——	can	——
new	——	tiny	——	fun	——

[ŋ]

S ___ S		___ #	
hanger	——	hang	——
singing	——	sing	——
finger	——	bang	——
winging	——	wing	——
clanging	——	king	——

Consonant Clusters

[l] Clusters

[pl]

# ___	S ___ S
play	airplane
plate	apply
please	applaud
place	
plane	

[kl]

___ #	# ___
clock	
cloud	
clue	
class	
clap	

[bl]

# ___	S ___ S	___ #
duckling	bloom	ably
ticklish	blind	cobbler
weekly	blood	wobbling
	blow	
	blank	

[gl]

# ___	S ___ S
glue	giggling
glow	ugly
gloomy	burgler
glass	
glad	

[fl]

# ___	S ___ S
flag	cornflake
fly	snowflake
floor	stiffly
flower	
flip	

[sl]

# ___	S ___ S
slam	wrestler
sleep	asleep
slow	nicely
slip	
sleigh	

(continued)

Consonant Clusters (continued)

[r] Clusters

[pr]

# ___	S ___ S	
pretty	___	suprise	___
print	___	supreme	___
prune	___	apron	___
pray	___		
praise	___		

[br]

# ___	S ___ S	
brain	___	umbrella	___
branch	___	fabric	___
break	___	library	___
broom	___		
bright	___		

[tr]

# ___	S ___ S	
trout	___	country	___
truck	___	subtract	___
tree	___	pantry	___
tray	___		
treat	___		

[dr]

# ___	S ___ S	
dry	___	address	___
drink	___	laundry	___
drop	___	raindrop	___
drum	___		
dress	___		

[kr]

# ___	S ___ S	
crib	___	secret	___
crow	___	across	___
cry	___	recruit	___
crowd	___		
cream	___		

[gr]

# ___	S ___ S	
grin	___	regret	___
grill	___	agree	___
grow	___	photograph	___
great	___		
grass	___		

[r] Clusters

[fr]

#___

fruit ___

free ___

fried ___

great ___

freeze ___

S___S

defrost ___

afraid ___

refreshment ___

[θr]

#___

three ___

throw ___

thread ___

[w] Clusters

[tw]

#___

twin ___

twice ___

twig ___

twilight ___

twirl ___

[kw]

#___

quit ___

queen ___

quake ___

quiet ___

quick ___

[sw]

(see [s] clusters)

(*continued*)

Consonant Clusters (continued)

[s] Clusters

[sp]

# ___	S ___ S	___ #
spill	whisper	wasp
space	inspect	lisp
spy	gospel	crisp
spark		
spin		

[st]

# ___	S ___ S	___ #
stove	mustard	most
stew	rooster	last
star	faster	lost
storm		
stop		

[sk]

# ___	S ___ S	___ #
sky	basket	ask
skip	scooter	mask
ski	risky	task
skunk		
skate		

[sw]

# ___	S ___ S
swamp	upswing
wim	high swing
sweet	carpet sweeper
sweater	
swell	

[sm]

# ___	S ___ S
smell	iceman
smoke	goldsmith
smile	basement
small	
smart	

[sn]

S ___ S	S ___ S
snow	unsnap
snail	closeness
snap	looseness
snake	
snack	

[sl]

(see [l] clusters)

[spr]

___
spray
spread
spring
sprint
sprinkle

[str]

___
strap
straw
stream
strange
street

[skr]

___
scream
scratch
screen
screw
scrap

[skw]

___
squirrel
square
squad
squeak
squirt

[spl]

___
splash
splendid
splatter
split
splurge

(continued)

189

Consonant Clusters (continued)

[ʃr] Clusters

#_____

shrimp _____

shrew _____

shred _____

shrug _____

shriek _____

APPENDIX 4D
Word Probes for Error Patterns

A. Introduction

The following error probes test 23 error patterns that, together, account for most error patterns found in the speech of clients in Stages 2 and 3. The most common error patterns are indicated with triple stars (***). The error probes are primarily used during the initial elicitation or during follow-up hypothesis testing. Error probes can also be used to test for stimulability, keyahonetic environments, key words (see Section V in Chapter 5), and for pre- and post-testing (see Chapter 6). If the clinician wishes, additional error probes can be developed. either to test different error patterns or to test an error pattern in more depth. To illustrate the latter situation, the error probes for the Lisping pattern test alveolar fricatives but not postalveolar fricatives which sometimes also are affected. To determine if a particular client's lisping pattern also affects postalveolar fricatives (and other consonants as well, if warranted), the clinician could develop words containing fricatives produced at other places of production. A form to help summarize information from error probes is provided in Appendix 5L.

B. Procedures

The speediest procedure to elicit the words is through delayed imitation or imitation, which allows stimulability to be determined at the same time the words are elicited (see Chapter 5 for a discussion of stimulability). If the words are elicited through naming or sentence completion, stimulability can be determined afterwards by asking the client to imitate words displaying the error patterns.

The examples on the following pages illustrate how word probes for error patterns might be utilized to assess Fronting. Delayed imitation was used to elicit the words, and therefore, additional stimulability testing was not undertaken.

Example: Fronting***

Definition: Substitution of an alveolar stop for a velar or postalveolar consonant.

Focus: Listen to the velar and postalveolar consonants. If they are said as alveolar consonants, the client likely has a Fronting pattern.

Word	Transcription	Yes/No	(Stimulable)
	t		
<u>k</u>ey	ƙi	X	NA*
<u>ch</u>eap	tʃip	—	NA
	d		
bu<u>g</u>	bʌǥ	X	NA
bu<u>sh</u>	bʊʃ	—	NA
i<u>tch</u>	ɪtʃ	—	NA
pi<u>ck</u>	pɪk	—	NA
	s		
<u>sh</u>eep	ʃip	X	NA
<u>j</u>ump	dʒʌmp	—	NA
<u>g</u>o	goʊ	—	NA
e<u>dge</u>	ɛdʒ	—	NA
Total		3/10	

***Triple stars indicate the most common error patterns.
*NA = not applicable.

---

1. **Definition.** The error probe begins with a definition of the error pattern.

2. **Focus.** The focus statement indicates the particular aspects of the client's speech to which the clinicians should attend.

3. **Word.** The words used to elicit the error pattern are listed on the left. The sounds that the error pattern may affect are underlined.

4. Transcription. The transcription is listed in the column next to the elicited words. Sounds affected by the error pattern are crossed out, and the client's production is indicated above the crossed out sound.

5. Yes/No. A check mark indicates that the pattern was elicited and a dash indicates the pattern was not elicited. The checks are totaled at the bottom, being careful to total only errors that result from the error pattern. Error patterns occurring approximately 40% of the time (2 or more times out of 5 opportunities or 4 out of 10 opportunities) are likely short-term treatment goals (see Chapter 6).

6. Stimulability. If the words are not elicited through delayed or immediate imitation, the client's stimulability for the sound is indicated through a check mark in the last column.

Word Probes for Error Patterns

A. Changes in Place of Production

1. Fronting***

Definition: Substitution of an alveolar stop for a postalveolar or velar consonant.

Focus: Listen to the underlined postalveolar and velar consonants. If they are said as alveolar consonants, the client likely has a Fronting pattern.

Word	Transcription	Yes/No	(Stimulable)
<u>k</u>ey	ki	_____	_____
<u>ch</u>eap	tʃip	_____	_____
bu<u>g</u>	bʌg	_____	_____
bu<u>sh</u>	bʊʃ	_____	_____
i<u>tch</u>	ɪtʃ	_____	_____
pic<u>k</u>	pɪk	_____	_____
<u>sh</u>eep	ʃip	_____	_____
<u>j</u>ump	dʒʌmp	_____	_____
<u>g</u>o	goʊ	_____	_____
e<u>dg</u>e	ɛdʒ	_____	_____
Total:		_/_	_____

2. Lisping***

Definition: Alveolar consonants (especially fricatives) are pronounced either on or between the teeth. They may also be produced with air flowing over the sides of the tongue, in which case it is called a lateral lisp.

Focus: Listen to the underlined alveolar fricatives. If they are pronounced either on or between the teeth, the client likely has a Lisping pattern. If the air flows over the sides of the tongue, the client has a Lateral Lisping pattern.

Word	Transcription	Yes/No	(Stimulable)
zoo	zu	_____	_____
bus	bʌs	_____	_____
zero	zirou	_____	_____
ozone	ouzoun	_____	_____
sun	sʌn	_____	_____
sneeze	sniz	_____	_____
asleep	əslip	_____	_____
see	si	_____	_____
maze	meiz	_____	_____
easy	izi	_____	_____
Total:		_/_	_____

3. Velar Assimilation***

Definition: Consonants assimilate to the place of production of a velar consonant.

Focus: Listen to the underlined non-velar consonants. If they are said as velar consonants, the client likely has a Velar Assimilation pattern.

Word	Transcription	Yes/No	(Stimulable)
bug	bʌg	_____	_____
cup	kʌp	_____	_____
duck	dʌk	_____	_____
poke	poʊk	_____	_____
goat	goʊt	_____	_____
pig	pɪg	_____	_____
beak	bik	_____	_____
dig	dɪg	_____	_____
kite	kaɪt	_____	_____
tag	tæg	_____	_____
Total:		_____/_____	_____

4. Labial Assimilation***

Definition: Consonants assimilate to the place of production of a labial consonant.

Focus: Listen to the underlined non-labial consonants. If the consonants are said as labial consonants, the client likely has a Labial Assimilation pattern.

Word	Transcription	Yes/No	(Stimulable)
bug	bʌg	_____	_____
cup	kʌp	_____	_____
tape	teɪp	_____	_____
dip	dɪp	_____	_____
deep	dip	_____	_____
bite	baɪt	_____	_____
cape	keɪp	_____	_____
pig	pɪg	_____	_____
beak	bik	_____	_____
cab	kæb	_____	_____
Total:		__/__	_____

5. Backing

Definition: Alveolar (and sometimes postalveolar) consonants are pronounced as velar stops.

Focus: Listen to the underlined alveolar and postalveolar consonants. If they are said as velar stops, the client likely has a Backing pattern.

Word	Transcription	Yes/No	(Stimulable)
t̲ie	taɪ	_____	_____
bu̲s	bʌs	_____	_____
ki̲d	kɪd	_____	_____
bu̲s̲h	bʊʃ	_____	_____
d̲ay	deɪ	_____	_____
s̲ee	si	_____	_____
i̲t̲c̲h	ɪtʃ	_____	_____
ea̲t	it	_____	_____
z̲oo	zu	_____	_____
j̲ump	dʒʌmp	_____	_____
Total:		_/_	_____

6. Glottal Replacement

Definition: Replacement of a consonant with a glottal stop.

Focus: Listen to the underlined consonants. If they are said as glottal stops, the client likely has a Glottal Replacement pattern.

Word	Transcription	Yes/No	(Stimulable)
bug	bʌg	_____	_____
up	ʌp	_____	_____
little	lɪɾl	_____	_____
key	ki	_____	_____
baby	beɪbi	_____	_____
beetle	biɾl	_____	_____
funny	fʌni	_____	_____
jet	dʒɛt	_____	_____
package	pækɪdʒ	_____	_____
egg	eɪg	_____	_____
Total:		__/__	_____

B. Changes in Manner of Production

1. Stopping***

Definition: Substitution of a stop for a fricative or affricate.

Focus: Listen to the underlined fricatives and affricates. If an underlined consonant is said as a stop, the client likely has a Stopping pattern.

Word	Transcription	Yes/No	(Stimulable)
sun	sʌn	_____	_____
fun	fʌn	_____	_____
bus	bʌs	_____	_____
thin	θɪn	_____	_____
joke	dʒoʊk	_____	_____
zoo	zu	_____	_____
dive	daɪv	_____	_____
maze	meɪz	_____	_____
chimp	tʃɪmp	_____	_____
ship	ʃɪp	_____	_____
Total:		_/_	_____

2. Gliding***

Definition: Substitution of a glide for a liquid.

Focus: Listen to the underlined liquid consonants. If they are said as glides, the client likely has a Gliding pattern.

Word	Transcription	Yes/No	(Stimulable)
rain	reɪn	_____	_____
light	laɪt	_____	_____
run	rʌn	_____	_____
row	roʊ	_____	_____
log	lɔg	_____	_____
leaf	lif	_____	_____
ring	rɪŋ	_____	_____
low	loʊ	_____	_____
ray	reɪ	_____	_____
late	leɪt	_____	_____
Total:		__/__	_____

3. Lateralization***

Definition: Sounds typically produced with central air emission (most commonly [s] and [z], but sometimes [ʃ], [ʒ], [tʃ], and [dʒ]) are pronounced with lateral air emission.

Focus:
Listen to the underlined consonants. If they are pronounced with lateral air emission, the client likely has a Lateralization pattern.

Word	Transcription	Yes/No	(Stimulable)
zoo	zu	_____	_____
bus	bʌs	_____	_____
cheap	tʃip	_____	_____
zero	ziroʊ	_____	_____
sun	sʌn	_____	_____
beach	bitʃ	_____	_____
show	ʃoʊ	_____	_____
sneeze	sniz	_____	_____
bush	bʊʃ	_____	_____
joke	dʒoʊk	_____	_____
Total:		__/__	_____

4. Affrication

Definition: Stops or fricatives (both usually alveolars) are pronounced as affricates.

Focus: Listen to the underlined stops and fricatives. If they are pronounced as affricates, the client likely has an Affrication pattern.

Word	Transcription	Yes/No	(Stimulable)
<u>s</u>un	sʌn	_____	_____
ma<u>t</u>	mæt	_____	_____
<u>c</u>i<u>t</u>y	sɪɾi	_____	_____
<u>b</u>us	bʌs	_____	_____
<u>d</u>ay	deɪ	_____	_____
to<u>e</u>	toʊ	_____	_____
ma<u>ze</u>	meɪz	_____	_____
ma<u>d</u>	mæd	_____	_____
dai<u>sy</u>	deɪzi	_____	_____
<u>z</u>oo	zu	_____	_____
Total:		_/_	_____

5. Nasalization

Definition: Non-nasal consonants (usually oral stops) are pronounced as nasal stops.

Focus: Listen to the underlined oral stops. If they are said as nasal stops, the client likely has a Nasalization pattern.

Word	Transcription	Yes/No	(Stimulable)
bug	bʌg	_____	_____
bee	bi	_____	_____
pie	paɪ	_____	_____
go	goʊ	_____	_____
kite	kaɪt	_____	_____
lid	lɪd	_____	_____
sheep	ʃip	_____	_____
day	deɪ	_____	_____
coat	koʊt	_____	_____
peek	pik	_____	_____
Total:		__/__	_____

6. Denasalization

Definition: Nasal consonants are pronounced as oral consonants (usually oral stops).

Focus: Listen to the underlined nasal consonants. If they are said as oral stops, the client likely has a Denasalization pattern.

Word	Transcription	Yes/No	(Stimulable)
mud	mʌd	_____	_____
song	sɔŋ	_____	_____
nap	næp	_____	_____
may	meɪ	_____	_____
name	neɪm	_____	_____
wing	wɪŋ	_____	_____
lamb	læm	_____	_____
new	nu	_____	_____
moon	mun	_____	_____
sun	sʌn	_____	_____
Total:		_/_	_____

C. Changes in the Beginning of Syllables or Words

1. Prevocalic Voicing***

Definition: Consonants are voiced when occurring before a vowel.

Focus: Listen to the underlined, word-initial consonants. If they are said with voicing, the client likely has a Prevocalic Voicing pattern.

Word	Transcription	Yes/No	(Stimulable)
<u>p</u>ie	paɪ	_____	_____
<u>sh</u>ow	ʃoʊ	_____	_____
<u>t</u>oe	toʊ	_____	_____
<u>th</u>in	θɪn	_____	_____
<u>k</u>ey	ki	_____	_____
<u>t</u>op	tɑp	_____	_____
<u>s</u>ee	si	_____	_____
<u>f</u>un	fʌn	_____	_____
<u>c</u>old	koʊld	_____	_____
Total:		__/__	_____

2. Initial Consonant Deletion

Definition: The initial consonant in the word is deleted.

Focus: Listen to the underlined, word-initial consonants. If they are deleted, the client likely has an Initial Consonant Devoicing pattern.

Word	Transcription	Yes/No	(Stimulable)
bee	bi	_____	_____
zoo	zu	_____	_____
cow	kaʊ	_____	_____
sun	sʌn	_____	_____
kite	kaɪt	_____	_____
fun	fʌn	_____	_____
pea	pi	_____	_____
go	goʊ	_____	_____
sheep	ʃip	_____	_____
thin	θɪn	_____	_____
Total:		_____/_____	_____

D. Changes at the End of Syllables or Words

1. Final Consonant Devoicing***

Definition: Obstruents are voiceless at the ends of words.

Focus: Listen to the underlined, word-final consonants. If they are said without voicing, the client likely has a Final Consonant Devoicing pattern.

Word	Transcription	Yes/No	(Stimulable)
bu<u>zz</u>	bʌz	_____	_____
pi<u>g</u>	pɪg	_____	_____
su<u>b</u>	sʌb	_____	_____
mu<u>d</u>	mʌd	_____	_____
ca<u>ve</u>	keɪv	_____	_____
e<u>dge</u>	ɛdʒ	_____	_____
brea<u>the</u>	brið	_____	_____
mu<u>g</u>	mʌg	_____	_____
bi<u>d</u>	bɪd	_____	_____
ro<u>be</u>	roʊb	_____	_____
Total:		__/__	_____

2. Final Consonant Deletion***

Definition: Deletion of a consonant at the end of a syllable or word.

Focus: Listen to the underlined, word-final consonants. If they are deleted, the client likely has a Final Consonant Deletion pattern.

Word	Transcription	Yes/No	(Stimulable)
sto<u>p</u>	stɑp	_____	_____
bu<u>s</u>	bʌs	_____	_____
ca<u>ve</u>	keɪv	_____	_____
bi<u>g</u>	bɪg	_____	_____
bi<u>b</u>	bɪb	_____	_____
ki<u>ng</u>	kiŋ	_____	_____
bu<u>zz</u>	bʌz	_____	_____
smo<u>ke</u>	smoʊk	_____	_____
bu<u>sh</u>	bʊʃ	_____	_____
bea<u>ch</u>	bitʃ	_____	_____
Total:		__/__	_____

E. Changes in Syllables

1. Reduplication***

Definition: Repetition of a syllable.

Focus: Listen to the underlined syllables. If they are repeated, the client likely has a Reduplication pattern.

Word	Transcription	Yes/No	(Stimulable)
<u>wa</u>ter	wɑɾɚ	_____	_____
<u>ca</u>rrot	kɛrɪt	_____	_____
<u>ki</u>tty	kɪɾi	_____	_____
<u>ba</u>by	beɪbi	_____	_____
<u>su</u>nny	sʌni	_____	_____
<u>bu</u>nny	bʌni	_____	_____
<u>ye</u>llow	jɛloʊ	_____	_____
<u>bu</u>tter	bʌɾɚ	_____	_____
<u>do</u>ggy	dɔgi	_____	_____
<u>co</u>okie	kʊki	_____	_____
Total:		_____/_____	_____

2. Syllable Deletion***

Definition: Deletion of an unstressed syllable.

Focus: Listen to the underlined syllables. If they are deleted, the client likely has a Syllable Deletion pattern.

Word	Transcription	Yes/No	(Stimulable)
<u>ba</u>nana	bənænə	_____	_____
<u>ba</u>lloon	bəlun	_____	_____
mo<u>ney</u>	mʌni	_____	_____
<u>a</u>fraid	əfreɪd	_____	_____
<u>be</u>low	bilou	_____	_____
wa<u>ter</u>	wɑɹɚ	_____	_____
kit<u>ty</u>	kɪɾi	_____	_____
<u>spa</u>ghetti	spəgɛɾi	_____	_____
bu<u>nny</u>	bʌni	_____	_____
ye<u>llow</u>	jɛlou	_____	_____
Total:		__/__	_____

F. Changes in Consonant Clusters

1. Cluster Reduction***

Definition: Deletion of a consonant in a consonant cluster.

Focus: Listen to the underlined consonant clusters. If one of the consonants is deleted, the client likely has a Cluster Reduction pattern.

Word	Transcription	Yes/No	(Stimulable)
stop	stɑp	_____	_____
bright	braɪt	_____	_____
slide	slaɪd	_____	_____
fix	fɪks	_____	_____
burnt	bɚnt	_____	_____
queen	kwin	_____	_____
spray	spreɪ	_____	_____
pride	praɪd	_____	_____
twin	twɪn	_____	_____
mist	mɪst	_____	_____
Total:		___/___	_____

Which Consonant Remains?

When a consonant cluster is reduced, which consonant remains? Typically, but not always, the consonant that remains is the one that is acquired earlier, according to age norms (see Chapter 5). For example, [st] is likely to be reduced to [t] and [br] is likely to be reduced to [b]. The same principle applies to clusters with three consonants. For example, [spr] is likely to be reduced to either [p] or [sp], whereas the [r], being acquired latest in the development of the three sounds, is the consonant most likely to be deleted.

2. Epenthesis (ePENthesis)***

Definition: Insertion of a vowel between consonants in a consonant cluster.

Focus: Listen to the underlined consonant clusters. If a schwa appears between the consonants, the client likely has an Epenthesis pattern.

Word	Transcription	Yes/No	(Stimulable)
smile	sməɪl	_____	_____
please	pliz	_____	_____
fry	fraɪ	_____	_____
drain	dreɪn	_____	_____
pray	preɪ	_____	_____
queen	kwin	_____	_____
stop	stɑp	_____	_____
sleep	slip	_____	_____
train	treɪn	_____	_____
spray	spreɪ	_____	_____
Total:		_____/_____	_____

G. Sound Reversals

1. Metathesis (meTAthesis)

Definition: The reversal of two sounds in a word, for example, saying *pet* as *tep*.

Focus: Listen to the underlined consonants. If the consonants are reversed in word-position, the client likely has a Metathesis error.

Word	Transcription	Yes/No	(Stimulable)
bug	bʌg	_____	_____
open	oʊpɪn	_____	_____
sun	sʌn	_____	_____
kite	kaɪt	_____	_____
goat	goʊt	_____	_____
deep	dip	_____	_____
sheep	ʃip	_____	_____
comb	koʊm	_____	_____
fun	fʌn	_____	_____
big	bɪg	_____	_____
Total:		__/__	_____

Influence of Dialect

Many persons who speak African American dialects pronounce [sk] in *ask* as [ks]. This pattern is the result of dialect, not a metathesis pattern.

H. Changes in Vowels and Syllabic Consonants

1. Vowel Neutralization***

Definition: A vowel is replaced with a neutral vowel (schwa, [ʊ], or [ɪ]).

Focus: Listen to the underlined words. If the vowels are said as a neutral vowel (schwa, [ʊ], or [ɪ]), the client likely has a Vowel Neutralization pattern.

Word	Transcription	Yes/No	(Stimulable)
b<u>ee</u>	bi	_____	_____
c<u>a</u>t	kæt	_____	_____
k<u>i</u>te	kaɪt	_____	_____
d<u>o</u>g	dɔg	_____	_____
s<u>a</u>t	sæt	_____	_____
sh<u>ee</u>p	ʃip	_____	_____
b<u>i</u>g	bɪg	_____	_____
c<u>o</u>mb	koʊm	_____	_____
g<u>oa</u>t	goʊt	_____	_____
gr<u>a</u>pe	greɪp	_____	_____
Total:		__/__	_____

2. Vocalization***

Definition: A syllabic consonant is replaced by a neutral vowel (schwa, [ʊ], or [ɪ]).

Focus: Listen to the underlined syllabic consonants. If they are said as a neutral vowel (schwa, [ʊ], or [ɪ]), the client likely has a Vocalization pattern.

Word	Transcription	Yes/No	(Stimulable)
zipp<u>er</u>	zɪpɚ	_____	_____
sadd<u>en</u>	sædn	_____	_____
teach<u>er</u>	titʃɚ	_____	_____
bott<u>le</u>	bɑrl	_____	_____
bigg<u>er</u>	bɪgɚ	_____	_____
sadd<u>le</u>	sædl	_____	_____
bott<u>om</u>	bɑrm	_____	_____
catt<u>le</u>	kærl	_____	_____
butt<u>on</u>	bʌrn	_____	_____
ratt<u>le</u>	rærl	_____	_____
Total:		__/__	_____

APPENDIX 4E
Multiple Error Patterns

A. Introduction

More than one error pattern can affect a sound. Three common error patterns often involved in multiple error patterns are Stopping, Prevocalic Voicing, and Final Consonant Devoicing. The following tables illustrate how these patterns combine with each other and with three other common error patterns—Fronting, Cluster Reduction, and Epenthesis. Sounds typically affected by the patterns appear on the left, and the pronunciations of the sound as it undergoes various patterns are depicted on the right. An example is included in each table to illustrate the effects of multiple patterns on words.

B. Stopping and Prevocalic Voicing

Sounds	Stopping	+	Prevocalic Voicing
feet [fit]	pit		bit
θ	t		d
s	t		d
ʃ	t		d
tʃ	t		d

C. Stopping and Final Consonant Devoicing

Sounds	Stopping	+	Final Consonant Devoicing
eve [ivl	ib		ip
ð	d		p
z	d		p
ʒ	d		p
dʒ	d		p

D. Fronting, Stopping, and Prevocalic Voicing

Sounds	Fronting	+	Stopping	+	Prevocalic Voicing
keep [kip]	tip		—		dip
ʃ	s		t		d
tʃ	s or t		t		d

E. Consonant Cluster Reduction, Stopping, and Prevocalic Voicing

Sample Clusters	Cluster Reduction	+	Stopping	+	Prevocalic Voicing
fleet [flit]	fit		pit		bit
fr	f		p		b
sl	s		t		d

F. Epenthesis, Stopping, and Prevocalic Voicing

Sample Clusters	Epenthesis	+	Stopping	+	Prevocalic Voicing
speak [spikl	səpik		təpik		dəbik
fr	fər		pər		bər
sm	səm		təm		dəm
sl	səl		təl		dəl

APPENDIX 4F
Sample Transcription Sheet

Word	Transcription	Environments				Other Environments		
		#___	V___V	___#		___	___	___

APPENDIX 4G

Sample Case History Questions for Preschoolers

In this example the case history is divided into four categories: communication development, birth/medical history, social development, and educational history (Bleile, 2002). Questions might easily be organized into other categories, and questions and categories need not be asked in the order given here.

A. Communication History

Questions:

• When did the child first babble on a regular basis?

• When did the child first speak three different words? What were they?

• When did the child start saying two and three word sentences on a regular basis?

• When did the child begin to speak in sentences, even though some of the words in the sentence may have been missing?

Rationale:

The purpose of the questions in the communication history is to determine if a child has evidenced delay in the attainment of major communication milestones. Ask about babbling because research indicates it is important for later speech and language development (Locke, 1993b). Similarly, the second question addresses an important, often well recalled milestone in the development of expressive vocabulary, while the third and fourth questions focus on significant, often recalled milestones in the development of syntax (Brown, 1973; Paul, 2001).

B. Birth/Medical History

Questions:

• Were there any complications during the pregnancy?

• Was the baby full-term?

• How long did the baby remain in the hospital after delivery?

• Does the child have any diagnosed medical conditions?

• Does the child take medications on a regular basis?

• Has the child ever been hospitalized?

- Has the child ever had an ear infection?

- How is the child's present health?

Rationale:

The questions in the birth/medical history are designed to discover any medical factors that might have affected communication development. For the birth history, ask if there were any complications during the pregnancy or delivery. Also ask if the baby was born full-term, and how long mother and child were in the hospital after the child was born. The latter question gives a sense of whether there were medical difficulties sufficiently great to require extended hospitalization. A stay of more than two or three days may signal an area that needs to be explored in more depth. Ask if the child has ever been hospitalized, which tells if there have been any serious health problems. Also ask if the child has had any ear infections, and, if so, how many, since some data indicate a connection between middle-ear problems and language development. Because medications and a wide range of medical conditions impact communication development, ask if the child formerly has been on or is currently on any medications other than antibiotics, and if he or she has any identified syndromes or medical conditions.

C. Social History

Questions:

- Who are the members of the child's family?

- Who are the main people with whom the child interacts?

Rationale:

The purpose of asking about the social history is to determine if a child has had opportunities to communicate and if he or she resides within an environment sufficiently stable to foster healthy communication development. The question is of stability rather than of composition. A stable environment can be maintained by any kind of family grouping—a mother and father, grandparents, same gender couples, or single parents. Questions to ask might be, who in the immediate family does the child interact with regularly? Does the child play with children outside the immediate family? How many times a week? Depending on the results of the medical part of the interview, you might also ask if the child has ever been hospitalized for any lengthy periods of time in the past. Hospitals, while good places to recover physically, are not ideally suited to nurture a child's social and communication needs. Due to the busy schedules of the hospital staff, a child is often required to communicate on someone else's schedule rather than when he or she has something to say. This type of social isolation may result in later behavior problems as well as delays in communication development (Fridy & Lemanek, 1993).

D. Educational History

Questions:
- Has the child ever attended any type of day care or preschool? Did he or she receive any special services?

- Is the child currently enrolled in any educational program? Does he or she receive any special services?

Rationale:
The goal in obtaining an education history is to discover if a child has received formal schooling, including special services. Both types of information may give valuable insights into a child's communication development, or, at the least, keep the evaluator from making recommendations for services that he or she may already be receiving.

APPENDIX 4H
Sample Oral Cavity Assessment Form

A. Instructions

The oral cavity assessment requires gloves, a mirror, a penlight, and a tongue depressor. The evaluator should be gloved, and universal health precautions should be followed. Score each item as "pass" (P) if no abnormal findings are shown, and as "no pass" (NP) if an abnormal finding is discovered. Make comments in the space provided after each item. The following is an example of how an abnormal finding might be indicated.

Example:

P ☐ **NP** ☒ **1. Face.** Sit at eye level across from the client and observe the face. Muscle weakness or spasticity might suggest cerebral palsy. Muscle weakness or drooping of one-half the face might suggest paralysis.

Comments: drooping left side of face

Sample Oral Cavity Assessment Form

P ☐ NP ☐ **1. Face.** Sit at eye level across from the client and observe the face. Muscle weakness or spasticity might suggest cerebral palsy. Muscle weakness or drooping of one-half the face might suggest paralysis.

Comments: _____

P ☐ NP ☐ **2. Breathing.** Observe the client breathing. Mouth breathing might indicate blockage of the nasal airway. If a problem is suspected, ask the client to close his or her mouth and breathe onto a mirror placed under the nose. An unfogged mirror or inability to breathe through the nose would be additional evidence that the nasal airway is not open.

Comments: _____

P ☐ NP ☐ **3. Lips.** Observe the client's lips for drooling, which might indicate the presence of dysarthria or another oral motor deficiency. Ask the client to perform the following activities to test for movement disorders:

Comments: _____

P ☐ NP ☐ **a. Spreading.** Ask the client to say [i] (to test lip spreading).

Comments: _____

P ☐ NP ☐ **b. Rounding.** Ask the client to say [u] (to test lip rounding).

Comments: _____

P ☐ NP ☐ **c. Rapid Movements.** Ask the client to say [pʌpʌpʌ] (to test rapid movements of the lips).

Comments: _____

P ☐ NP ☐ **4. Jaw.** Turn the client's head to each side, observing for gross retrusions or protrusions of the maxilla or mandible.

Comments: _____

P ☐ **NP** ☐   5. **Teeth.** Ask the client to open the mouth so you can examine the teeth.

P ☐ **NP** ☐   a. **Missing Teeth.** Look for missing teeth. Missing front teeth have the most direct effect on speech through [s] and [z].

Comments: _____

P ☐ **NP** ☐   b. **Bite.** To observe the client's bite, instruct the client to bite down lightly on the back teeth and to open the lips. In a normal overbite, the upper front teeth are about one quarter inch in front of the lower teeth and cover about one third of the top of the lower teeth.

Comments: _____

P ☐ **NP** ☐   c. **Overbite.** Note whether the client has an excessive overbite or an open bite (i.e., the upper teeth do not cover part of the lower teeth at any point along the dental arch).

Comments: _____

P ☐ **NP** ☐   6. **Tongue.** Observe the client's tongue.

P ☐ **NP** ☐   a. **Size.** Determine that the tongue is not grossly large or small. A tongue that appears shriveled either on one or both sides might indicate paralysis.

Comments: _____

P ☐ **NP** ☐   b. **Reach.** Ask the client to touch the alveolar ridge with the tongue tip. A client whose tongue tip cannot reach the alveolar ridge may have a short lingual frenum (i.e., the attachment under the tongue).

Comments: _____

P ☐ **NP** ☐   c. **Laterality.** Instruct the client to move the tongue laterally to test mobility.

Comments: _____

P ☐ NP ☐   **7. Hard Palate.** Instruct the client to extend the head back.

P ☐ NP ☐   **a. Clefts.** Observe the hard palate for signs of repaired or unrepaired clefts, fistulas, and fissures.

Comments: _____

P ☐ NP ☐   **b. Coloration.** Observe the midline, using a penlight if needed. Normal coloration of the midline is pink and white. A blue tint in the midline could indicate a submucous cleft. A blue tint lateral to the midline is not a cause for alarm. If a blue line is found at the midline, gently rub the posterior portion of the hard palate, feeling for a cleft.

Comments: _____

P ☐ NP ☐   **8. Soft palate.** Instruct the client to open his or her mouth three quarters of maximum to get the best velar elevation.

P ☐ NP ☐   **a. Clefts.** Observe the soft palate for signs of repaired and unrepaired clefts, fissures, and fistulas.

Comments: _____

P ☐ NP ☐   **b. Coloration.** Look for a normal pink and white coloration at the midline. As with the hard palate, a blue tint at midline may indicate a submucous cleft. A blue tint lateral to the midline is not a cause for concern.

Comments: _____

P ☐ NP ☐   **c. Nasality.** Ask the client to say a sustained "ah." A nasal sounding "ah" may indicate difficulty closing the nasal tract. Observe to see whether the velum can be elevated to the plane of the hard palate.

Comments: _____

P ☐ **NP** ☐ **9. Uvula.** Ask the client to say a sustained "ah" and observe his or her uvula. A bifid uvula (it looks like two uvula) might indicate the presence of other anatomical problems.

Comments: _____

P ☐ **NP** ☐ **10. Fauces.** Ask the client to say a sustained "ah" and look for signs of redness and inflammation or movement of the faucial pillars that might indicate infection.

Comments: _____

P ☐ **NP** ☐ **11. Pharynx.** Ask the client to say a sustained "ah" and look at the back of the throat. Presence of a Passavant's pad might indicate a possible velopharyngeal valving problem.

Comments: _____

CHAPTER

5

Analysis

The following topics are discussed in this chapter:

I. OVERVIEW

Almost all published assessment instruments provide guidelines to help evaluate information obtained during screenings and assessments. Most clinicians, however, prefer to perform their own analyses in addition to those prescribed by standardized tests. The sections in this chapter describe nonstandardized measures of severity, intelligibility, prespeech vocalizations, phonetic inventories, error patterns, individual consonants and consonant clusters, stimulability, phonetic placement and shaping, adjusted and developmental age, dialect, and communication strategies. Each section describes specific measures and concludes with brief summary comments. The clinical uses of these types of analysis are summarized in Table 5–l.

Table 5–1. Clinical purposes of five forms of analysis.

Type of Analysis	Clinical Purposes
Severity	A primary means used to establish the need for clinical services
Intelligibility	A possible means to establish the need for clinical services, also a possible means to help select treatment targets
Age norms	A primary means to help select treatment targets, also used to establish the need for clinical services
Better abilities	A primary means to help select treatment targets
Related analyses	A primary means to identify client characteristics important to the articulation and phonological analysis (adjusted age, developmental age, dialect, acquisition strategies)

II. SEVERITY

Severity is a measure of the degree of a client's articulation and phonological disorder. Severity of involvement is a primary measure used to justify providing or refusing clinical treatment. The most frequently used measurement tools assess severity through either clinical judgment scales or percentages.

A. Clinical Judgment Scales of Severity

1. **Appropriate Clients.** Clinical judgment scales are used with clients in all stages to establish the need for treatment, but are most applicable with clients in Stages 3 and 4 for whom clinicians require a quick means to assess large numbers of potential clients.

2. **Description.** The measures used most frequently to assess severity of involvement are clinical judgment scales, which assess severity through the use of judges familiar with the client's speech. The judges typically are one or more speech language clinicians who are asked to rank the client's articulation and phonological development compared to persons of similar age or level of cognitive development. Sample clinical forms to test for severity using 3- and 4-point scales of clinical judgments are provided in Appendixes 5A and 5B, respectively.

B. Percentage of Consonants Correct (PCC)

1. Appropriate Clients. The PCC is used to establish the need for treatment with clients whose speech contains multiple substitutions and deletions. Typically, these clients are in Stage 3.

2. Description. As its name suggests, the PCC measures severity as a function of the percentage of consonants the client produces correctly out of the total number of consonants the client attempts (Shriberg & Kwiatkowski, 1982). A sample clinical form and scoring instructions to test for severity using the PCC is provided in Appendix 5C.

C. Articulation Competence Index (ACI)

1. Appropriate Clients. The ACI is intended to establish the need for treatment in clients whose speech contains many distortions. Clients include selected children in Stages 3 and 4.

2. Description. The ACI is a new measure that was developed to assess the percentage of consonant distortions out of the total number of speech sounds that the client attempts (Shriberg, 1993). Results of a normative study comparing children aged 3;0–5;11 who were without articulation and phonological disorders ($N = 199$) to children with such disorders ($N – 117$) indicated that the mean ACI scores of the nondelayed group were under 50%, and the mean scores of the delayed group were near 70% or higher (Shriberg, 1993). A sample clinical form and detailed scoring instructions to test for severity using the ACI are provided in Appendix 5D.

Will My Child Speak?

Some children with developmental disabilities may not learn to speak for many years. A question that often haunts parents of children with this most severe form of articulation and phonological impairment is, will my child ever speak? The general rule of thumb is that if a child is going to speak, he or she will do so by 5 years of age. Every experienced speech-language clinician, however, can point to exceptions to this general rule, remembering children who achieved their first words at somewhat later ages. Further, speech is not all or none. Many more children with disabilities are able to use speech in conjunction with sign language and augmentative communication than do not speak at all (Bleile, 1991a).

D. Percentage of Development

1. **Appropriate Clients.** Percentage of development is used to establish the need for treatment in clients at all levels of articulation and phonological development, but is most useful with clients in Stages 1 through 3.

2. **Description.** Percentage of development is the difference between a client's chronological age and the age equivalent corresponding to his or her level of articulation and phonological development. A child 3 years of age, for example, whose articulation and phonological development approximated that of a child 2 years of age would have a delay of 33%. States differ in the specific cutoff criteria they use to establish the need for articulation and phonological treatment. The state of New Jersey, for example, uses a delay of 33% in one area of development to establish the need for developmental services (Kitley & Buzby-Hadden, 1993). A sample clinical form to test for severity using percentage of development is provided in Appendix 5E.

E. Summary Comments

Severity of involvement is often used to establish the need for articulation and phonological treatment. Unfortunately, severity is determined differently by counties, school districts, and sometimes even by clinicians in the same clinical setting, leading to situations in which a client might be deemed eligible for articulation and phonological services in one community but not in another. Severity of articulation and phonological involvement is measured by various means, each with its own strengths and limitations. Clinical judgment scales, the most widely used severity assessment instruments, are simple and quick to use, but are highly subjective. The best researched procedure is the PCC, which is intended primarily for use with clients with multiple substitutions and deletions. The value of the PCC is limited somewhat by its dependence on spontaneous speech samples, which makes its use problematic in clinical settings that cannot afford the time needed for data collection and analysis.

The ACI is a new measure of severity intended for use with clients whose speech contains many distortions. A limitation of the ACI is that, as its author notes, reliable data bases do not exist to identify various types of distortions (Shriberg, 1993). As with the PCC, the ACI requires a spontaneous speech sample, which limits its potential usefulness in clinical settings that cannot afford the time needed to perform data collection and analysis.

Percentage of development offers a relatively quick means to calculate severity using information that is obtained as part of the evaluation. The developmental theory on which the calculation is based, however, seems somewhat odd, because it is probably more accurate to say that a client's speech is similar to a younger child's speech in some respects rather than saying that the client's speech is a certain percentage younger than a child's chronological age. Percentage of development also appears to ignore individual differences in children's rate of articulation and phonological development.

III. INTELLIGIBILITY

Intelligibility is the factor most frequently cited by both speech-language clinicians and lay persons in deciding the severity of a client's articulation and phonological disorder (Gordon-Brannan, 1994; Shriberg & Kwiatkowski, 1983). Three means used to assess intelligibility are clinical judgment scales of intelligibility, frequency of occurrence, and effects of error patterns on intelligibility.

A Clinical Rule of Thumb

By 3 years of age a child's spontaneous speech should be more than 70% intelligible to unfamiliar adults. By 4 years of age a child's spontaneous speech should be intelligible to unfamiliar adults, even though some articulation and phonological differences between the child's speech and that of the adult community are likely to be present.

A. Clinical Judgment Scales of Intelligibility

1. **Appropriate Clients.** Judgment scales of intelligibility are used with clients in Stages 2 through 4. Like severity scales, intelligibility scales are most useful in clinical settings where clinicians need to perform large numbers of assessments to identify clients in need of treatment.

2. **Description.** Clinical judgment scales of intelligibility are similar in purpose and method to the clinical judgment scales of severity (see Section II). As with severity judgment scales, a judge or judges (typically,

speech-language clinicians) familiar with the client are asked to rank the client's speech compared to persons of similar chronological or developmental age (see Section VI for a discussion of developmental age). Two sample clinical forms for use in testing intelligibility using clinical judgments are provided in Appendixes 5F and 5G.

B. Frequency of Occurrence

1. Appropriate Clients. A frequency of occurrence analysis is used with clients in Stages 2 through 4 to help select treatment targets (see Chapter 6).

2. Description. Frequency of occurrence refers to the relative frequency of sounds in the language of the client's community. Frequency of occurrence is related to intelligibility based on the hypothesis that, all other matters being equal, the higher a sound's relative frequency of occurrence the greater the sound's impact on intelligibility. A sample clinical form used to test a client's intelligibility using relative frequency of American English consonants is provided in Appendix 5H.

C. Error Patterns

1. Appropriate Clients. Assessment of the effects of error patterns on intelligibility is typically undertaken with clients in Stage 3 to help select short-term goals (see Chapter 6).

2. Description. Although clinicians have speculated about the effects of error patterns on intelligibility (Hodson, 1986a), the relationship between error patterns and intelligibility has only recently begun to be studied (Leinonen-Davies, 1988; Yavas & Lamprecht, 1988). A sample error pattern analysis used to assess a client's intelligibility is provided in Appendix 5I. Additionally, research suggests that speakers are more likely to be judged unintelligible as the number of patterns increase, deletion and assimilation patterns increase, unusual patterns occur, patterns co-occur, and variability of patterns increases (Yavas & Lamprecht, 1988).

D. Summary Comments

Intelligibility, although a critical concept in the study of articulation and phonological disorders, is notoriously difficult to measure in clinical settings (Kent, Miolo, and Bloedel, 1994). This is because intelligibility does not directly reflect the number of sounds produced correctly. In fact, the correlation between number of consonants produced correctly and perceived intelligibility is relatively low (r = .42) (Shriberg & Kwiatkowski, 1982). Factors that affect intelligibility include number of errors, types of errors, consistency of errors, speaking rate, and frequency of the error sound in the language. Intelligibility is also affected by variables that are difficult to control, for example, the listener's familiarity with the speaker and the nature of the social environment in which the speech occurs.

Of the three measures discussed in this section, frequency of occurrence has been studied the most. As with clinical judgment scales of severity, clinical judgment scales of intelligibility are simple and quick to use, but they are highly subjective. The relationship between error patterns and intelligibility has only recently been investigated, and the number of subjects studied to date remains relatively small (Leinonen-Davies, 1988; Yavas & Lamprecht, 1988).

IV. AGE NORMS

Age norms show the average ages at which children without developmental delays acquire articulation and phonological behaviors. Age norms are used to select treatment targets and to establish the age corresponding to the client's articulation and phonological development. A child 4 years of age, for example, whose major articulation and phonological abilities correspond to those of a child 2 years of age, would likely be assessed as having approximately the articulation and phonological skills of a child 2 years of age. In certain treatment approaches, articulation and phonological behaviors that a client is most delayed in acquiring would likely be selected as early treatment targets (see Chapter 6). The areas of development for which age norms are most frequently obtained in clinical settings are prespeech vocalizations, phonetic inventories, error patterns, and consonants and consonant clusters.

A. Prespeech Vocalizations

1. Appropriate Clients. Analysis of prespeech vocalizations is undertaken with clients in Stage 1 to help select short-term goals and treatment targets (see Chapter 6) and to establish the age that best approximates the level of the client's articulation and phonological development.

Realistic Criteria

Is a vocalization established if it occurs once? Or does it need to occur three times? Or five times? Or even seven times? Obviously, a criterion of three is likely to identify more vocalizations as established than a criterion of seven. Similarly, in how many words does a sound need to occur before we say it is established in a client's phonetic inventory? Once? More than once? Time permitting, I employ three occurrences as my establishment criterion, because I have observed that most clients who produce a vocalization or sound three times can produce it more frequently in more lengthy evaluations. Realistically, however, time does not always permit three productions to be obtained. If I use fewer than three occurrences to establish a vocalization or sound, I indicate this in my clinical report, using a phrase such as, "The sound was considered established based on two occurrences."

---

2. **Description.** Prespeech vocalizations are utterances without apparent meaning that are produced by infants from shortly after birth to around 11 or 12 months of age (see definition of independent analysis in Chapter 2). Many researchers believe that prespeech vocalizations provide "practice" in making the speech mechanism "go where the infant wants it to go" (Bleile, Stark, & Silverman McGowan, 1993; Locke, 1983a; Locke & Pearson, 1992; Oller, 1980; Stark, 1980; Vihman, Ferguson, & Elbert, 1986). The client's level of vocal development is the highest age at which a vocalization occurs three or more times during the evaluation session. A sample clinical form used to determine the age level that best approximates the client's prespeech vocalizations is provided in Appendix 5J.

B. Phonetic Inventories

1. **Appropriate Clients.** Analysis of phonetic inventories is undertaken with clients in Stage 2 and less advanced clients in Stage 3 to help establish treatment targets (see Chapter 6) and to determine the age that best approximates the level of the client's articulation and phonological development.

2. Description. Phonetic inventories describe the client's ability to produce speech sounds, regardless of whether or not the sounds are produced correctly relative to the language of the client's community (see definition of independent analysis in Chapter 2). A phonetic inventory analysis, for example, might indicate a client's consonant inventory as containing [t], [k], and [s] but would not indicate whether [t] was produced for [t] in *two* or for [z] in *zebra*. The greatest clinical value of a phonetic inventory analysis is that it provides information on the number and types of consonants in phonetic inventories of children during the second and third year of life (Dyson, 1988; Stoel-Gammon, 1985).

The phonetic inventories of children's intelligible utterances are relatively well-documented. However, information that includes both intelligible and unintelligible utterances is based on a smaller number of subjects ($N = 7$) (Robb & Bleile, 1994). Sample clinical forms used to perform a phonetic inventory analysis of consonants are provided in Appendix 5K. The developmental level of the client's phonetic inventory is the age that most closely approximates the number and type of the client's established consonants. For an analysis restricted only to intelligible words, a consonant is considered established when it occurs in at least two different words (the criterion used in the original studies). For an analysis of both intelligible and unintelligible words, a consonant is considered established when it occurs in at least three different words (the criterion used in the original study).

C. Error Patterns

1. Appropriate Clients. Analysis of error patterns is performed with clients in Stages 2 and 3 to help select short-term goals (see Chapter 6) and to determine the age level that best approximates the client's level of articulation and phonological development.

2. Description. Error patterns describe the client's accuracy in producing sound classes in the language of the client's community (see definition of relational analysis in Chapter 2). Error patterns encompass both what are traditionally called phonological processes and certain types of articulation errors (those affecting sound classes). As described in Chapter 4, the term *error pattern* is used in this book to avoid biasing the discussion to either an articulation or phonological perspective. A scale used to determine the frequency with which an error pattern occurs in a client's speech is provided in Table 5–2. The

Table 5–2. Percentage and whole number criteria for disappearance of error patterns.

Categories	Percentages	Whole Numbers[a]	
		(5 Opportunities)	(10 Opportunities)
Highly frequent	75–100%	4/5–5/5	8/10–10/10
Frequent	50–74%	3/5	5/10–7/10
Present	25–49%	2/5	3/10–4/10
Disappearing	1–24%	1/5	1/10–2/10
Disappeared	0%	0/5	0/10

[a]Whole numbers refer to the number of different words. For example, 3/5 means the error pattern occurred in 3 out of 5 words.

categories in the scale are used to help select short-term treatment goals. The most likely candidates for short-term treatment goals are error patterns within the "present" category (see Chapter 6). A sample clinical form used to summarize the analysis of a client's error patterns is provided in Appendix 5L, and a sample clinical form showing when selected major error patterns are eliminated is presented in Appendix 5M.

D. Consonants and Consonant Clusters

1. Appropriate Clients. Analysis of consonants and consonant clusters is undertaken with clients in Stages 2 through 4 to help select treatment targets (see Chapter 6) and to establish the age that best approximates the level of the client's articulation and phonological development.

2. Description. Analysis of consonants and consonant clusters describes the client's ability to produce the individual consonants and consonant clusters in the language spoken in the client's community (see definition of relational analysis in Chapter 2). Analysis of consonants and consonant clusters is the longest established and still one of the most frequently used procedures in the care of clients with articulation and phonological disorders. A scale used to determine the frequency with which a consonant and consonant cluster occurs in a client's speech is provided in Table 5–3. The categories in the scale are used to help select treatment targets. The most likely candidates for treatment targets are error patterns within the "emerging" category

Table 5–3. Percentage and whole number criteria for acquisition of consonants and consonant clusters.

Categories	Percentages	Whole Numbers[a]	
		(5 Opportunities)	(10 Opportunities)
Mastered	90–100%	5/5	9/10–10/10
Acquired	75–89%	4/5	8/10
Present	50–74%	3/5	5/10–7/10
Emerging	10–49%	1/5 and 2/5	1/10–4/10
Rare	9%	1/5	—
Absent	0%	0/5	0/10

[a]Whole numbers refer to the number of different words. For example, 4/5 means the sound was produced correctly in 4 out of 5 words.

(see Chapter 6). The ages at which consonants and consonant clusters are typically acquired are listed in Tables 5–4 and 5–5, respectively (Smit, Hand, Frelinger, Bernthal, & Byrd, 1990). For the present purposes, to be considered acquired a sound needed to meet two criteria: (1) both males and females correctly produced the sound and (2) the percentage of subjects correctly producing the sound never dropped below 50% (for 50% criteria) or 75% (for 75% criteria) at any subsequent age level. A sample clinical form used to analyze consonants and consonant clusters using a 50% acquisition criteria is provided in Appendix 5N.

E. Summary Comments

Age norms are extremely useful clinically but several factors limit their value.

1. Normal Variation. The ages cited in age norms are averages. Some children fall above the average and others fall below. For example, a child might acquire a certain sound at 2 years, 4 months that age norms indicate should be acquired at 2 years. Is the child delayed or is this normal variation? The answer depends on the average variation (standard deviation) for acquiring the speech behavior being considered. If the average variation is, for example, 2 months, then a

Table 5–4. Age of acquisition (50% to 75% correct) of American English consonants averaged across both word-initial and word-final positions.

Consonant	50%	75%	Consonant	50%	75%
m	<3;0	<3;0	f	<3;0	3;6
n	<3;0	<3;0	v	3;6	4;6
ŋ	<3;0	<7;6[a]	θ	4;6	6;0
h	<3;0	<7;6	ɚ	4;6	5;6
w	<3;0	<3;0	s	3;6	5;0
j	<3;0	3;6	z	4;0	6;0
p	<3;0	<3;0	ʃ	3;6	5;0
t	<3;0	<3;0	tʃ	3;6	6;0
k	<3;0	<3;0	dʒ	3;6	4;6
b	<3;0	<3;0	r	3;6	6;0
d	<3;0	<3;0	l	3;6	6;0
g	<3;0	<3;0			

[a]Transcriber difficulties may have resulted in this sound being acquired at 7:6.

Source: Adapted from "The Iowa articulation normjs project and its Nebraska replication" by A. Smit, L. Hand, J. Frelinger, J. Bernthal, & A. Byrd (1990), *Journal of Speech and Hearing Disorders, 55,* 779–798.

Table 5–5. Age of acquisition (50% to 75% correct) of American English consonants clusters in word initial positions.

Consonant	50%	75%	Consonant	50%	75%
tw	3;0	3;6	pr	4;0	6;0
kw	3;0	3;6	br	3;6	6;0
sp	3;6	5;0	tr	5;0	5;6
st	3;6	5;0	dr	4;0	6;0
sk	3;6	5;0	kr	4;0	5;6
sm	3;6	5;0	gr	4;6	6;0
sn	3;6	5;6	fr	3;6	6;0
sw	3;6	5;6	θr	5;0	7;0
sl	4;6	7;0	skw	3;6	7;0
pl	3;6	5;6	spl	5;0	7;0
bl	3;6	5;0	spr	5;0	8;0
kl	4;0	5;6	str	5;0	8;0
gl	3;6	4;6	skr	5;0	8;0
fl	3;6	5;6			

Source: Adapted from "The Iowa articulation norms project and its Nebraska replication" by A. Smit, L. Hand, J. Frelinger, J. Bernthal, & A. Byrd (1990), *Journal of Speech and Hearing Disorders, 55,* 779–798.

4-month delay may signify an actual delay in articulation and phonological development. If, however, the average variation is 4 months,
then the child's articulation and phonological development is within
expected age limits. Unfortunately, information on average variation
is often lacking, which makes it difficult to interpret results from
clients with mild delays in articulation and phonological development.

2. **Ethnic and Class Biases.** Most age norms are derived from studies of Caucasian, middle-class children. It is not known at present
how useful this information is in interpreting assessment data from
clients from other socioeconomic classes and ethnic and racial
groups. Equally important, virtually no information exists on the pri-
orities that members of non-Caucasian ethnic and racial groups
assign to remediating various types of articulation and phonological
disorders (Bleile & Wallach, 1992; Taylor & Peters-Johnson, 1986).

3. **Language Biases.** Almost all age norms are based on English-
speaking children. At present, little is known about how children
acquire speech in languages other than English. This gives our field a
narrow, ethnocentric view of articulation and phonological development. Additionally, this lack of normative information about other
languages makes it almost impossible to evaluate the speech of non-
English-speaking clients.

V. BETTER ABILITIES (STIMULABILITY)

Better abilities (stimulability) are a client's more advanced articulation and
phonological skills, and are a primary means used to select treatment targets
(see Chapter 6). Several procedures help identify a client's better abilities:
imitation, key environments, key words, and phonetic placement and shaping.

A. Imitation

1. **Appropriate Clients.** Imitation is used routinely with clients in
Stages 2 through 4 to help select treatment targets (see Chapter 6).

2. **Description.** Imitation is the ability to say a treatment target correctly during delayed or immediate modeling. A client who pronounces
[k] correctly during imitation, for example, is considered stimulable
for [k]. The logic behind this type of stimulability testing is that sounds
that can be produced correctly during imitation are easier for clients to

acquire than treatment targets that cannot be imitated. Many times, hypotheses about stimulability are tested while collecting the speech sample. A clinician, for example, might ask the client to name pictures, and then ask the client to imitate words that the client pronounced incorrectly. Hypotheses about stimulability can also be tested using the same procedure during the course of eliciting speech through word probes for sounds and error patterns. Another option to test for stimulability is to present the client with a word list specially developed for this purpose. Such a word list is provided in Appendix 50.

B. Key Environments

1. **Appropriate Clients.** Analysis of key environments is performed with clients in Stages 2 through 4 to help select treatment targets (see Chapter 6).

2. **Description.** A key environment is a phonetic environment in which the client is able to successfully produce a sound or class of sounds. Key environments often are syllable and word positions, but may also include the presence of other sounds. An example of a word (and syllable) key environment is a client who can produce velar stops only at the ends of words. An example of a key environment that includes the presence of another sound is a client who can produce a labial consonant only at the beginning of a word if the word also ends in a labial consonant, or a client who can produce [t] only when followed by a front vowel in the same syllable. Key environments vary by client, so that, for example, word-final position may be a key environment for velar stops for one client, but not for another. The speech of yet another client may not contain any key environments, containing, instead, sounds that are produced with some success across several environments.

To discover whether a key environment exists for a sound, the clinician should ask him- or herself, "Is there any phonetic environment in which the client is successful in producing the sound?" Key environments are often first discovered during the collection of the initial speech sample. Typically, hypotheses about possible key environments are tested using word probes such as those presented in Chapter 4. More uncommon key environments are tested using word probes developed by the clinician (Bleile, 1991b).

Although individual differences in key environments are extensive, the following is a list of 12 "best bets."* See Table 6–4 for a similar list of key environments in which to establish sounds.

Consonants
1. All other things being equal, the best bet for consonants is the beginning of a word, as in *do.*

Multiple Consonants
2. A best bet for a consonant made at a given place of production is a word with another consonant made at the same place of production, as in *king* and *beep.*

Voicing
3. A best bet for voiced consonants is before a vowel, as in *bee.*
4. Another best bet for voiced consonants (especially voiced fricatives) is between vowels, as in *diver.*

Word-initial Position
5. A best bet for word-initial consonants is a two-word phrase in which the first word ends with a consonant and the second word begins with a vowel, as in *it is.* In this context, the final consonant of the first word tends to "migrate" to the beginning of the next word, as in the pronunciatyion of *it is* as *i tis.*
6. A best bet for a word beginning with a vowel without a hard glottal stop is a word beginning with "h" and "silent h," as in *heat.*
7. A best bet for voiceless consonants is at the end of a syllable or word, as in *bit.*

Nasal Consonants
8. A best bet for nasal consonants is before a low vowel, as in *mad.*

Alveolar Consonants
9. A best bet for alveolar consonants is before front vowels in the same syllable, as in *tea.*
10. A best bet for [s] and [z] is after [t] and [d], respectively, and before [i], as in [*tsi*] and [*dzi*].

---

*Adapted from: *Articulation and phonological disorders: A book of exercises for students (Second Edition),* by Ken M. Bleile (1996), San Diego, Singular Publishing Group.

Velar Consonants

11. A best bet for velar consonants is at the end of a syllable or word, as in *peak.*
12. Another best bet for velar consonants is before back vowels in the same syllables, as in *go.*

C. Key Words

1. **Appropriate Clients.** Analysis of key words is performed with clients from Stage 2 through Stage 4 to help select treatment targets (see Chapter 6).

2. **Description.** Key words occur when a client's success in producing a sound is limited to a few specific words. Many times key words are of special importance to the client. During the years when the *Star Wars* movies were at the height of their popularity, for example, the name of the movies' villain, Darth Vader, was a key word for [v] for many children. Names of favorite friends and characters in television series are also "first bets" when trying to find key words. Key words need not be special to the client and, in fact, any word can be a key word. Key words are typically discovered while collecting the initial speech sample or performing hypothesis testing. Because key words are often useful in treatment, the clinician should circle key words as they are discovered or in other some manner indicate that a key word exists.

D. Phonetic Placement and Shaping

1. **Appropriate Clients.** Brief trials using phonetic placement and shaping are performed with more mature and cognitively advanced clients in Stage 3 and clients in Stage 4 to help select treatment targets (see Chapter 6).

2. **Description.** Phonetic placement and shaping techniques physically direct a client to produce a sound. A phonetic placement technique for [t], for example, might involve directing the client to touch his or her tongue tip to the alveolar ridge. The logic behind including brief trials of phonetic placement and shaping techniques in the assessment is to determine if they provide the client a means to produce a difficult sound. A relatively complete description of phonetic placement and shaping techniques is presented in Appendix 7C.

E. Summary Comments

When analyzing a client's speech, it is equally (or more) important to determine the client's areas of strength as it is to establish the client's deficit areas. The analysis of better abilities is undertaken to identify the client's more advanced articulation and phonological skills. The information gained from these analyses is often useful in selecting treatment targets.

The primary types of analyses of better abilities involve imitation, key environments, key words, and phonetic placement and shaping. A natural question raised by stimulability testing is whether a client who is stimulable for a treatment target would make progress even if treatment was not provided. Research on this question is equivocal (Diedrich, 1983; Madison, 1979; Powell, Elbert, & Dinnsen, 1991). More studies are needed before the predictive value of stimulability is known. Until then, stimulability provides a quick method for choosing treatment targets that are likely to meet with success. Key environments and key words provide important means for selecting treatment targets for clients in Stages 2 through 4. Brief trials using phonetic placement and shaping techniques provide useful methods to determine if selected clients in Stage 3 and clients in Stage 4 might benefit from use of these techniques during treatment.

VI. RELATED ANALYSES

Several analyses are performed in conjunction with the above assessments. Some analyses are performed with virtually all clients; others are restricted to clients in selected clinical populations. Because the analyses described in this section are united only by their "related" status, summary comments are provided after each subheading rather than at the end of the section.

A. Adjusted Age

1. **Appropriate Clients.** Adjusted age is determined for infants and toddlers born prematurely to determine the client's potential for articulation and phonological development.

2. **Description.** Adjusted age is the client's chronological age adjusted for prematurity. Adjusted age is calculated for clients 24 months or younger who were born prematurely to establish the

client's best potential for articulation and phonological development. For example, a client with a chronological age of 22 months and an adjusted age of 20 months is expected to have the articulation and phonological skills of a child 20 months of age, not a child 22 months of age. A sample clinical form used to determine adjusted age is provided in Appendix 5P.

3. Summary Comments. Adjusted age is not calculated for clients older than 24 months, because by that age children born prematurely are thought to have "caught up" in development.

B. Developmental Age

1. Appropriate Clients. Developmental age is calculated for clients with intellectual or cognitive impairments to establish the client's potential for articulation and phonological development.

2. Description. Developmental age (also called mental age) is the age that most closely corresponds to the client's level of cognitive development. For example, a client whose chronological age is 9 years, but whose developmental age is 6 years, is expected to have the articulation and phonological development commensurate to a child 6 years of age. A sample clinical form used to determine developmental age is provided in Appendix 5Q.

3. Summary Comments. Developmental age is best calculated using a verbal intelligence quotient (verbal IQ). In clinical practice, the standard score from the *Peabody Picture Vocabulary Test—Revised* (PPVT-R) (Dunn & Dunn, 1981) is sometimes used to determine developmental age, because PPVT-R scores are positively correlated with verbal intelligence. It should be noted, however, that the correlation between a client's PPVT-R score and his or her verbal intelligence is not always reliable (Dunn & Dunn, 1981); therefore, determination of a person's verbal intelligence based on a PPVT-R score must be made with caution. With younger clients, the level of the client's language reception abilities is often used to approximate developmental age.

C. Dialect

1. Appropriate Clients. The influence of dialect is identified in all appropriate clients in Stages 2 through 4 to differentiate dialect from speech characteristics that signify a possible articulation and phonological disorder.

Dialect Reduction

Techniques used to treat articulation and phonological disorders can also be used to reduce dialect. I have some concern about providing dialect reduction, because such treatment may confirm the impression of some persons (including the client) that dialect is a type of disorder. Nonetheless, I occasionally provide this clinical service, because in my opinion the client's right to clinical care for what he or she perceives to be a problem outweighs other considerations. I accompany treatment for dialect reduction with an educational program on the nature of dialects.

---

2. **Description.** Dialect is a variation in language resulting from the influence of a region, social group, racial group, or ethnic group. Sample clinical forms used to help identify possible dialect characteristics in two major ethnic dialects, African American English (AAE) and Hawaiian Island Creole (HC), are provided in Appendixes 5R and 5S, respectively.

3. **Summary Comments.** Dialects are a natural part of language, and dialect characteristics need to be identified in all appropriate clients so that they will not be diagnosed as articulation and phonological disorders.

Limited English Proficiency

Discussion of speakers with limited English proficiency lies beyond the scope of this book. The reader is referred to Cheng (1987) and Goldstein (2000) for excellent discussions of assessing speech and language in Asian and Spanish populations, respectively.

D. Communication Strategies

1. Appropriate Clients. Analysis of acquisition strategies is undertaken with clients in Stage 2 and less advanced clients in Stage 3 to identify the possible influence of learning style on assessment and treatment.

2. Description. Communication strategies were described in Chapter 2. Possible clinical implications of communication strategies are described in this section, and major strategies and their hallmarks are summarized in Table 5–6. Although a child's communication strategies are often readily identifiable by clinicians attuned to their possible presence, in-depth analyses can be extremely time consuming and typically are not performed in clinical settings. Differing from other sections in this chapter, the following discussion is intended to facilitate identification rather than describe specific analytic procedures.

a. Selectivity. A client following a communication strategy based on selectivity "picks and chooses" words that contain speech elements a child already pronounces. A client, for example, may have an expressive vocabulary containing words beginning with [t] and [k] and only attempt new words that begin with those sounds. Selectivity is used to choose treatment targets, increasing the likelihood that a client will attempt to pronounce words (see Chapter 6).

Table 5–6. Communication strategies and their hallmarks.

Strategies	Hallmark
Selectivity	A child "picks and chooses" words that contain speech elements already produced.
Word-based learning	A child's pronunciation of a speech element varies depending on the word in which it occurs.
Favorite sounds and word recipes	A child uses a few favorite sounds and recipes to pronounce all words.
Homonym seeking or avoiding	A child either seeks or avoids homonyms.
Gestalt learning	A child knows "the tune before the words."

b. **Word-based Learning.** A client following a word-based strategy pronounces a speech element differently depending on the word in which it occurs. Although this, along with the other communication strategies, is a form of disability, persistent use of a word-based strategy results in extensive variability in the production of sounds. Reduction in variability is a possible treatment goal in selected clients (see Chapter 6).

c. **Favorite Sounds and Word Recipes.** A client whose communication strategy is based on favorite sounds and word recipes uses a few phonetic formulas to pronounce all words. Extensive use of favorite sounds may result in increased homonyms and may signify difficulty in acquiring a repertoire of diverse speech elements. A client whose communication strategies include favorite sounds and word recipes may more easily acquire words that follow their preferred patterns. On the negative side, the speech of such a client often is highly unintelligible, because only a few means are used to pronounce a large number of sounds and syllables.

d. **Homonym Seeking and Avoiding.** A client whose communication strategy is based on homonym seeking or avoiding either seeks or avoids words that sound alike but mean different things. Homonym avoiding seldom is a clinical problem. Reduction in homonyms is a possible short-term treatment goal (see Chapter 6).

e. **Gestalt Learning.** A client whose communication strategy is based on gestalt learning "knows the tune before the words"—that is, pronounces intonation of phrases and sentences more accurately than individual speech elements. Sometimes a client who pronounces the intonation of sentences better than the sounds in the sentence is said to speak "jargon." A client with "jargoning" is often difficult to understand, because sounds within words are highly inaccurate.

3. **Summary Comments.** Communication strategies remind us a client is actively engaged in speech development. Many clients are highly selective in the words they say; others follow a word-based strategy in which how a sound is pronounced depends on the word in which it occurs. Other clients may have favorite sounds or develop simple "word recipes" to pronounce almost all words. Homonym seekers simplify the task of pronunciation, but often pay a price in intelligibility. Lastly, some clients appear to focus less on the pronunciation of words and more on the intonation patterns within which words occur.

APPENDIX 5A
4-Point Clinical Judgment Scale of Severity

A. Instructions

Ask one or more speech-language clinicians familiar with the client's speech to independently mark the number on the assessment scale below that, in their professional judgment, best describes the client's severity of articulation and phonological involvement. If more than one judge is used, add the judges' scores and divide the total by the number of judges to obtain an average score. An average score of between 3 and 4 is commonly needed to receive articulation and phonological services, although a less stringent criterion is possible with clients who have risk factors for future articulation and phonological development.

B. Assessment Scale

- ☐ 1   No disorder
- ☐ 2   Mild disorder
- ☐ 3   Moderate disorder
- ☐ 4   Severe disorder

APPENDIX 5B

3-Point Clinical Judgment Scale of Severity

A. Instructions

Ask one or more speech-language clinicians familiar with the client to independently check the statements on the assessment scale below that in their professional judgment describe the client's speech. Each statement is rated 1 or 0. Typically, an average score of 1 or more is needed to justify articulation and phonological services.

B. Assessment Scale

☐   The client's speech has or in the future is likely to have an adverse affect on his or her social development and educational progress.

☐   The client's speech calls attention to itself.

☐   The client's speech is delayed relative to developmental age norms.

APPENDIX 5C
Percentage of Consonants Correct (PCC)

A. Instructions

Calculate the client's PCC percentage using the procedures described below and on the following pages. The level of severity needed to obtain articulation and phonological services varies by clinical setting. A score of 50–65% or less is recommended for most client populations. A less stringent criterion—65% or higher—is recommended for clients at risk for future articulation and phonological difficulties.

B. Step 1: Collect Data and Identify Utterances

The following data collection procedures are used:

Obtain a continuous speech sample of between 50 to 100 utterances.

Determine the meaning of the utterances.

Identify any dialect characteristics (example: *aks* or *ask* in African American English)

Identify casual speech pronunciations (example: *Cheat yet?* for *Did you eat yet?*)

Identify allophones (example: [ɾ] for [t] in *butter*).

C. Step 2: Exclusion Criteria

Exclude the following data from analysis:

Exclude all unintelligible and partially intelligible utterances.

Exclude vowels (including [ɝ]).

Do not count the addition of consonants in front of vowels (example: *hit* for *it*) because the target is a vowel.

Exclude consonants in the third or more repetition of the same word, if the pronunciation does not change (example: count only the first two instances of [b] in three or more repetitions of *bee* [bi bi bi]).

Exclude beyond the second consonant in successive utterances with the same pronunciation, but score all consonants if the pronunciation changes.

D. Step 3: Identify Errors in the Remaining Data

Follow these criteria to identify consonant errors:

Score dialect, casual speech, and allophones based on the consonant the client intended (example: *aks* for *ask* is correct in AAE, but *ats* is incorrect).

Score a consonant as incorrect if in doubt about whether it is correct or incorrect.

Score consonant deletions as incorrect (example: *be* for *bed*).

Score consonant substitutions as incorrect (example: *bee* for *pea*).

Score partial voicing of initial consonants as incorrect.

Score distortions (no matter how mild) as incorrect.

Score additions of a sound to consonant as incorrect (example: *mits* for *miss*).

Score initial [h] and [n/ŋ] substitutions in stressed syllables as incorrect, but not in unstressed syllables (example: *swin* for *swing* is incorrect, but *jumpin* for *jumping* is correct).

E. Step 4: Calculate PCC

Perform the following calculation to determine PCC:

1. Formula

$$\frac{\text{total number of correct consonants}}{\text{total number of intended consonants}} \times 100 = \text{PCC}$$

2. Example

$$\frac{70 \text{ consonants correct}}{100 \text{ consonants attempted}} \times 100 = 70\%$$

F. Step 5: Determine Level of Severity

Indicate the client's level of severity using the following scale:

85%	= Normal development	☐
65–85%	= Mild to moderate disorder	☐
50–65%	= Moderate to severe disorder	☐
<50%	= Severe disorder	☐

APPENDIX 5D
Articulation Competence Index (ACI)

A. Instructions

Calculate the client's ACI using the procedures described below and on the following pages. A score of 70% or higher suggests the need for articulation and phonological services. A lower score might indicate the need for services if the client was judged at risk for future articulation and phonological difficulties.

B. Step 1: Collect Data

Follow the data collection procedures as for the PCC (Appendix 5C).

C. Step 2: Exclude Nonclinical Distortions from Analysis

Exclude all nonclinical distortions due to regional, ethnic, or socioeconomic influence.

D. Step 3: Identify Clinical Distortions

The following are scored as clinical distortions:

[l] or [r] with lip rounding

[l] or [r] made in the velar position

[r] and r-colored vowels produced as vowels

Lateralized sibilant fricatives or affricates

Lisped sibilant fricatives or affricates

Weakly produced consonants

Imprecise consonants and vowels

Failure to maintain oral/nasal contrasts (nasal emissions, denasalized nasal consonants, nasalized oral consonants, and nasalized vowels and diphthongs)

Notable failure to maintain appropriate voicing (nonaspiration of prevocalic voiceless stops, voicing of voiceless obstruents, and partial devoicing of voiced obstruents)

E. Step 4: Calculate Percentage of Consonants Correct (PCC)

Calculate the PCC using the following formula:

1. Formula

$$\frac{\text{total number of correct consonants}}{\text{total number of intended consonants}} \times 100 = \text{PCC}$$

2. Example

$$\frac{70 \text{ consonants correct}}{100 \text{ consonants attempted}} \times 100 = 70\%$$

F. Step 5: Calculate Relative Distortion Index (RDI)

Calculate RDI using the following formula:

1. Formula

$$\frac{\text{total number of distortion errors}}{\text{total number of speech errors}} \times 100 = \text{RDI}$$

2. Example

$$\frac{60 \text{ distortions}}{70 \text{ speech errors}} \times 100 = 85.71\% \ (86\%)$$

G. Step 6: Calculated ACI

Calculate ACI using the following formula:

1. Formula

$$\frac{\text{PCC} + \text{RDI}}{2} \times \text{ACI}$$

2. Example

$$\frac{70 + 86}{2} = 78\%$$

APPENDIX 5E
Percentage of Development

A. Instructions

Determine the age equivalent corresponding to the client's articulation and phonological development using the formula described below. Next, divide the age equivalent score (in months) by the client's age (in months). Use adjusted age rather than chronological age with clients 24 months or younger who were born prematurely. The specific percentage needed to qualify for articulation and phonological services varies by state. New Jersey, for example, uses a 33% delay as the criteria for developmental services.

1. Formula

$$\frac{\text{developmental age in months}}{\text{chronological age in months}} = \text{percentage of delay}$$

2. Example

$$\frac{24 \text{ months}}{36 \text{ months}} = 33\% \text{ delay in development}$$

APPENDIX 5F
3-Point Clinical Judgment Scale
of Intelligibility

A. Instructions

Ask one or more speech-language clinicians familiar with the client to place a check mark next to the statements on the assessment scales below that in their professional judgment describe the client's intelligibility during conversation. If more than one judge is used, add the judges' scores and divide the total by the number of judges. The score needed to obtain service for a possible articulation and phonological disorder varies by setting and age of the client.

B. Assessment Scale

☐ 1 Readily intelligible

☐ 2 Intelligible if topic is known

☐ 3 Unintelligible even with careful listening

APPENDIX 5G

5-Point Clinical Judgment Scale
of Intelligibility

A. Instructions

Ask one or more speech-language clinicians familiar with the client to place a check mark next to the statements on the assessment scales below that in their professional judgment describe the client's intelligibility during conversation. If more than one judge is used, add the scores and divide the total by the number of judges to obtain an average score. The score needed to obtain service for a possible articulation and phonological disorder varies by setting and age of the client.

B. Assessment Scale

☐ 1   Completely intelligible

☐ 2   Mostly intelligible

☐ 3   Somewhat intelligible

☐ 4   Mostly unintelligible

☐ 5   Completely unintelligible

APPENDIX 5H

Percentage of Occurrence
of American English Consonants

A. Instructions

Identify the client's consonant errors and place a check mark next to consonants listed on the assessment scale that the client produces incorrectly. The list is arranged in descending order from greatest to least frequent in occurrence.

B. Assessment Scale[a]

Percentage of Occurrence of American English Consonants

Consonant	Rank	Percentage	Consonant	Rank	Percentage
t ____	1	13.7	p ____	13	3.9
n ____	2	11.7	b ____	14	3.5
s ____	3	7.1	z ____	15	3.0
k ____	4	6.0	ŋ ____	16	2.5
d ____	5	5.8	f ____	17	2.4
m ____	6	5.6	j ____	18	2.2
l ____	7	5.6	ʃ ____	19	1.5
r ____	8	5.2	v ____	20	1.2
w ____	9	4.8	θ ____	21	0.9
h ____	10	4.2	tʃ ____	22	0.7
ð ____	11	4.1	tʒ ____	23	0.6
g ____	12	4.1	ʒ ____	24	0.0

[a] The data source for this assessment scale is Shriberg and Kwiatkowski (1983).

APPENDIX 5I

Effects of Error Patterns
on Intelligibility

A. Instructions

Identify the client's error patterns and place a check mark next to any patterns on the assessment form on the scale below that occur in the client's speech. The list of error patterns is arranged in descending order from most to least effect on intelligibility.

B. Assessment Scale[a]

Beginning of Word	**End of Word**
Most to least effect:	Most to least effect:
Fronting _____	Final Consonant Deletion _____
Gliding _____	Fronting _____
Initial voicing _____	Word Final Devoicing _____
Stopping _____	
Cluster reduction _____	

---

[a] The data source for this assessment scale is Leinone-Davies (1988).

APPENDIX 5J
Prespeech Vocalizations[a]

A. Instructions

Obtain a speech sample following the procedures described in Chapter 4. Place check marks next to the age levels corresponding to the client's vocalizations on the assessment scale below. The age equivalent of the clients vocal development is the most advanced age at which an established vocalization occurs.

B. Assessment Scale

Prespeech Vocalization

Present	Approximate Age	Milestones
___ ___ ___	0–6 weeks	Crying, fussing, vegetative sounds
___ ___ ___	2–3 months	Begins to produce cooing behaviors
___ ___ ___	2–4 months	Begins to produce pleasure sounds such as "mmmm"
___ ___ ___	3–4 months	Cooing behavior is well established, babbling behavior (repetition or consonants and vowels) begins to appear
___ ___ ___	4 months	Produces some intonation during sound making and may engage in vocal play when playing with toys; vocalizations begin to be dominated by sounds produced at the front of the mouth, including raspberries and trills
___ ___ ___	7–8 months	Produces babbling (repetition of syllable)

---

[a] The data source for this appendix is Stark (1980). The checklist was adapted from J. Vannucci (1994).

APPENDIX 5K
Phonetic Inventories[a]

A. Instructions

Obtain a speech sample following the procedures described in Chapter 4. Tally the client's consonants using the forms on the following pages, placing a hash mark above each consonant the client produces. For example, if the client says [bi], [bu], and [ip], place two hash marks above [b] on the word-initial form and one hash mark above [p] on the word-final form. Circle consonants that the client produces in two or more different words (if analyzing only intelligible speech) or three or more different words (if analyzing both unintelligible and intelligible speech). Next, compare the client's consonant development to the inventories listed in either Phonetic Inventories (Intelligible Speech) or Phonetic Inventories (Intelligible and Unintelligible Speech). Look for the closest match between the client's consonant inventory and that listed on the phonetic inventory forms, expecting that your client's consonant inventory is not likely to exactly match the number and types of consonants shown on the phonetic inventory forms.

---

[a] The data sources for this appendix are Stoel-Gammon (1985), Dyson (1988), and Robb and Bleile (in press).

B. Sample Form for Determining Phonetic Inventories in Word-Initial Position

Manner of Production	Place of Production						
	Bilabial	Labiodental	Interdental	Alveolar	Postalveolar	Palatal	Velar	Glottal
Oral Stop	p b			t d			k g	
Fricative		f v	θ ð	s z	ʃ			
Affricate					tʃ dʒ			
Nasal Stop	m			n				
Liquid Central				r				
Lateral				l				
Glide	w					j		h

C. Sample Form for Determining Phonetic Inventories in Word-Final Position

Manner of Production	Place of Production						
	Bilabial	Labiodental	Interdental	Alveolar	Postalveolar	Palatal	Velar	Glottal
Oral Stop	p b			t d			k g	
Fricative		f v	θ ð	s z	ʃ ʒ			
Affricate					tʃ dʒ			
Nasal Stop	m			n			ŋ	
Liquid Central				r				
Lateral				l				

D. Phonetic Inventories (Intelligible Speech)

Highest Level	Age (in mos.)	Position	Number of Consonants	Typical Consonants
_____	15	Initial	3	b d h
_____		Final	none	ø
_____	18	Initial	6	b d m n h w
_____		Final	1	t
_____	24	Initial	9	b d g t k m n h w f s
_____		Final	6	p t k n r s
_____	29	Initial	14	b d g p t k m n h w j f s l
_____		Final	11	d p t k m n ŋ f s ʃ tʃ

E. Phonetic Inventories (Intelligible and Unintelligible Speech)

Highest Level	Age (in mos.)	Position	Number of Consonants	Typical Consonants
_____	12	Initial	5	b d h g m h
_____		Final	1	m
_____	18	Initial	6	b d m n h w
_____		Final	2	t s
_____	24	Initial	10	b d p t k m n h s w
_____		Final	4	t k n s

APPENDIX 5L
Summary Form for Error Probe Analysis

A. Instructions

Obtain a speech sample during the initial assessment using either standardized or nonstandardized procedures. Next, perform error probes for
the error patterns you consider most likely to be treatment targets, post-
poning consideration of more minor and infrequent error patterns. Use
either the error probe forms themselves or, if desired, the form below to
tabulate the results of the error probe analysis. The following example
shows how the form is used to summarize the error probe for Fronting
and Lisping. Whole numbers refer to the number of different words in
which the error pattern occurred. For example, 8/10 means the error pattern occurred in 8 of 10 words.

B. Example

Error Patterns	Occurrence	Stimulability
Fronting	8/10	Yes (words: key, go)
Lisping	10/10	No

C. Summary Form for Error Probe Analysis

Error Patterns	Occurrence	Stimulability
Changes in Place of Production		
Fronting***	_____	_____
Lisping***	_____	_____
Velar Assimilation***	_____	_____
Labial Assimilation***	_____	_____
Backing	_____	_____
Glottal Replacement	_____	_____

(continued)

Summary Form (*continued*)

Error Patterns	Occurrence	Stimulability
Changes in Manner of Production		
Stopping***	_____	_____
Gliding***	_____	_____
Lateralization***	_____	_____
Affrication	_____	_____
Nasalization	_____	_____
Denasalization	_____	_____
Changes in the Beginning of Syllables or Words		
Prevocalic Voicing***	_____	_____
Initial Consonant Deletion	_____	_____
Changes at the End of Syllables or Words		
Final Consonant Devoicing***	_____	_____
Final Consonant Deletion***	_____	_____
Changes in Syllables		
Reduplication***	_____	_____
Syllable Deletion**	_____	_____
Changes in Consonant Clusters		
Cluster Reduction***	_____	_____
Epenthesis***	_____	_____
Sound Reversals		
Metathesis	_____	_____
Changes in Vowels and Syllabic Consonants		
Vowel Neutralization***	_____	_____
Vocalization***	_____	_____

APPENDIX 5M

Typical Ages at Which Selected Major Error Patterns Disappear

A. Instructions

Obtain a speech sample using either error probes (Appendix 4B) or through some other method. Next, identify the error patterns on the assessment scale on the next page that are expected to have disappeared below the client's chronological or developmental age.

B. Typical Ages at Which Selected Major Error Patterns Disappear[a]

Disappear Before 3;0

_____ Prevocalic Voicing

_____ Velar Assimilation

_____ Labial Assimilation

_____ Reduplication

_____ Final Consonant Deletion

_____ Fronting

_____ Syllable Deletion

Disappear After 3;0

_____ Epenthesis

_____ Gliding

_____ Cluster Reduction

_____ Final Consonant Devoicing

_____ Stopping

---

[a] The data source for this appendix is Stoel-Gammon and Dunn (1985).

APPENDIX 5N

Acquisition of American English Consonants and Consonant Clusters[a]

A. Instructions

Obtain a speech sample following either the standardized or nonstandardized procedures described in Chapter 4. Place a check mark next to consonants and consonant clusters that the client produces correctly. If using the information for children under 3 years old, consonants must be produced correctly in at least two of three word positions (initial, medial, final). If using the information for older children, consonants must be produced correctly in both word-initial and word-final position and consonant clusters must be produced correctly in word-initial position.

B. Acquisition of American English Consonants

Consonant	Age	Consonant	Age
m	<2;0 _____	f	<3;0 _____
n	<2;0 _____	v	3;6 _____
ŋ	2;0 _____	θ	4;6 _____
h	<2;0 _____	ð	4;6 _____
w	<2;0 _____	s	3;6 _____
j	<3;0 _____	z	4;0 _____
p	<2;0 _____	ʃ	3;6 _____
t	2;0 _____	tʃ	3;6 _____
k	2;0 _____	dʒ	3;6 _____
b	<2;0 _____	r	3;6 _____
d	2;0 _____	l	3;6 _____
g	2;0 _____		

[a] The data sources for this appendix are Sander (1972) and Smit, Hand, Frelinger, Bernthal, & Byrd (1990). Data from Sander (1972) are for children under 3 years of age. Data from Smit et al. (1990) met two criteria: (1) at least 50% of both males and females correctly produced the sound in word initial and word final positions (consonants) or word initial position (consonant clusters), and (2) the percentage of subjects correctly producing the sound at subsequent age levels never dropped below 50%.

C. Acquisition of American English Consonant Clusters

Cluster	Age	Cluster	Age
tw	3;0 _____	pr	4;0 _____
kw	3;0 _____	br	3;6 _____
sp	3;6 _____	tr	5;0 _____
st	3;6 _____	dr	4;0 _____
sk	3;6 _____	kr	4;0 _____
sm	3;6 _____	gr	4;6 _____
sn	3;6 _____	fr	3;6 _____
sw	3;6 _____	θr	5;0 _____
sl	4;6 _____	skw	3;6 _____
pl	3;6 _____	spl	5;0 _____
bl	3;6 _____	spr	5;0 _____
kl	4;0 _____	str	5;0 _____
gl	3;6 _____	skr	5;0 _____
fl	3;6 _____		

APPENDIX 5O
Stimulability

A. Instructions

Determine which sounds you wish to test, and then ask the client to imitate the appropriate words. Place a check mark next to consonants and consonant clusters for which the client is stimulable. The assessment scale in this appendix is organized according to the typical age of acquisition of consonants and consonant clusters. Stimulability is tested in three word positions (initial, medial, and final) for sounds acquired under 3 years of age. Consonants acquired at 3 years or older are tested in two word positions (initial and final). Consonant clusters are tested in word-initial position. Readers wishing to test stimulability in a greater number of word positions are referred to Appendix 4B for a word list not organized according to age of acquisition.

---

[a] The data sources for this appendix are Sander (1972) and Smit, Hand, Frelinger, Bernthal, & Byrd (1990). Data from Sander (1972) are for children under 3 years of age. The consonants were produced correctly in 2 of 3 word positions (initial, medial, and final). Data from Smit et al. (1990) met two criteria: (1) at least 50% of both males and females correctly produced the sound in word-initial and word-final positions (consonants) or word-initial position (consonant clusters), and (2) the percentage of subjects correctly producing the sound at subsequent age levels never dropped below 50%. The Smit et al. data does not contain information for [ʃr] consonant clusters.

B. Stimulability Assessment Scale[a]

<2;0

[w]

#___		S___	
wind	___	flower	___
wet	___	tower	___
win	___	shower	___

[m]

#___		S__S		___#	
moon	___	mama	___	game	___
mop	___	gummy	___	boom	___
mud	___	hammer	___	swim	___

[p]

#___		S__S		___#	
pan	___	puppy	___	ape	___
pot	___	diaper	___	map	___
pie	___	sleepy	___	hop	___

[h]

#___	
home	___
hat	___
help	___

[n]

#___		S__S	
nice	___	honey	___
new	___	rainy	___
knife	___	tiny	___

[b]

#___		S__S		___#	
bee	___	baby	___	crab	___
bat	___	hobby	___	bib	___
book	___	tuba	___	tub	___

2;0

[ŋ]

S___S	___#
singing	sing
winging	king
hanger	hang

[t]

#___	S___S	___#
tea	twenty	ate
tag	water	bat
toe	waiter	boat

[d]

#___	S___S	___#
dive	soda	kid
dog	daddy	mud
doll	birdie	bed

(continued)

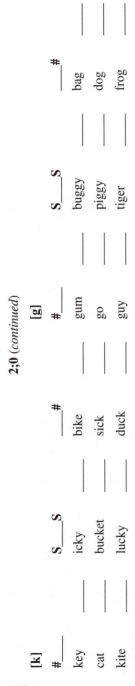

2;0 (continued)

[g]

#		S__S		__#	
gum	——	buggy	——	bag	——
go	——	piggy	——	dog	——
guy	——	tiger	——	frog	——

3;0

[k]

#		S__S		__#	
key	——	icky	——	bike	——
cat	——	bucket	——	sick	——
kite	——	lucky	——	duck	——

[f]

#		__#	
fun	——	safe	——
feet	——	hoof	——
fog	——	cough	——

[j]

#	
yes	——
yard	——
yell	——

[tw]

twin	——
twice	——
twig	——

[kw]

quit	——
queen	——
quick	——

276

3;6

[v]

# ___		___ #	
vine	___	dove	___
van	___	move	___
vote	___	wave	___

[ʃ]

# ___		___ #	
shoe	___	dish	___
sheep	___	crash	___
shell	___	wash	___

[tʃ]

# ___		___ #	
chair	___	watch	___
cheese	___	peach	___
chain	___	witch	___

[s]

# ___		___ #	
sun	___	bus	___
soap	___	kiss	___
sit	___	face	___

[dʒ]

# ___		___ #	
jump	___	judge	___
jet	___	huge	___
juice	___	page	___

(*continued*)

3;6 (*continued*)

[l]

\# _____	\# _____
light	ball
laugh	fall
left	eel

[sk]

\# _____
---
sky
skip
ski

[r]

\# _____	\# _____	_____
rain	car
row	air
root	chair

[sp]

\# _____
---
spin
space
SPY

[st]

\# _____
---
stove
stew
stop

[sw]

\# _____
---
swamp
swim
sweet

[sm]

\# _____
---
smell
smoke
small

[pl]

\# _____
---
play
plate
please

[fl]

\# _____
---
flag
fly
floor

[bl]		[gl]		[br]		[fr]		[skw]	
# ___		# ___		# ___		# ___		# ___	
bloom	___	glue	___	brain	___	fruit	___	squeak	___
blind	___	glow	___	broom	___	free	___	square	___
blood	___	glass	___	break	___	frog	___	squad	___

4;0

[z]					
___ #					
zoo	keys	___			
zero	please	___			
zip	buzz	___			

[pr]		[kr]		[dr]		[kl]	
# ___		# ___		# ___		# ___	
pray	crib	___	dry	___	clock	___
print	crow	___	drum	___	cloud	___
prune	cry	___	drop	___	clue	___

(continued)

4;6

[θ]
#_____ think _____
thief _____
thick _____

#_____ teeth _____
broth _____
north _____

[ð]
#_____ that _____
this _____
them _____

[gr]
#_____ grin _____
grass _____
grow _____

[sl]
#_____ slam _____
sleep _____
slow _____

5;0

[tr]
#_____ trout _____
truck _____
tree _____

[θr]
#_____ three _____
throw _____
thread _____

[spr]
#_____ spray _____
spread _____
spring _____

[str]
#_____ street _____
straw _____
stream _____

[skr]
#_____ screw _____
scratch _____
screen _____

[spl]
#_____ splash _____
split _____
splurge _____

280

APPENDIX 5P
Calculation of Adjusted Age (AA)

A. Instructions

Use the formula below to calculate adjusted age for clients 24 months or younger who were born prematurely.

1. Adjusted Age Formula
Chronological age – Prematurity in weeks = Adjusted age

2. Example
5 months – 3 weeks premature = 4 months, 1 week old

APPENDIX 5Q
Calculation of Developmental Age (DA)

A. Instructions

Use the formula below to calculate developmental age for clients with possible cognitive or intellectual limitations.

1. Verbal IQ or Standard Score

a. Client's verbal intelligence

b. Standard score (PPVT-R)

2. Developmental Age Formula

$$\frac{\text{Client's IQ or PPVT-R Standard Score} \times \text{CA in months}}{100} = \text{Developmental Age Level}$$

3. Example

$$\frac{82 \times 36}{100} = 29.52 \text{ months (30 months)}$$

APPENDIX 5R
African American English (AAE)[a]

A. Instructions

Transcribe the client's speech. Place a check mark next to the client's AAE patterns on the assessment form that follows. AAE patterns are excluded from analysis of articulation and phonological disorders.

B. Assessment Scale for African American English (AAE)

Patterns	Examples
☐ Stopping	
[θ] → [t]	*thought* is *tought*
[ð] → [d]	*this* is *dis*
☐ Place changes between vowels and word finally	
[θ] → [f]	*bath* is *baf*
[ŋ] → [n]	*swing* is *swin*
[ð] → [v]	*bathing* is *baving*
☐ Devoicing at ends of words	
[b] → [p]	*slab* is *slap*
[d] → [t]	*bed* is *bet*
[g] → [k]	*bug* is *buk*
☐ Lowering of [I] before nasals	
[ɪ] → [ɛ]	*pin* is *pen*
☐ Deletion	
V + [r] → V + ø	*more* is *mo*
CC# → Cø#	*nest* is *nes*
☐ Vowel nasalization and nasal deletion	
V + N → nasalized vowel	*tame* is *tã*

---

[a] The data source for this appendix is Cole and Taylor (1990).

APPENDIX 5S
Hawaiian Island Creole (HC)[a]

A. Instructions

Transcribe the client's speech. Place a check mark next to the client's Hawaiian Island Creole patterns on the assessment form that follows. Exclude Hawaiian Island Creole patterns from analysis of articulation and phonological disorders.

B. Assessment Scale for Hawaiian Island Creole

Patterns	Examples
☐ Stopping	
[θ] → [t]	*thick* is *tick*
[ð] → [d]	*this* is *dis*
☐ Backing in environment of [r]	
[θr] → [tʃr]	*three* is *chree*
[tr] → [tʃr]	*tree* is *chree*
[str] → [ʃtrʒ]	*street* is *shtreet*
☐ Deletion	
V + [r] → V + schwa	*here* is *hea*
CC# → Cø#	*nest* is *nes*

---

[a] The data source for this appendix is Lyons (1994).

CHAPTER

6

Treatment Principles

The following topics are discussed in this chapter:

I. OVERVIEW OF TREATMENT

Four treatment principles are discussed in this chapter: purposes of treatment, goals (long- and short-term), treatment targets, and administrative decisions. In each section an introductory discussion is followed by a discussion of clients at specific stages in articulation and phonological development. The chapter concludes with brief summaries of complete intervention programs and a discussion of methods to evaluate treatment effectiveness.

II. PURPOSES OF TREATMENT

As discussed in Chapter 2 and Chapter 5, a client's stage of articulation and phonological development is more important than chronological age when making decisions about clinical care. For convenience, ways in which the general purpose of treatment changes depending on a client's stage of articulation and phonological development are presented in Table 6–1.

Table 6–1. Primary purposes of care at four different stages in articulation and phonological development.

Stages	Age Range in Typically Developing Children	Treatment Goals
Stage 1	Birth–12 months	Facilitate development of vocal skills that underlie later speech development
Stage 2	12–24 months	Facilitate development of a functional vocabulary for purposes of communication
Stage 3	24 months to 5 years	Facilitate acquisition of major speech elements
Stage 4	5 years through adolescence	Facilitate development of literacy and eliminate errors affecting late-acquired speech items

---

Early Intervention

Younger clients almost always receive articulation and phonological treatment within the framework of an early intervention program with a strong emphasis on language development (Bleile & Miller, 1994). Several studies have demonstrated the effectiveness of early intervention on later developmental skills (Infant Health and Development Program, 1990; Bricker, Bailey, & Bruder, 1984; Ramey & Campbell, 1984; White, Mastrapierl, & Casto, 1984; Mantovani & Powers, 1991). The Infant Health and Development Program (1990), for example, after studying preterm at-risk infants in eight different clinical settings, found that the children who received early intervention had intelligence quotients (IQs) from 6.6 to 13.2 points higher than preterm children who received only routine follow-up care. The smaller gains in intelligence were obtained by children with the lowest birthweights, perhaps reflecting reduced potential for learning. A striking finding of the study was that preterm children who did not receive early intervention were 2.7 times more likely to have IQ scores in the mentally retarded range at 3 years of age than preterm children who did receive early intervention.

III. LONG-TERM GOALS

Long-term goals are the articulation and phonological behaviors that the clinician desires for the client to exhibit by the end of treatment or after a designated time period, such as a semester or school year.

A. Stage 1

The most common long-term treatment goal is for articulation and phonological development to be appropriate compared to chronological or developmental age. Adjusted age should be used instead of chronological age for clients 2 years or younger who were born prematurely (see Chapter 5). Success or failure to achieve long-term goals typically is measured using age norms, although clinical judgment scales of severity represent a second possibility (see Chapter 5).

B. Stage 2

The most common long-term treatment goal is for articulation and phonological development to be appropriate compared to chronological or developmental age. Adjusted age should be used instead of chronological age for clients 2 years or younger who were born prematurely (see Chapter 5). Success or failure to achieve long-term goals is measured using age norms and/or judgments of severity of involvement (see Chapter 5).

C. Stage 3

The long-term treatment goal is for articulation and phonological development to be appropriate compared to chronological or developmental age. Success or failure to achieve long-term goals typically is measured using age norms and measures of either severity of involvement or intelligibility (see Chapter 5).

D. Stage 4

The most common long-term treatment goal typically is for articulation and phonological development to be appropriate compared to chronological or developmental age (see Chapter 5). Success or failure to achieve long-term goals may be measured using age norms, severity of involvement, and/or degree of intelligibility. Another possible long-term goal is to eliminate articulation and phonological errors that affect a person's happiness or social and educational development. Such a long-term goal would be appropriate, for example, for a client who was teased because of a [w] for [r] substitution or who experienced embarrassment when speaking to groups because of a frontal lisp. The success or failure to achieve this long-term goal might be determined at a client and/or family interview at the conclusion of treatment.

IV. SHORT-TERM GOALS

Short-term goals are the steps, each typically lasting from a few weeks to several months, through which long-term goals are achieved. The major short-term goals for clients in each of the four stages in articulation and phonological development are listed in Table 6–2.

Table 6–2. Short-term goals for clients at four different stages in articulation and phonological development.

Stages	Short-term Goals
Stage 1	Increase opportunities to vocalize
	Acquire developmentally advanced vocalizations
	Teach functional, high-frequency words in familiar contexts
	Facilitate conversational turn-taking
Stage 2	Stimulate expressive vocabulary development
	Encourage speech for communication
	Reduce homonyms
	Reduce variability
	Maximize established speech skills
Stage 3	Reduce or eliminate errors affecting classes of speech elements
	Facilitate speech in phrases and sentences
	Encourage use of speech in settings outside the home
Stage 4	Facilitate mastery of late-acquired consonants and consonant clusters
	Teach pronunciation of literary and scientific vocabulary
	Increase phonological awareness
	Encourage use of speech in social and educational settings

A. Stage 1

Short-term goals for a client in Stage 1 include:

- Increase opportunities to vocalize

- Acquire developmentally advanced vocalizations

- Teach functional, high-frequency words in familiar contexts

- Facilitate conversational turn-taking

1. Increase Opportunities to Vocalize. This short-term goal seeks to increase opportunities for a child to vocalize. It is appropriate for a hospitalized client and for a victim of environmental neglect or abuse. Increasing vocalizations can be pursued as early as the first few months of life, as a client awakens more frequently and becomes more alert. A possible short-term goal, for example, might be to provide opportunities for a hospitalized client to vocalize on waking or before napping, and/or to train a parent how to better interact with their child. In most settings, vocal stimulation is carried out by a family member, although in a hospital setting this task might be undertaken by a speech-language clinician, an aide, or a nurse.

2. **Acquisition of Developmentally Advanced Vocalizations.** This short-term goal facilitates acquisition of developmentally advanced vocalizations. It is appropriate for a client either at risk for or already experiencing delays in articulation and phonological development. As above, this short-term goal can be pursued as early as the first months, as a client awakens more frequently. A short-term goal, for example, might be to facilitate babbling for a client whose most developmentally advanced vocalization is squealing and making raspberries.

3. **Teach Functional, High-frequency Words in Familiar Contexts.** This short-term goal facilitates acquisition of receptive vocabulary. It is appropriate for a client either at risk or already experiencing difficulty learning correspondences between sound and meaning (vocabulary learning). Word acquisition is facilitated in highly familiar contexts within which a small number of words occur frequently (see Chapter 3). For example, a child with a delay in vocabulary acquisition might be exposed to food names in the context of eating lunch.

4. **Facilitate Conversational Turn-taking.** This short-term goal facilitates acquisition of "my turn, your turn" aspects of sound making (Chapter 3). It is appropriate for a client developmentally 4 to 6 months or older. To facilitate turn-taking, for example, a caretaker might be encouraged to engage a child in games of peek-a-boo or so-big.

B. Stage 2

Short-term goals for a client in Stage 2 include:

- Stimulate expressive vocabulary development
- Encourage speech for communication
- Reduce homonyms

- Reduce variability

- Maximize established speech skills

1. **Stimulate Expressive Vocabulary Development.** This short-term goal facilitates acquisition of words for purposes of communication. It is appropriate for all clients in Stage 2, but especially for those with an expressive vocabulary of less than 50 words. Articulation and phonological problems are thought to be major factors in limiting expressive vocabulary development in such diverse populations as children with Down syndrome and otherwise typically developing children with expressive language delay (Miller, 1992; Paul, 1991). One approach to facilitate expressive vocabulary development is experimental. It consists of the following four steps.

   a. **Step 1:** Determine size of expressive vocabulary. Before beginning to teach news words, it is important to know what words a child already says. The MacArthur communicative development inventories (Fenson, Dale, Reznick, Thal, Bates, Hartung, Pethick, & Reilly, 1993) provides an excellent standardized measure to assess expressive vocabulary. A simple nonstandardized approach is to ask a caregiver what words a child says, and then list the words. Two cautions are needed in a nonstandardized assessment. First, many caregivers are inclined to only identify words that the child "speaks well." To counter this tendency, let a caregiver know you are interested in identifying all words a child says, regardless of how they are pronounced. Second, caregivers typically do not recall all of a child's spoken words when first asked. This problem can be countered by acknowledging the difficulty in recalling all words a child says, and then asking the caregiver to let you know additional words as they are recalled. An additional technique that frequently helps is to let a caregiver know beforehand to bring a list of all the words a child says to the assessment.

   b. **Step 2:** Analyze phonetic inventory. A phonetic inventory analysis identifies speech elements a child is capable of producing (see Chapters 3 and 5). Inventories of consonants, vowels, syllables, and stress (if a child's speech contains multisyllabic words) are useful. If a child's expressive vocabulary is small, many times a phonetic inventory is determined after a quick glance at a phonetically transcribed word list.

c. **Step 3:** Select words to teach. Selection of words to teach is based on three principles:

(1) Selectivity. As discussed in Chapter 3, research indicates a child is more likely to attempt to pronounce words that contain speech elements already mastered. Clinically, this means that words selected for teaching must contain speech elements within a child's phonetic inventory, either as produced spontaneously or through stimulability testing. To illustrate, if a clinician's goal is to facilitate development of word-initial consonants, selected words should begin with consonants that a child already produces spontaneously or during stimulability testing.

(2) Inventory expansion. Most often, a clinician seeks to expand a Stage 2 child's speech abilities to include more developmentally advanced speech elements. Practically, this entails selection of words containing speech elements that increase a child's phonetic inventory. When analyzing a child's phonetic inventory, special attention is given to likely treatment targets, especially emerging places and manners of production and appearance of consonants in new syllable positions. To illustrate, if a child's speech contains twelve words beginning with bilabial consonants and one beginning with an alveolar consonant, a likely treatment target would be a word beginning with an alveolar consonant. Additional discussion of selection of treatment targets in Stage 2 is contained in Section X of this chapter.

(3) Child's interests. The team who selects words to teach consists of three members: a clinician, a caregiver, and a child. A clinician's role is to develop a word list that meets the selectivity and inventory expansion criteria, a caregiver's role is to consider which words a child is likely to attempt, and a child's role is to say the words. Being a child, the third member of the team has veto power over the decisions of the other two. Practically, this means a clinician and caregiver generate a longer word list than will be used. To illustrate, a clinician might generate a list of 10 possible words, 3 of which a caregiver believes a child will say, and 1 or 2 of which a child actually says.

d. **Step 4:** Teach words. Words are taught within one of several highly functional, naturalistic clinical approaches. Bombardment is used to increase the frequency with which a child hears words (see Chapter 7). To illustrate, suppose a clinician wished to teach a child the word *bed* in a half-hour session in a clinic setting. The room would contain one or more toy beds, dolls, and other toys that might be utilized in activities involving getting ready for bed. During the treatment session, the clinician and child would engage in bedtime activities with the dolls, perhaps brushing teeth, putting on pajamas, and tucking in. During these activities, the clinician would frequently model bed, sometimes without expecting a child response and other times asking for one. For example, the clinician might say, "Look at the bed." Or, "It's getting time for bed. Bed time is so much fun." Or, "What should the baby sleep on? Can you tell me in words?"

No single rule exists regarding how many different words to teach within a given time period. A child with better cognitive abilities would be taught more words, and a cognitively less advanced child would be taught fewer. Typically, a child with relatively intact cognitive abilities receiving therapy 30 to 45 minutes per session twice weekly is exposed to 2 or 3 different words per session, and the same words are continued for two weeks. During this time, a home program is maintained. At the end of two weeks, words that have not been attempted by the child are discarded and replaced. New words may either continue to contain the same speech elements as the discarded words, or, if new speech abilities are emerging, may contain newly emerging speech elements. For example, while teaching *bed* a clinician might hear the client say [du] for *dog*, and decide to introduce words with initial [d], such as *dog* or *day*.

e. Monitoring Progress. Results of any clinical program should be monitored, especially an experimental one. Important aspects of expressive vocabulary development to monitor include:

- Is a child acquiring the words being taught?

- Are words taught by a therapist being used outside the therapy setting?

- Does the child's speech contain new and emerging speech elements?

- Is a child acquiring words other than those taught by a therapist?

- Is a child generally becoming more verbal?

My experience is that during the first weeks of treatment a caregiver often reports slow progress, but then a child starts using more "therapy words" at home. As therapy proceeds, a caregiver often reports the pace of vocabulary growth quickens, with a child acquiring both "therapy words" and words not taught in therapy. Often a caregiver also reports that a child is generally more verbal than prior to beginning therapy.

2. **Encourage Speech for Communication.** This short-term goal encourages a client to use vocal means to communicate wants and needs. It is appropriate for all clients in Stage 2, especially for a child who appears frustrated. A child early in Stage 2 might be encouraged to use any type of vocalization as part of a communication repertoire; as a child proceeds through Stage 2, vocalizations are replaced with words. For example, a child prone to tantrums might be encouraged to use his words to communicate instead of his legs.

3 **Reduce Homonyms.** This short-term goal seeks to reduce percentage of homonyms (words that sound alike, but have different meanings) in the client's speech. Presence of homonyms is normal in both children's and adult's speech, but unusual numbers of homonyms in small expressive vocabularies may severely interfere with communication. For example, a client with a 10-word expressive vocabulary, seven of which are pronounced as [bi], is likely to experience difficulty communicating, especially when speaking to unfamiliar adults. There are two general approaches to reducing homonyms: eliminate errors causing homonyms and "flooding."

a. **Eliminate Errors Causing Homonyms.** This approach eliminates error patterns or sound class errors causing homonyms (Ingram, 1989). A client, for example, who pronounces *cookie*, *Tom*, *kite*, and *toe* as [di] might have reduction of Fronting as a short-term goal, so that *cookie* and *kite* would then be pronounced with initial [k] and *Tom* and *toe* would be pronounced with an initial [t].

b. **Flooding.** This approach reduces the number of homonyms by putting communicative pressure on a child (Bleile & Miller, 1994). Somewhat ironically, flooding creates more homonyms in a client's speech, resulting in communicative breakdown and frustration, inducing speech changes as the client is forced to attempt new pronunciations in order to communicate. A client whose expressive vocabulary was dominated by words pronounced as [di], for example, would be taught words that the assessment indicated would also be pronounced [di]. A clinician would then engage the client in the type of request for clarification activities described in Chapter 7. To illustrate, a client might say [di] to request a cookie, and a clinician might then give a spoon, key, or plate, or other object that the client also pronounces as [di].

4. **Reduce Variability.** This short-term goal reduces a client's alternate word pronunciations. Reduction in variability is appropriate for clients in Stage 2 and some less advanced clients in Stage 3 whose pronunciation of words is extremely variable. Two types of variability exist: intra-word variability and inter-word variability. *Intra-word variability* is variation in the pronunciation of speech in the same word. A client whose speech showed intra-word variability, for example, might say the initial sound in *bee* as [b], [p], or [mb]. *Inter-word variability* is variation in the pronunciation of speech elements in different words. A client whose speech showed inter-word variability, for example, might say [b] as [b] in *bee*, as [d], in *bay*, and [p] as in *boo*.

Intra- and inter-word variability both interfere with communication. More positively, however, variability suggests that better pronunciation of a sound lies within a client's phonetic abilities, even though the client may not yet be able to produce it correctly on all occasions. When the short-term goal is to reduce variability, a general clinical strategy is to encourage a client to produce the most developmentally advanced variant of the sound.

When the Goal Is Nothing New

At least three situations exist in which the short-term goal of treatment is to extend a client's use of existing articulation and phonological abilities rather than to facilitate the acquisition of new sounds and syllables. The first situation is when a clinician affords opportunities to vocalize to a client in Stage 1 who may have experienced either deprivation through neglect or as a result of lengthy hospitalizations. The second situation is when the expressive vocabulary of a client in Stage 2 or 3 contains many homonyms and a clinician "floods" the vocabulary with words that result in increased numbers of homonyms. The third situation is when a clinician helps construct a larger expressive vocabulary for a client in Stage 2 or 3 using existing articulation and phonological skills.

5. **Maximize Established Speech Abilities.** This short-term goal seeks to maximize the client's existing articulation and phonological abilities (Bleile & Miller, 1994). It is appropriate for clients in Stage 2 for whom the major treatment goal is vocabulary building and less advanced clients in Stage 3 who are temporarily "stalled" in articulation and phonological development. This short-term goal increases use of existing abilities to pronounce speech elements. Use of established speech abilities facilitates word acquisition through eliminating unfamiliar speech elements. It is especially useful with a client whose major communication strategies include word recipes or selectivity (see Chapter 5). Constructed words should be pragmatically useful and contain well-established speech elements. If a client's established phonetic inventory, for example, contained the CV syllables, [k] and [i], a clinician would discuss with a client's caregivers whether the word *key* has functional value for the client. If so, *key* would receive special emphasis during treatment and the client's family would attempt to facilitate use of the word at home.

Why Distinctive Features and Error Patterns?

Distinctive feature and error pattern approaches were developed to speed remediation through generalization of treatment results from a treated sound to untreated sounds. A distinctive feature approach organizes sounds into classes based on shared acoustic and articulatory features; the hoped-for result of treatment is that generalization will occur from the treated sounds to other sounds that share similar features. Facilitating acquisition of [f], for example, may facilitate the client's acquisition of other fricatives. An error pattern approach organizes sounds according to the errors they typically undergo; the hoped-for result of treating one sound is that the results will generalize to other sounds that undergo the same error. Which approach facilitates better generalization—use of distinctive features or error patterns? I do not believe there is yet sufficient research to answer that important question.

C. Stage 3

Short-term goals for a child in Stage 3 include:

• Reduce or eliminate errors affecting classes of speech elements

• Facilitate speech in phrases and sentences

• Encourage use of speech in settings outside the home

Additionally, many short-term goals useful for a child in Stage 2 may also be appropriate for a child in early Stage 3.

1. Reduce or Eliminate Errors Affecting Classes of Speech Elements. This short-term goal seeks to eliminate errors affecting classes of speech elements, including consonants and vowels, syllable shapes, stress patterns, and intonation. The most frequent clinical short-term goal for a client in Stage 3 focuses on errors involving sound classes (consonants and vowels). Two closely related approaches eliminate errors affecting sound classes: distinctive feature approaches and error pattern approaches.

a. Distinctive Feature Approaches. In a distinctive feature approach, sounds receive remediation based on membership in a sound class. Sound classes most often used for this purpose are place, manner, and voicing categories found in a consonant chart.

Some clinicians remediate all sounds in a sound class (Blodgett & Miller, 1989). For example, a clinician might treat all velar consonants in the speech of a client who pronounced velar consonants as alveolar consonants. Other clinicians recommend treating fewer sounds within a sound class (Elbert, Powell, & Swartzlander, 1991; Williams, 1991). I remediate from two sounds up to 50% of the sounds in a sound class in the hope that the treatment results will generalize to other sounds sharing the distinctive feature. For example, a client who pronounced [k] and [g] as alveolar consonants in the beginning of syllables might receive treatment for [k], the hope being that the results would generalize to other velar consonants. Providing remediation to selected sounds in a sound class appears to help some clients generalize, and costs no additional time for those who do not. Word probes such as those described in Appendix 4A are used to determine whether generalization has occurred.

b. **Error Pattern Approaches.** An error pattern approach eliminates mispronunciations that affect a sound class. As with a distinctive feature approach, some clinicians provide treatment to all sounds affected by an error pattern, whereas others, the author included, provide remediation to from two sounds up to 50% of sounds affected by an error pattern in the hope that the treatment results will generalize to other sounds affected by the error pattern. A client, for example, might have a Fronting error pattern in the beginning of syllables, and treatment might focus on remediating [k] in that syllable position in the hope that the results will generalize to [g] and [ŋ].

An important issue concerns which error patterns should be selected for remediation. I typically select error patterns that are either frequent (50%–75% of all possible occurrences) or present (25%–49% of all occurrences) (see Table 5–2 for categories based on whole numbers rather than percentages). I tend to avoid error patterns that are highly frequent (75%–100% of all possible occurrences), because their remediation often is too time-consuming and frustrating for younger clients. I also tend to avoid remediating error patterns that are disappearing (1%–24%), because in most situations the client appears to be overcoming them without treatment.

2. **Facilitate Speech in Phrases and Sentences.** This short-term goal facilitates use of syntactic and morphological means to express feelings and thoughts. It is appropriate for a child who pronounces a speech element correctly in an isolated word but is unable to do so in longer connected speech. For example, a child may say [s] in *see* and *sun*, but may pronounce [s] as [t] in a phrase such as, "The sun is shining."

3. **Encourage Use of Speech in Settings Outside the Home.** This short-term goal encourages speech development through exposure to less familiar persons in settings outside the home. As discussed in Chapter 3, a child in Stage 3 increasingly comes into contact with a range of persons in various social and educational contexts. Such contact both challenges and extends a child's speech abilities because more speech is required to communicate. Encouragement of speech use outside the home is appropriate for a child who is medically stable and sufficiently advanced developmentally. The former requirement is important because, while a setting outside the home often is a catalyst for speech development, contact with larger numbers of people may result in increased numbers of illnesses.

D. Stage 4

Short-term goals for a child in Stage 4 include:

• Facilitate mastery of late-acquired consonants and consonant clusters

• Teach pronunciation of literary and scientific vocabulary

• Increase phonological awareness

• Encourage use of speech in social and educational settings

1. **Facilitate Mastery of Late-acquired Consonants and Consonant Clusters.** A central short-term goal for clients in Stage 4 is to eliminate errors affecting late-acquired consonants and consonant clusters. Most often, emerging (25–49% correct) consonants are selected as short-term goals (see Table 5–3 for categories based on whole numbers rather than percentages). However, rare (1–24% correct) consonants are sometimes selected as short-term goals with clients who do not become frustrated easily, and acquired (50–74% correct) consonants are sometimes selected with clients who do not appear to be improving without treatment. Absent (0% correct) sounds are seldom selected as short-term goals because they often prove extremely challenging for clients; mastered (75–100% correct) sounds and syllables are seldom selected because they appear well on the way to being acquired already.

2. **Teach Pronunciation of Literary and Scientific Vocabulary.** This short-term goal eliminates speech errors affecting literary and scientific vocabulary. During the course of learning to read, a Stage 4 child is exposed to and must learn to pronounce many complex syllable and stress patterns (see Chapter 3). Elimination of speech errors affecting such words is appropriate for a child who may otherwise have no—or few—speech difficulties. My clinical impression is that difficulty pronouncing literary and scientific vocabulary has a higher prevalence among those diagnosed with learning problems than among those without such problems.

3. **Increase Phonological Awareness.** This short-term goal increases conscious awareness of speech elements and the ability needed to succeed in segmentation and identification tasks often encountered in learning to read. Phonological awareness is an appropriate short-term goal within a broader articulation and phonological treatment program for a child in late Stage 3 and in early Stage 4.

4. Encourage Use of Speech in Social and Educational Settings. This short-term goal encourages use of speech in social and educational settings. Increased and more sophisticated use of speech in such contexts is expected as a child advances through the school setting. Use of speech in social and educational settings is appropriate for a Stage 4 child both to permit more complete participation in society and to act as a catalyst for further speech development.

V. OVERVIEW OF TREATMENT TARGETS

Although long- and short-term goals give direction to clinical endeavors, treatment targets are the actual sounds and syllables through which change in a client's articulation and phonological systems is facilitated. For example, a long-term goal might be, "Articulation and phonological development will be appropriate for the client's age," and the short-term goal might be, "Elimination of Fronting in the beginning of syllables." The treatment target is the sound (or sounds) through which the restriction on velar consonants (Fronting) in syllable-initial position is eliminated. To illustrate, a client who pronounced [s] and [z] as stops might receive treatment for [s], the hope being that the results would generalize to [z] and other fricatives. The major issues that arise in considering treatment targets include: selecting appropriate targets, determining how many targets should be treated, changing treatment targets, and choosing linguistic levels and phonetic environments.

VI. SELECTING TREATMENT TARGETS

Most often, a clinician selects treatment targets that a client demonstrates some capacity to produce—that is, the treatment target is a better ability (stimulable). Because the client already has some capacity to produce the treatment target, the clinician can more quickly generalize the treatment target to other words or phonetic environments, rather than focusing treatment on the often frustrating and time-consuming task of teaching the client to pronounce a treatment target that the client shows no capacity to produce in any circumstance. Four possible methods to determine whether a client is able to produce a treatment target are listed in Table 6–3 and described below.

Table 6–3. Four methods to select treatment targets.

Criteria	Definitions
Imitation	A client produces the treatment target during imitation
Emerging sound	A client produces the treatment target in either several phonetic environments or one key phonetic environment
Key word	A client produces the treatment target in one or a few selected words
Phonetic placement and shaping	A client produces the treatment target through phonetic placement or through shaping an existing sound

A. Imitation

Imitation, as the name implies, is a client's ability to imitate a treatment target (see Section V in Chapter 5 for assessment procedures). Imitation indicates that a client is physically able to produce the sound. Treatment seeks to generalize use of the sound from imitation to spontaneous speech.

B. Emerging Sound

An emerging sound is one that is produced correctly on 10% to 49% of all occasions in one or more phonetic environments (the phonetic environment is called a key environment if the client is only able to produce the treatment target in a single phonetic environment). An example of an emerging sound is [k] in the speech of a client who correctly produced [k] in word-initial position in 2 of 10 words (20%). If the client is able to produce a treatment target in several phonetic environments, treatment seeks to increase the frequency with which the sound is produced. If the client is only able to produce the sound in one key environment treatment seeks to generalize success from that phonetic environment to other phonetic environments.

C. Key Word

A key word is a word in which the client successfully produces the treatment target. Although any word can be a key word, many times key words have special significance for a client such as being the name of a favorite toy or person. Treatment based on a key word seeks to generalize success in producing the sound to other words (see Section XIII for discussion of the Paired-stimuli [key word] treatment program).

D. Phonetic Placement and Shaping

Phonetic placement involves the physical placement of a client's articulators into position to produce a sound. Phonetic placement of [t], for example, entails detailed instructions that guide the client to quickly touch the alveolar ridge with the tongue tip. Shaping involves developing a new sound from a sound already in the client's phonetic inventory. Shaping techniques, for example, provide a series of steps through which a [t] might be shaped into [s]. Treatment seeks to generalize success in performing phonetic placement and shaping techniques to spontaneous speech. Phonetic placement and shaping techniques are provided in Appendix 7C.

E. Stage 1

The most appropriate treatment targets for clients in Stage 1 are those that are emerging and for which the client is stimulable.

F. Stages 2 and 3

The most appropriate treatment targets for clients in Stages 2 and 3 are those that are stimulable and emerging. The next most-preferred treatment targets are those that are either emerging, stimulable, or in key words or key environments. Treatment targets may also be rarely produced sounds, although the likelihood exists that the client will find such targets more frustrating. For this reason, the preferred clinical strategy is to monitor rarely occurring sounds and treat them after they are produced correctly more frequently.

G. Stage 4

As with clients in earlier stages of articulation and phonological development, the most appropriate treatment targets for clients in Stage 4 are treatment targets that are stimulable, emerging, or in key words. Unlike clients in earlier stages, the clinician can also target more rarely produced sounds, because many clients in Stage 4 are able to tolerate less immediate treatment success. The often greater cognitive maturation of clients in Stage 4 also allows the clinician to utilize shaping and phonetic placement techniques. Even so, such techniqu require more patience and attention than is possible for clients in stage 4 who are immature or who experience behavioral problems, intellectual deficits, or cognitive impairments.

VII. MOST AND LEAST KNOWLEDGE METHODS

Most often, treatment targets require the client to acquire new sounds and syllables. Two methods can be used to determine how similar treatment targets should be compared to the client's current articulation and phonological abilities: the most knowledge method and the least knowledge method.

A. Most Knowledge Method

The most knowledge method is a traditional criterion used to choose treatment targets. In this method, treatment targets differ minimally from the sounds the client already produces (Elbert & Gierut, 1986). This means that the client has a great deal of knowledge about the treatment target, because he or she already is producing many features of the treatment target in other sounds. For example, within the most knowledge method the treatment target for a client whose phonetic inventory contained one oral stop ([p]) and no fricatives would likely be another oral stop—perhaps a sound that differed only in voicing (e.g., [b]) or in place of production (e.g., [t] or [k]). The close similarity between the client's existing abilities and the treatment target is intended to ensure that the new sound will be acquired without great frustration for the client (Van Riper, 1978). A possible limitation of a most knowledge method is that treatment must proceed in small increments, which proves time-consuming with clients who have multiple articulation and phonological errors. To acquire the entire set of oral stops, for example, the above client's treatment targets would include [b], [t], [d], [k], and [g].

Least Knowledge:
Distinctive Features or Error Patterns?

The least knowledge method is closely associated with the use of a distinctive feature approach, but it might also be undertaken within an error pattern framework. For example, a client's speech might contain the following characteristics: stopping, a well-established

(continued)

[b], no alveolar consonants, and stimulability for [f] and [s]. In a more traditional most knowledge method, the likely treatment target in this situation is [f], because that sound is most similar to [b] (a labial consonant). In a least knowledge method, the likely treatment target is [s], because [s] facilitates the acquisition of a new place of production.

B. Least Knowledge Method

In a least knowledge method, treatment targets differ from the client's existing abilities by multiple features (Elbert & Gierut, 1986; Powell, 1991). The client described above whose speech contained one oral stop ([p]) and no fricatives, for example, might have [z] as a treatment target. The essential idea underlying a least knowledge method is that treatment targets should afford the client the opportunity to acquire skills needed to produce more than single sounds. In acquiring [z], for example, the client also acquires a new contrast in place of production (bilabial and alveolar), a new voicing contrast (voiceless and voiced), and a new manner of production (stop and fricative).

C. Stage 1

Although in principle a least knowledge method is possible for clients in Stage 1, all the clients I have treated have only responded to a more traditional most knowledge method.

D. Stage 2

I typically use an approach for a client in Stage 2 midway between a most and least knowledge method. My clinical experience is that a strict most knowledge method limits a Stage 2 client's ability to generalize, and a strict least knowledge method is too frustrating for a young child. For this reason, a simple two step procedure is used to select treatment targets for Stage 2 clients:

1. **Within Capacity.** Select treatment targets based on the criteria listed in Section VI (imitation, key word, or emerging in at least one key phonetic environment). This assures a client has the capacity to pronounce the treatment target.

2. **Promote Expansion.** If more than one treatment target meets the above criteria, select the one least similar and most developmentally advanced compared to what the client currently produces. This expands a client's speech-making abilities.

3. **Illustration.** To illustrate the selection process, suppose a client's speech showed a preponderance of V and CV words, the consonant was [b], and that stimulability testing indicated the client could pronounce several additional word-initial consonants and no word-final consonants.

   a. **Step 1 (Within Capacity).** If a clinician wished to focus on consonant development, selection of treatment targets would be made from among those for which the client was stimulable. Thus, word-final consonants would not be a treatment target, since the client does not yet show capacity to pronounce consonants in that environment. Not until later in development, when consonants begin to emerge word-finally, would they be likely treatment targets.

   b. **Step 2 (Promote Expansion).** Treatment targets are selected to expand the range of speech elements that a client shows some capacity to pronounce. For purposes of illustration, suppose the word-initial consonants for which the client is stimulable are [p], [t], and [s]. If a clinician wished only to select one treatment target, the following would play a role in the consideration: [p] would introduce voiceless consonants into the client's phonetic inventory, [t] would introduce voiceless consonants and a new place of production, and [s] would introduce voiceless consonants and a new place and manner of production. Wishing to maximally expand the client's speech-making capacities, the likely treatment target selection would be [s], [t] would be the next most likely, and [p] would be the least likely (again, for purposes of illustration it is assumed that a clinician was limited to selecting only one treatment target).

E. Stage 3

The same method used to select treatment targets for a client early in Stage 3 is often used for a client in Stage 2. This method is useful throughout Stage 3 for clients with more limited attention and cognitive skills. A least knowledge method sometimes succeeds well with a client in later Stage 3 who has relatively intact cognitive and attention abilities.

F. Stage 4

A least knowledge approach becomes less clinically relevant for clients in Stage 4, because generalization to untreated sounds is less relevant when errors arise only in a few late-acquired consonants, consonant clusters, and unstressed syllables in more difficult multisyllabic words.

VIII. NUMBER OF TREATMENT TARGETS

Typically, only one treatment target is facilitated per session. This is because many clients find it confusing to receive treatment on more than one target in a single session. The exceptions to this general rule are clients who require a flexible approach (see next section) or when a clinician chooses a multiple phoneme approach (see discussion of articulation programs later in this chapter).

More than one treatment target can be facilitated over the same period of weeks or months. Two general strategies are used to help decide how many treatment targets to facilitate simultaneously: training deep and training wide (Elbert & Gierut, 1986). *Training deep* provides intensive treatment on one or two treatment targets, which allows proportionally more attention to be devoted to each treatment target than is the case when a greater number of treatment targets are selected. *Training wide* provides treatment on three or more treatment targets, which offers the client more opportunities to discover relationships between targets than if a training deep strategy is selected. A client who receives treatment on [p], [d], and [s], for example, is being exposed to contrasts in place of production (bilabial and alveolar), voicing (voiced and voiceless), and manner (stop and fricative).

A. Stages 1 through 3

Training wide is appropriate with clients in the first three stages of articulation and phonological development due to these clients' greater number of errors and shorter attention spans.

B. Stage 4

Although training wide is appropriate for all clients, a training deep approach often appears better suited to clients in Stage 4 who have sufficient attention spans to concentrate on a treatment target for an extended time period.

IX. CHANGING TREATMENT TARGETS

An important consideration is determining when to change from one treatment target to another during the course of treatment. In this book, three criteria for changing treatment targets are flexibility, time, and percentage.

A. Flexibility

If a flexible criterion is used, a treatment target is facilitated until the client becomes disinterested, at which point another treatment target is introduced. An illustration of a flexible criterion is the statement: "Treatment for [b] will continue for as long as the client's interest is sustained."

B. Time

If a time criterion is used, a certain amount of treatment time (typically, 60 minutes) is devoted to each target (Hodson, 1989). After that time is completed, treatment shifts to another treatment target. After treatment for all targets is completed (called a cycle), the treatment targets are treated again (a second cycle). Cycles are repeated until all treatment targets are remediated, which typically requires from three to four cycles (approximately 1 year of treatment). An illustration of a time criterion is the statement, "Treatment for [t] will be provided for 1 hour in cycle 1."

C. Percentage

If a percentage criterion is used, a treatment target is facilitated until a certain percentage of correct production is reached. An illustration of a percentage criterion is the statement: "Correct production of [s] in word initial position 75% of the time."

D. Stage 1

A flexible approach can be extremely useful with clients in Stage 1 and other clients whose cognitive abilities do not permit successful performance using more structured criteria. For example, the short-term goal might be to facilitate reduplicated babbling, and the possible treatment targets might be reduplicated CV syllables that begin with [b], [d], or [m]. The clinician would then come to each treatment session ready to facilitate any of the treatment targets, depending on the client's inclinations.

E. Stage 2

A time approach is an appropriate criterion for many clients in Stage 2. For example, a clinician might provide 1 hour of treatment for each treatment target. Clients who lack the cognitive and attention abilities for a time criterion are treated using a flexible approach. For example, the client's short-term goal might be to eliminate Prevocalic Voicing, and the possible treatment targets might be [t] in *tea* and *toe*, [p] in *pie*, and [f] in *food*. The clinician would then come to each treatment session ready to facilitate any of the treatment targets.

F. Stage 3

Time is an appropriate criterion for changing treatment targets with the vast majority of clients in Stage 3. For example, the speech of a client in transition between Stages 3 and 4 might contain Gliding and errors affecting several individual sounds, including Stopping of [s] and Devoicing of word-final [b]. A cycle for such a client might include an hour each of treatment for [l], [r], [s], and word-final [b]. Lastly, clients in Stage 3 who lack the cognitive and attention abilities needed for a time criterion are provided treatment using the flexible approach described for clients in Stages 1 and 2. Clients in Stage 3 with exceptionally good attention skills are provided treatment using a percentage criterion.

G. Stage 4

A percentage criterion is appropriate for most clients in Stage 4, although a time criterion may be needed for clients in Stage 4 who have limited attention and cognitive abilities. For example, a cycle for a client in Stage 4 might include an hour each of treatment for [s], [r], and unstressed syllables in multisyllabic words.

X. LINGUISTIC LEVEL AND PHONETIC ENVIRONMENTS

Treatment targets typically are introduced in a single linguistic level in either one or two phonetic environments. The possible linguistic levels are isolated sounds, nonsense syllables, words, phrases, sentences, and spontaneous speech; the possible phonetic environments are word positions (initial, medial, final) and syllable positions (syllable initial, final, intervocalic, stressed and unstressed syllable, etc.).

A. Stage 1

Information in this section is not appropriate for clients in Stage 1.

B. Stages 2 through 4

1. Linguistic Level. The preferred level for introducing treatment targets for clients in Stages 2 through 4 is the isolated word, because it is the lowest linguistic level that most closely approximates the skills the client uses outside the clinic setting. The exception to this general rule occurs when phonetic placement and shaping techniques are employed to introduce a treatment target to a client in Stage 4. More often, however, isolated sounds and nonsense syllables serve best as prompts during treatment for selected clients in Stage 3 and with most clients in Stage 4 who experience failure at the word level. If the client, for example, experiences failure with [d] in *dog,* the clinician might prompt, "This is the [di] sound. Say [di]. Good. Now say [dog]."

If a client already successfully produces a treatment target at the word level, treatment targets can be introduced at the level of the phrase, sentence, or spontaneous speech. A client, for example, might be asked to tell a story based on characters whose names contain the treatment target. Alternately, a client and clinician might play a barrier game in which the objects contain the treatment target (see Chapter 7 for additional suggestions for activities to facilitate treatment targets in phrases, sentences, and spontaneous speech).

2. Phonetic Environments. Phonetic environment (syllable position, word position, and nearby sounds) is critically important to the production of many sounds. The most likely phonetic environments in which to introduce treatment targets are listed in Table 6–4. However, as with most clinical enterprises, the clinician does best to follow the client's lead in selecting both the number and types of phonetic environments in which to introduce treatment targets. If, for example, the client is more successful producing velar stops between vowels, then treatment should begin by facilitating velar stops in that position. Similarly, if the client appears stimulable for [t] in both word-initial and word-final positions, the clinician may consider beginning treatment in both positions.

Table 6–4. "Best bets" for environments within which to establish treatment targets.

Treatment Targets	Environments
All treatment targets	Establish in CV, CVCV, or VC syllables
All treatment targets	Establish in stressed syllables
Consonants	Except for the instances noted below, establish consonants in the beginning of words
Voiced	Establish either between vowels or in the beginning of words and syllables
Voiceless	Establish at the end of syllables and words
Velar stops	Establish at the end of words or at the beginning of words before a back vowel
Alveolar stops	Establish at the beginning of words before front vowels
Voiced fricatives	Establish between vowels

Source: From *Child Phonology: A Book of Exercises for Students* (p. 78) by K. Bleile, (1991b), San Diego, CA: Singular Publishing Group, with permission.

XI. GENERALIZATION AND MAINTENANCE

Treatment targets are selected based on a clinician's treatment philosophy in conjunction with the clinician's perception of the nature of the client's articulation and phonological disorder. For example, a clinician who believes that intelligibility is of primary importance is likely to select treatment targets that have the greatest impact on that aspect of articulation and phonological development. (See Chapter 5 for the effects of consonants and error patterns on perceived intelligibility.) Similarly, a clinician who believes that degree of developmental delay is of primary importance is likely to select treatment targets that have the greatest impact on the client's development delay (see Chapter 5 for age norms). Finally, a clinician who believes that the social and educational impact of articulation and phonological disorders is of primary importance is likely to select treatment targets with the greatest effect on the client's social and educational well-being.

A common concern to all clinical philosophies is treatment target generalization and maintenance.

A. Generalization

Two types of generalization exist: linguistic generalization, and generalization to other persons and settings.

1. Linguistic Generalization. Some clients easily generalize results of treatment to untreated sounds, linguistic levels, and words. For most clients, however, generalization happens more slowly and less completely. Although no procedures are guaranteed to promote generalization in all clients, distinctive feature approaches, error pattern approaches, least knowledge methods, and training wide maximize the chance that generalization will occur to other sounds. When the short-term goal is reduction of Fronting, for example, the hope is that the results of success on one sound will generalize to other sounds affected by the Fronting pattern. If, however, generalization does not occur, a clinician needs to treat the individual sounds affected by the Fronting pattern.

2. Generalization to Other Settings and Persons. Generalization to other persons and settings is facilitated through treatment activities that reflect real-life situations and use real words of high functional value to a client. The following ideas help promote generalization to other settings and persons:

- Hold frequent meetings with caregivers and other professionals to keep them informed about treatment goals and progress.

- Have a client's caregivers occasionally attend and assist in treatment sessions.

- With clients in Stages 3 and 4, give the caregiver a list of 10 words containing a target sound and ask that 2 minutes a day be spent having the client say each word. To avoid the caregiver becoming "a teacher," do not provide this suggestion until the client is approximately 80% correct in the clinic setting in producing the treatment target at the word level.

- With clients in Stages 3 and 4, prepare a 2-minute audio tape of words containing the client's treatment targets and ask the client's parent to play it to the client.

- With clients in Stages 3 and 4, ask the caregiver to place stickers around the house as reminders of treatment targets.

B. Maintenance

Two important issues in maintenance of clinical gains are changing linguistic levels and family involvement.

1. Changing Linguistic Levels. Generally, treatment continues at one linguistic level until a client produces the treatment target correctly 75% of the time before beginning treatment on the next linguistic level. A client, for example, should produce word-initial [t] correctly 75% of the time at the level of the isolated word before beginning treatment for the sound at the phrase level is begun. The criterion of 75% is chosen because at that point the sound is acquired and, in most cases, is likely to progress to 100% correct without additional treatment. When a client is able to produce all treatment targets correctly 75% to 90% of the time in spontaneous speech, treatment is generally discontinued; the higher percentage is used if the clinician is concerned that the client will regress after treatment is ended, as happens too frequently over the long months of summer vacation.

2. Family Involvement. Sometimes treatment success does not last after the client is discharged. With younger clients, the most important means of maintaining hard-won treatment successes after discharge is securing the cooperation of the client's family. This is accomplished through frequent meetings during which the purposes and goals of treatment are carefully explained and, if needed, home programs are developed. With clients in later stages of articulation and phonological development, both family involvement and ongoing exercises designed to develop the client's self-monitoring skills throughout treatment are the best guarantees that treatment gains will not be lost.

XII. ADMINISTRATIVE DECISIONS

Treatment requires the clinician to make administrative decisions about the organization of treatment sessions, including whether to provide treatment individually or in groups, the frequency and length of sessions, types of activities, and length of individual treatment activities.

A. Types of Sessions

Treatment can be provided either in individual or group sessions. Individual sessions consist of a single client and are often preferred during the early stages of treatment when the clinician is introducing new treatment targets. Group sessions typically consist of three to five clients of similar ages and developmental levels and are often preferred in the middle and late stages of therapy, when goals shift from introducing new treatment targets to helping the client to generalize and maintain what has been learned.

B. Frequency of Sessions

Treatment for clients at all levels of articulation and phonological development typically is provided from two to five times a week. Some evidence exists that intensive therapy (four to five times a week) is slightly more efficient for clients in Stage 4 than less intensive therapy (twice a week) for a longer number of weeks (Bernthal & Bankson, 1998).

C. Length of Sessions

Individual therapy sessions range from 10 to 15 minutes to 1 hour. Group sessions typically range from 30 to 45 minutes.

D. Length of Activities in Sessions

Individual activities in sessions may last from less than a minute to nearly 30 minutes.

E. Format of Activities

There are four basic types of activities: drill, drill play, structured play, and play (Shriberg & Kwiatkowski, 1982).

1. *Drill* involves the clinician presenting material for mass practice by the client in activities such as repeating lists of words, naming pictures, and so on.

2. *Drill play* involves drills presented in the context of games such as spinning wheels, game boards, and so on.

3. *Structured play* is drill play presented in play-like activities such as playing house, shopping, parking toy cars in a garage, and so on.

4. *Play* is child-oriented activity during which acquisition of targets is facilitated.

F. Stage 1

Decisions about treatment sessions are arrived at in conjunction with the client's caregivers. The options for treatment sessions and activities are to provide treatment on an individual or group basis from two to five times a week. Individual sessions typically last from 5 to 15 minutes, and group sessions typically last approximately 30 minutes. The client's attention for specific activities in treatment sessions typically ranges from a few seconds to 1 to 2 minutes. The preferred format for activities is play.

G. Stage 2

Decisions about treatment sessions are arrived at in conjunction with the client's caregivers. The options for treatment sessions and activities are to provide treatment individually or in early intervention groups from two to five times a week. Individual sessions typically last from 20 to 30 minutes, and early intervention sessions typically last from approximately 30 to 45 minutes. The client's attention for specific activities in treatment sessions typically ranges from a few minutes to 10 minutes. The preferred format for activities is play.

H. Stage 3

Decisions about treatment sessions are arrived at in conjunction with the client's caregivers. The options for treatment sessions and activities are to provide treatment in individual or group sessions from two to five times a week. Individual and group sessions typically last from 30 to 45 minutes. Individual activities in treatment sessions may last up to 10 minutes. The preferred formats for activities are structured play and drill play. Research indicates that drill play is more effective and efficient with clients in Stage 3 than structured play and is equally as effective as drill (Shriberg & Kwiatowski, 1982).

I. Stage 4

The options for treatment sessions and activities are to provide treatment from two to five times a week in individual or group sessions. Individual sessions typically last from 30 to 45 minutes, and group sessions typically last approximately 45 minutes to 1 hour. Individual activities in treatment sessions are likely to last 10 to 15 minutes. The preferred formats for activities are drill play and, with more mature clients, drill.

XIII. COMPLETE INTERVENTION PROGRAMS

A number of complete intervention programs have been developed to treat clients with articulation and phonological disorders. Although these programs are sometimes used in their entirety, more often clinicians borrow an idea here and adapt a procedure there as clinical need arises. The following is a summary of the major intervention programs presently in use in English-speaking countries. The programs are organized into two subsections: articulation (motor) and phonology (language) (Bernthal & Bankson, 1998). Before attempting any of the programs summarized below, the reader is referred to the references for detailed explanations of principles and procedures.

Articulation and Phonological Programs

Although there are crucial differences between articulation and phonological programs, few would debate that speech involves both motor control (articulation) and language knowledge (phonology). Instead, the debate in our field is over the relative importance of these two concepts in the remediation of speech disorders.

A. Articulation Programs

Articulation programs share the assumption that speech problems are largely motoric in origin—a reasonable assumption, considering that these programs were largely developed to treat school-age children with errors affecting individual, late-acquired consonants and consonant clusters. The most influential articulation programs are the Van Riper approach, the Paired-stimuli program, the Sensory-motor program, Multiple Phoneme program, and the Motoric Automatization of Articulatory Performance Program.

1. Van Riper Approach (Traditional Approach)

a. **Reference.** Van Riper, C. (1978). *Speech correction: Principles and methods* (6th ed.). Englewood Cliffs, NJ: Prentice-Hall.

b. **Overview.** The Van Riper approach (also called the Traditional Approach), first published in the mid-1930s, is a compilation of clinical ideas developed during the early years of the 20th century. The assumptions underlying the Van Riper approach are that articulation and phonological errors may result from both faulty perception abilities and inadequate oral motor skills. Treatment consists of both perceptual and production training. Production training often begins with isolated sounds or nonsense syllables in order to avoid interference with existing "speech habits." Treatment proceeds in small increments (a most knowledge method), so that the client may experience as much success as possible.

c. **Comment.** Throughout most of the 20th century the Van Riper approach was the most widely accepted clinical model for treating articulation and phonological disorders, but it declined in popularity as clinical populations grew ever younger and more intensely involved. Still, the Van Riper approach remains a viable clinical alternative with many clients in Stage 4, the clinical population for which it was chiefly intended. The Van Riper approach is less successful with clients in Stages 2 and 3, both as a model of articulation and phonological disorders and as a set of practical treatment procedures.

2. Paired-stimuli (Key Word) Program

a. **Reference.** Irwin, J., & Weston, A. (1975). The paired-stimuli monograph. *Acta Symbolica, 6,* 1–76.

Evolution of an Idea

The founders of our profession knew that sounds belonged to sound classes, although they tended not to emphasize this in clinical practice because it was not pertinent to the care of their clients, the vast majority of whom experienced speech problems affecting individual consonants and consonant clusters. Interest in sound classes grew in the late 1960s and

(continued)

1970s, as the caseloads of speech-language clinicans increasingly came to include preschoolers, the majority of whom had errors affecting entire sound classes. At that point, clinicians became concerned about the enormous amount of time required if each sound needed to be treated individually.

b. **Overview.** The Paired-stimuli program was developed based on principles of behavioral psychology. The assumption underlying the Paired-stimuli program is that success in producing a sound embedded in a word can be generalized to other words containing the sound. A key word contains a treatment target that is produced correctly 9 out of 10 times in either the initial or final position. If a key word is not found during the assessment the clinician facilitates the acquisition of the treatment target and then transfers it to a key word. The clinician then selects 10 words that have the same error in the same word position. A picture of the key word is placed in the center of the table and the training words are placed around it. The client is instructed to say the key word, which is then reinforced, followed by a training word, which is not reinforced unless it is produced correctly. Training proceeds until all of the training words are produced (called one training string). Three training strings are completed in one half-hour training session.

c. **Comment.** The most interesting aspect of the Paired-stimuli program is that it provides a means to generalize correct production of a treatment target in one word to other words. Although conceived as a behaviorist program, the Paired stimuli program might be modified by deemphasizing the reinforcement aspects of the program and offering the client instructions that rely more on his or her linguistic abilities. A session, for example, might begin with activities to facilitate the client's awareness of the treatment target and to help the client to identify the correct production of the treatment target in a key word, for example, [s] in *sun*. Next, the clinician might place pictures of the key word and training words in a circle, as described above, explaining, "Let's play a game. In the game, first you say *sun* and then one of the other words, going around the circle until we say all the words. Try to say the words on the outside with the same snake sound as *sun*." The instructions, of course, could be modified, simplified, or expanded based on the client's interests and level of cognitive development.

3. Sensory-motor Program

a. **References.** McDonald, E. (1964). *Articulation testing and treatment: A sensory-motor approach.* Pittsburgh, PA: Stanwix House.

Shine, R. (1989). Articulatory production training: A sensory-motor approach. In. N. Creaghead, P. Newman, & W. Secord (Eds.), *Assessment and remediation of articulatory and phonological disorders* (pp. 355–359). Columbus, OH: Charles E. Merrill.

b. **Overview.** The Sensory-motor program was developed in the mid-1960s. It remains influential today largely because of its contention that the syllable is the basic unit of speech production (a controversial but popular idea) and because of the importance it places on phonetic environments in assessment and treatment. Treatment consists of production practice of treatment targets in various syllable contexts in increasing levels of phonetic complexity. A client, for example, might be taught [t] before front vowels in nonsense CV syllables. Treatment might proceed to other vowel contexts, other syllable positions, and other speech levels, such as multisyllabic utterances. Practicing motor skills is believed by the authors to improve perceptual skills as well; therefore, perceptual training is not provided.

c. **Comment.** The emphasis that the Sensory-motor program placed on syllable and phonetic contexts foreshadowed later phonological approaches. The steps in a Sensory-motor program can be time-consuming to complete, and many clients are bored by its reliance on phonetic drills. Nonetheless, the program provides an option for use with more mature clients with intact cognitive skills.

4. Multiple Phoneme Program

a. **References.** McCabe, R., & Bradley, D. (1975). Systematic multiple phonemic approach to articulation therapy. *Acta Symbolica, 6,* 1–18.

Bradley, D. (1989). A systematic multiple-phoneme approach. In N. Creaghead, P. Newman, & W. Secord (Eds.), *Assessment and remediation of articulatory and phonological disorders* (pp. 305–322). Columbus, OH: Charles E. Merrill.

b. Overview. The Multiple Phoneme program is a behaviorally oriented treatment method originally developed for children with repaired cleft palates. The Multiple Phoneme program is similar to the Van Riper method, with the major exception that as its name implies, the Multiple Phoneme program allows more than one sound to be treated in a single treatment session. The authors place great emphasis on the need to collect ongoing data during treatment sessions.

c. Comments. The Multiple Phoneme program represents an early attempt to provide treatment to more than one sound at a time, an issue of primary importance for clients who have more severe articulation and phonological disorders. The program is rooted strongly in behaviorism and would be difficult to attempt without at least some acceptance of that theory. The program requires that the client know "letters" or phonetic symbols, which makes its use difficult with virtually all preschoolers. Finally, many younger school-age children find it confusing to receive treatment on more than one sound in a single treatment session.

5. Motoric Automatization of Articulatory Performance Program

a. Reference. Hoffman, P., Schuckers, G., & Daniloff, R. (1989). *Children's phonetic disorders: Theory and treatment.* Boston: Little, Brown.

b. Overview. This program (its somewhat cumbersome name is henceforth abbreviated MAP for Motoric Automatization Program) represents a recent attempt to provide treatment of speech problems from an articulation perspective. The primary goal of MAP is to provide practice in executing speech movements. This is achieved in two overlapping steps: stimulability and rehearsal. In the first step, the clinician elicits speech through imitation, which gives the client some experience of success as well as the opportunity to observe and imitate the clinician's demonstration. During this stage, the clinician also produces sounds with exaggeration (e.g., lots of lip rounding for labials) to give the client practice in manipulating the articulators in response to the clinician's model.

In the rehearsal step, the client practices treatment targets in increasingly complex linguistic levels and phonetic environments, including nonsense syllables, words and word pairs, sentences, and narratives. To help the client become aware of his or her speech errors, the clinician practices saying treatment targets as the client would. Other rehearsal activities include providing the client information on physiology and anatomy, viewing productions in a mirror, and listening to his or her speech on audio or video tapes.

c. Comment. MAP is an intelligent adaptation of an articulation approach to the treatment of clients with articulation and phonological disorders. As such, MAP offers a valuable treatment option for clients in Stage 4 with sufficient cognitive and attention abilities to reflect on their speech and to benefit from extensive motor practice.

B. Phonological Programs

Articulation approaches, which dominated the care of speech disorders for most of the 20th century, began to lose their appeal for many clinicians in the 1970s. The reason for this was that the primary tenets of articulation approaches—emphasis on individual sounds, phonetic drill, treatment of sounds in isolation and in nonsense syllables, improvements in small increments of change—although well suited to higher functioning clients with a few errors in late-acquired consonants and consonant clusters, proved far less useful with newer populations just appearing on the clinical horizon, many of whom were more severely involved preschoolers with speech problems affecting entire classes of sounds. Phonological approaches gained in popularity in the 1970s largely because their emphasis on sound as an aspect of language offered a means to treat the newer, more involved populations.

As indicated earlier in this chapter, currently two major types of phonological approaches exist: distinctive feature approaches (which attempt to encourage generalization based on the membership of sounds in sound classes) and phonological process approaches (which attempt to encourage generalization based on errors that classes of sounds undergo). Currently, the most influential distinctive feature program is that proposed by Blache (1989), and the most influential phonological process programs are the Cycles program, Metaphon, and Easy Does It For Phonology. An approach called contrast therapy is used in both some distinctive feature and phonological process programs. Contrast therapy activities are a loosely organized set of facilitative techniques rather than a treatment program and they are discussed in Section IV (Word Pairs) in Chapter 7. Appendix 7B contains a relatively extensive list of word pairs for use in contrast therapy activities. Appendix 6A contains a summary of recent approaches based on word pairs (minimal pairs), with special emphasis on a multiple opposition intervention approach.

1. Blache's Distinctive Feature Program

a. Reference. Blache, S. (1989). A distinctive feature approach. In N. Creaghead, P. Newman, & W. Secord (Eds.), *Assessment and remediation of articulatory and phonological disorders* (pp. 361–382). Columbus, OH: Charles E. Merrill.

b. Overview. Distinctive feature approaches represented a first attempt to apply linguistic theory to the treatment of persons with articulation and phonological disorders. Early distinctive feature programs (Costello & Onstein, 1976; McReynolds & Engmann, 1975; McReynolds & Bennett, 1972) were actually hybrids of phonological and articulation approaches—the distinctive features used to promote generalization were phonological, and the activities used in treatment were motor-based. Although pioneering in their efforts and influential in their time, the first distinctive feature programs are no longer in wide use.

The most influential distinctive feature program today is Blache's (1989). In Blache's approach, sounds are taught as contrastive units within words using contrast therapy activities (see Chapter 7, Section IV. Treatment proceeds in four major steps. In Step 1, the clinician assesses the client's knowledge of the meanings of the words that are to be used in treatment. A client whose treatment target was [p], for example, might be shown pictures of a pan and a man, and asked, "Point to the one you use to cook. Point to the one that is another word for boy." In Step 2, the client is tested to determine if he or she can discriminate between word pairs differing by a single sound. A client, for example, might be shown the pictures of the pan and man, and asked to point to the picture of the pan. In Step 3, the client is taught to distinguish between the word pairs in speech production. A client, for example, might be asked to say *pan,* and the clinician then picks up the picture card that matches the client's pronunciation. To illustrate, if the client pronounced pan as man, the clinician would pick up the picture of the man. In Step 4, after the client can pronounce the treatment target at the word level, the word is placed in increasingly complex linguistic contexts, such as after a definite article, in three-word sentences, four-word sentences, and so on.

c. Comment. Blache's distinctive feature program represents the most recent attempt to apply distinctive feature theory to intervention with persons with speech problems. Blache's program (as well as the other distinctive feature programs cited above) utilizes distinctive features borrowed from linguistic theory rather than the familiar place, manner, and voicing distinctions used in this book and elsewhere (Williams, 1993). As several authors have observed, linguistic-based distinctive feature systems are intended to describe cross-language universals, and they are not always ideally suited to describing the speech of persons with articulation and phonological disorders (Folkins & Bleile, 1990; Parker, 1976). Blache's distinctive feature program is appropriate for selected clients in Stage 3 and clients in Stage 4.

2. Cycles Program

a. Reference. Hodson, B., & Paden, E. (1991). *Targeting intelligible speech.* Austin, TX: Pro-Ed.

b. Overview. The Cycles program is the most widely used phonological process approach in the United States. As its name suggests, the primary concept underlying this program is the cycle, which is a time period during which all error patterns that need remediation are facilitated in succession. Cycles last from 5 to 16 weeks, and, typically, three to six cycles (30–40 hours at 40–60 minutes per week) are usually required for a client to become intelligible. Error patterns are targeted for remediation based on percentage of occurrence (40% or greater), effect on intelligibility, and stimulability. Sounds in error patterns are selected for treatment based on stimulability. Typically, each sound in an error pattern receives one hour of therapy per cycle before the clinician goes on to the next sound in the error pattern. All error patterns targeted for remediation receive treatment in each cycle. Only one error pattern is targeted during a treatment session. Treatment activities consist of auditory bombardment, therapeutic play, and drill play to encourage production; probes to test for improvement and generalization; and a short home program for families.

c. Comment. Perhaps the most important insight of the Cycles program is its proposal that time rather than percentage correct is a better criterion for when to change treatment targets for most clients in Stage 2 and clients in Stage 3. The use of a time criterion appears to better replicate the gradual nature of articulation and phonological acquisition; a time criterion also appears better suited to the attention skills of a client in Stage 3 than does keeping a client on a task until a certain percentage criterion is obtained. Typically, the Cycles program does not utilize contrast therapy activities, although nothing in principle forbids doing so (Hodson, 1989). Tyler (1993) suggests that contrast therapy activities—whether as part of a Cycles program or as part of another approach—are more appropriate for clients who have relatively intact cognitive skills.

3. Metaphon Therapy

a. References. Dean, E., & Howell, J. (1986). Developing linguistic awareness: A theoretically based approach to phonological disorders. *British Journal of Disorders of Communication, 1,* 223–238.

Dean, E., Howell, J., Hill, A., & Waters, D. (1990). *Metaphon resource pack.* Windsor, UK: NFER-Nelson.

b. Overview. Metaphon therapy (metaphon is an abbreviation of metaphonology) was developed in the mid-1980s, and although Metaphon is not yet well known to most American speech-language clinicians, it has already found a receptive audience in Ireland and Great Britain. The primary tenet of Metaphon therapy is that phonological learning involves the client becoming aware of the contrastive nature of phonemes (Dean, Howell, Waters, & Reid, 1995).

Metaphon therapy devotes great attention to teaching the client how to modify sounds to be more easily understood. Many activities used in Metaphon Therapy to achieve this result are already familiar to most speech-language clinicians, including the use of metaphors for sounds (e.g., [s] might be called the "hissing sound") and contrast therapy activities. The most unique aspects of Metaphon are its heavy reliance on facilitative techniques to increase metalinguistic awareness and its tying of metalinguistics with a phonological approach. Another noteworthy aspect of Metaphon therapy is that it allows the client and clinician to negotiate the choice of metaphors to be used in treatment.

c. Comments

Metaphon therapy offers an interesting treatment option for clients in Stage 3 and Stage 4. The authors of Metaphon therapy have conducted a number of single-subject design experiments to test the effectiveness of their program and presently are engaged in a large-scale study to demonstrate its efficacy (Dean, Howell, & Waters, 1993).

4. Easy Does It for Phonology

a. Reference. Blodgett, E., & Miller, V. (1989). *Easy Does It For Phonology.* East Moline, IL: LinguiSystems.

b. Overview. *Easy Does It For Phonology* (henceforth abbreviated EDIP) is a relatively new program that combines aspects of several articulation, distinctive feature, and phonological process approaches. The EDIP program consists of four steps: (1) The client is bombarded with stimulus items so he or she becomes aware of the distinctive feature being omitted or distorted; (2) the client is taught that the presence or absence of a distinctive feature makes a difference in meaning; (3) the client learns to produce the target feature in various activities; and (4) the client learns to produce the target feature and contrast it with his or her phonological process. A very worthwhile contribution of the authors is the development of simple metaphors to refer to consonant clusters, multisyllabic words, and word positions (see Table 7–3).

c. Comment. EDIP offers a treatment option for clients in Stages 3 and 4 with relatively intact cognitive skills. EDIP combines principles from articulation, distinctive feature, and phonological process approaches. EDIP's metaphors for consonant clusters, multisyllabic words, and word positions are likely to find wide clinical use.

XIV. ASSESSMENT OF TREATMENT PROGRESS

Assessing the effectiveness of treatment is essential in managing all clients, not least because periodic assessments of progress are required by law, in most workplaces, and for reimbursement by insurance companies. The need for information on treatment outcome was listed as the highest health care priority by a recent American Speech-Language-Hearing Association task force (Task Force on Health Care, 1993). The two major options to assess treatment progress are pre- and post-tests and ongoing information gathering.

Why Not Assess Progress Using Standardized Tests?

Standardized assessment instruments are seldom used to evaluate treatment progress, because the number of items that assess treatment targets is likely to be small. To illustrate, an assessment instrument testing 70 words is likely to contain only 3 or 4 words assessing [s], and only one of the words might assess [s] in word-initial position. If the clinician has spent a semester working on [s] in word-initial position, using the standardized assessment instrument will not show therapeutic gains.

A. Pre- and Post-tests

As the names suggest, pretests are administered prior to treatment (often as part of the assessment) and post-tests are administered at major junctures in treatment, often to determine if short- or long-term goals have been attained. Many clinicians prefer pre- and post-tests to assess treatment progress because they are quick and easy to administer and do not require attention to be directed away from the client during treatment sessions.

1. **Flexibility of Pre- and Post-tests.** Progress for any treatment target or treatment goal can be assessed using pre- and post-tests. A pre- and post-test for a client in Stage 1, for example, might assess the quantity or type of vocalizations produced during one or across several treatment sessions. Pre- and post-tests for a client in Stage 2, on the other hand, might assess the percentage of homonyms in the client's vocabulary or the number of sounds in the client's phonetic inventory. Similarly, a pre- and post-test for a client in Stage 3 might assess the percentage of occurrence of various error patterns, whereas a pre- and post-test for a client in Stage 4 might assess the percentage of correct productions of a sound on a picture naming task, or the number of correct productions of [sn] clusters in 1 minute of spontaneous speech describing a picture showing a "snow party." Results of pre- and post-tests are usually reported as percentage values. A

possible statement in a clinical report is, "The client was administered pre- and post-tests of [s] in word-initial position. The client scored 20% correct in the pre-test and 90% correct on the post-test."

2. **Examples.** Two quick and effective types of pre- and post-tests are word probes and judgment scales of severity and/or intelligibility. Many times a client receives both types of pre- and post-tests.

   a. **Word Probes.** The sound and error probes presented in Chapter 5 can easily be adapted into pre- and post-tests for clients in Stages 3 or 4. For example, a sound probe might indicate that a client was able to produce [s] 2 of 5 times word initially, and none of 5 times both between vowels and word-finally. This information could be used as the pre-test, and the probe would be given again at the completion of treatment as the post-test. (There is no "correct" number of words that should be included in a probe. A general rule of thumb is 10 words per treatment target.) Error probes also can be used as pre- and post-tests. For example, the client might demonstrate a Fronting pattern on 8 of 10 words (80%) during the pre-test and might demonstrate Fronting on 2 of 10 words (20%) on the post-test.

   b. **Intelligibility and Severity Testing.** Judgment scales of severity and intelligibility often serve as pre- and post-tests to assess treatment progress. Procedures to perform these measures were described in Chapter 5. If the judges are clinicians, three clinicians should be used, if possible. Clinical judgments of severity and intelligibility have the difficulties noted in Chapter 5, the chief of which is that the faster methods are highly subjective. Also, measures that show only a few degrees of disability may not be sufficiently sensitive to detect smaller increments of improvement. Results of intelligibility and severity judgment scales might be reported as, "Three of three trained speech-language clinicians judged the client to have a severe speech disorder before the onset of therapy. The client is now judged to have a mild speech disorder."

B. Ongoing Information Gathering

Although more time-consuming than pre- and post-tests, some clinicians collect ongoing information on the client's progress toward meeting a therapy objective. During each treatment session, for example, the clinician tabulates the client's rate of success, usually as a percentage value.

To illustrate, the clinician might tabulate that the client is 50% accurate in producing a treatment target during session 1, 58% accurate in session 2, 64% accurate in session 3, and so on. Ongoing information gathering has an important advantage over pre- and post-testing in that it allows the clinician to more closely monitor the client's treatment progress.

Consumer Interviews

In addition to the assessments described in this section, treatment progress is always assessed by asking the client (when applicable), family, and significant persons in the client's environment if they have noticed change. The results should be included in the clinical report.

C. Single-subject Design Experiments

Single-subject design experiments, while a type of ongoing information gathering procedure, are sufficiently complex to warrant separate consideration.

Single-subject design experiments constitute an attempt to put clinical endeavors on a more rigorous scientific footing. Although commonly employed in behavioral psychology, single-subject design experiments have not found their way into widespread clinical use in speech-language pathology, perhaps because they are time-consuming to perform and their use requires some specialized knowledge. The information below outlines the basic steps and logic behind one type of single-subject design experiment called a multiple baseline design. Before attempting such an experiment the reader is referred to the more complete discussions on this topic appearing in McReynolds and Kearns (1983).

1. **Introduction.** Single-subject design experiments provide a method to demonstrate that improvement in the client results from the clinician's treatment rather than from extraneous factors such as time and maturation.

2. **Multiple Baseline Design Experiments.** The type of single-subject design experiment that is most applicable to the clinical care of articulation and phonological disorders is called a multiple

baseline design. A multiple baseline design can be used to evaluate treatment if (1) the client has at least two potential treatment targets and (2) the client's treatment targets are not so closely related that, when the client treats one target, the other target will also improve. For example, [p] and [b] would probably not be suitable treatment targets in a single-subject design experiment, because in many cases when a clinician focuses on [p] (or [b]) the cognate also improves. Better treatment targets for a single-subject design experiment might be [p] and [s], because improving one would not be expected to improve the other.

3. **Components of Multiple Baseline Design Experiments.** Multiple baseline design experiments consist of two phases, called A (baseline) and B (treatment). During the baseline, no treatment on the treatment target is provided. The baseline and treatment phases each must be at least three intervals (usually treatment sessions) in length. For example, data are collected during baseline for at least three treatment sessions, and treatment is provided for at least the same (and most likely more) number of sessions. Changes in percentage values between the baseline and treatment phases are the means most frequently used to demonstrate treatment progress. The results of the experiment are usually displayed as a simple graph of the type shown in Figure 6–1.

4. **Steps in Carrying Out a Multiple Baseline Experiment.** The following steps are used during a multiple baseline experiment.

   a. **Selection.** Select at least two treatment targets that are not so closely related that the client's progress in achieving one target is likely to affect the other target.

   b. **Baseline.** Begin collecting baseline data on both targets during the first session. For example, ask the client to pronounce 20 words beginning with the first treatment target and 20 different words beginning with the second treatment target. Graph the data as percentage of correct productions. Continue to collect baseline data for both treatment targets during at least three sessions. If the client begins to show improvement on the first treatment target prior to the end of baseline, continue collection of baseline data until the percentage of correct productions is the same for two sessions in a row or until the last session of baseline shows fewer correct productions than the session that preceded it. The purpose of collecting the additional baseline data is to ensure that improvement is not

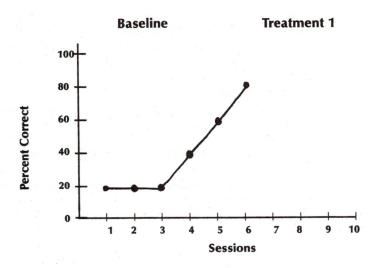

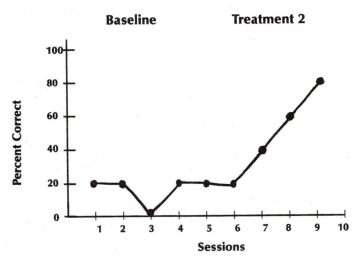

Figure 6–1. Example of a multiple baseline experiment.

due to factors other than treatment. If the client continues to improve without treatment, the clinician should abandon the experiment because the client may not need treatment for that treatment target.

c. **Treatment (First Treatment Target).** Begin treatment for the first treatment target while continuing to collect baseline data for the second treatment target.

d. **Treatment (Second Treatment Target).** After criterion (typically 75% correct) is reached for the first target, begin treatment for the second treatment target. Continue to provide treatment for the second treatment target until criterion is reached for it as well.

APPENDIX 6A
A Multiple Oppositions Intervention Approach

A. Lynn Williams

There have been several recent innovations in treatment approaches for children with articulation and phonological impairments. All are based on a contrastive model of intervention and therefore are variations of the minimal pair treatment approach that has been commonly used over the past several decades. These include maximal oppositions (Gierut, 1989; 1990); treatment of the empty set (Gierut, 1992); and multiple oppositions (Williams, 2000a; 2000b; 2003). These approaches differ with regard to the number of contrasts that are being trained at one time and the type of contrastive pairs that are constructed.

A comparison of the four contrastive approaches is provided in Table 6–5. The four approaches are compared with regard to the construction of sound contrasts, assumptions, and rationale. Williams (2002) presented this comparison for a child who substituted [g] for /d/.

As shown in this table, three of the treatment approaches utilize single contrastive sound pairs. The fourth approach, multiple oppositions, addresses the extensive loss of adult sounds that is common in severe speech disorders by utilizing multiple contrastive sound pairs. For multiple oppositions, the larger, integrated treatment sets result in intervention that addresses several error sounds from one rule set. This intervention model is based on holistic, systemic sound learning that can be accounted for by principles of distributed learning.

A number of divergent sources provide a theoretical rationale for implementing larger/integrated treatment sets for phonological disorders. For example, theories of learning, neural theory of attention and learning (cf., Milner, 1999), and cognitive science (cf., Lepore & Pylyshyn, 1999) can inform the structure of intervention for children with phonological impairments. Recent developments in neurosciences and computational frameworks suggest that learning and acquisition are interactive processes (cf., Elman, Bates, Johnson, Karmiloff-Smith, Parisi, & Plunkett, 1997).

Connectionist models also have been used to examine the ways in which change occurs and what drives mechanisms to change (cf., Judd, 1990). Within a connectionist framework, the smaller, less complex treatment sets of minimal pairs predict that learning is linear and constrained by generalization

Table 6–5. Comparison of Contrastive Phonological Intervention Approaches (Williams, 2002).

Minimal Pairs (Weiner, 1981)	Maximal Oppositions (Gierut, 1989; 1990)	Empty Set (Gierut, 1992)	Multiple Oppositions (Williams, 2000)
Single contrastive pairings of child's error with target sound	Single contrastive pairings of comparison sound with target sound (known ~ unknown)	Single contrastive pairings of two target sounds (unknown ~ unknown)	Multiple contrastive pairings of child's error with several target sounds from across a rule set
g ~ d / # ____	m ~ d / # ____	r ~ d / # ____	(see diagram)

g is contrasted with: d, f, tS, st

go ~ doe	moo ~ dew	row ~ doe	goo → dew, food, chew, stew
gate ~ date	more ~ door	ray ~ day	
gown ~ down	mate ~ date	rye ~ dye	

gore → door, four, chore, store

(continued)

Table 6–5. (*Continued*)

Minimal Pairs (Weiner, 1981)	Maximal Oppositions (Gierut, 1989; 1990)	Empty Set (Gierut, 1992)	Multiple Oppositions (Williams, 2000)
Assumptions:	Assumptions:	Assumptions:	Assumptions:
1. child will fill in the gap between what is trained and what still needs to be learned across the rule set 2. adult-based categories (e.g., backing) are the basis for the child's error and sound organization	1. phonemic distinctiveness (i.e., salience) of comparison sound will facilitate learning 2. child will fill in the gap of missing phonemic features (i.e., frication, voicing, coronal) based on distinctiveness of contrastive pairing	1. phonemic distinctiveness (i.e., salience) of two target sounds will facilitate learning 2. child will fill in the inventory gaps based on distinctiveness of contrastive pairings and learning two new sounds simultaneously	1. learning is facilitated by the size and nature of linguistic "chunks" presented to child (learning of the whole is greater than the sum of its parts) 2. learning is a dynamic interaction between child's unique sound system and intervention
Predicts target contrast will generalize to other phonetically similar sounds affected by child's error pattern	Predicts that target contrast will create system-wide change on basis of child filling in phonemic gaps	Predicts that target contrast will create greater system-wide change on basis of child filling in phonemic gaps and learning more than one phoneme at a time	Predicts learning will be generalized across a rule set (i.e., learning will generalize to obstruents and clusters collapsed to [g] in the 1:17 phoneme collapse) and result in system-wide restructuring

of similarity of input patterns. Conversely, the larger, more complex treatment sets of multiple oppositions predict that learning is a non-linear, dynamic, and interactive process. In this view, the child's sound system is represented as an entire configuration of connected, overlapping, and differentially weighted units. As a result, the whole is not merely the sum of the parts, but rather an entire configuration. This configuration is different from its component parts and therefore represents the fact that the child knows it as a unified network and not as a collection of discrete sounds. Multiple oppositions is based on the assumption that learning is facilitated by the size and nature of the linguistic "chunks" that are presented as input to the child's sound system. Thus, principles of distributed learning and activation of similar patterns of units create a cascading effect throughout the network by utilizing a variety of treatment exemplars (or "linguistic chunks"). The fact that the treatment exemplars are integrated across a rule set will serve to strengthen new representations and stabilize neural representations, thereby resulting in a change in the original network.

Differences in learning that result from differences in treatment approaches may relate to differences in the size of the linguistic "chunks" that are presented to children in treatment. The larger/integrated treatment sets of multiple oppositions involve intervention *across* a child's entire rule rather than to an isolated aspect of the child's system or rule. In addition, the larger/integrated treatment sets take into account the unique sound system and phonological organization that the child created to accommodate a limited system relative to the adult sound system. Therefore, not only are more sounds trained (i.e., larger treatment sets), but the integrated treatment sets comprise target sounds from across the child's error rule. Focusing the child's attention on their error pattern in this manner confronts them with the extent of phonologic change that must be achieved while exposing the child to the relatedness of all the target sounds to their error pattern. The distributed input of the larger/integrated treatment sets therefore enlarges the frame of relevant learning. In this regard, the larger/integrated treatment input represents the "gestalt" of learning that needs to occur. The assumption is that the whole of the learning task is greater than the sum of its parts.

Williams (2000a) proposed that the complexity of the input with regard to the size and nature of the treatment sets poses an interesting learnability question, as well as a question about the mechanisms of change. Specifically, is it easier to learn new sound contrasts and reorganize the sound system using the more complex input of larger/integrated treatment sets of the multiple oppositions approach or the less complex input of smaller/non-integrated treatment sets of the minimal pair approach? Two logical, though competing, hypotheses for the phonologic learnability associated with each approach can be considered.

The first hypothesis would indicate that smaller/non-integrated input is easier to learn. This is based on the fact that there is only a single contrast to be learned, therefore the focus in treatment is greater; there is less semantic load in terms of treatment exemplars; and there are less demands on attention and memory. Minimal pair therapy is based on the premise that the target contrast is generalizable to other phonetically similar sounds that are affected by the child's error pattern.

The opposing hypothesis would indicate that although the smaller/non-integrated treatment sets are less complex, the input would be relatively more difficult to learn and integrate phonemically. Although the child has only a single new contrast to learn, it is fragmented from a larger, more diverse rule pattern and therefore is more difficult to integrate into a new rule set. This second hypothesis suggests that larger/integrated treatment sets would present the child with the range and diversity of the new contrasts, which would facilitate rule discovery and increase generalization. The distributed input of the larger/integrated treatment sets therefore enlarges the frame of relevant learning. This assumption proposes that learnability of multiple sound contrasts across a rule will make it easier for a child to systematically reorganize his or her sound system than when intervention is provided on a single contrast that is isolated from the entire rule set. Thus, larger/integrated treatment sets would lead to greater generalization.

It is hypothesized that the larger and integrated treatment sets of the multiple opposition model will result in more new contrasts being added to the child's system and greater generalization than when single contrasts of minimal pairs are trained. Therefore, multiple oppositions has a potential advantage over the singular minimal pair model in terms of shortened length of treatment and improved intelligibility and teachability.

C H A P T E R

7

Facilitative Techniques

The following topics are discussed in this chapter:

I. OVERVIEW OF FACILITATIVE TECHNIQUES

The methods employed to effect change in a client's articulation and phonological development are called facilitative techniques. The term "facilitative" is usually preferred to "teaching" or "instruction" to emphasize that treatment is an interaction between the clinician's efforts and the client's capacity and willingness to learn. The major facilitative techniques employed in the treatment of articulation and phonological disorders include bombardment, metaphors, descriptions and demonstrations, touch cues, word pairs, building syllables and words, facilitative talk, and direct instruction.

II. BOMBARDMENT

Children typically acquire the sounds and syllables they hear most often. Bombardment is a well-established method used to increase the relative frequency of a treatment target in the client's environment (Nemoy & Davis, 1954). Typically, a client is not required to speak or vocalize during bombardment activities, only to listen. Some clinicians also recommend that the client wear a frequency modulated system during bombardment activities to increase the treatment target's saliency (Hodson, 1989). Depending on the client's age and the clinician's treatment philosophy, bombardment activities may last from a few minutes to 10 minutes. Some clinicians undertake bombardment only when introducing a new treatment target. Other clinicians include bombardment activities as part of each treatment session.

A. Stages 1 Through 3

Many clinicians begin each treatment session with clients in Stages 2 or 3 by bombarding the client with sounds, objects, and words containing the treatment target. (Bombardment might also be performed with clients in Stage 1, although it is not typical to do so.) Most commonly, the treatment target appears in the same position in all the words being used to bombard the client. Bombardment activities last from a few minutes up to approximately 10 minutes. A client in Stage 3 whose treatment target was [k], for example, might be exposed to objects beginning with [k] pulled out of a "magic box" or be asked to use a pretend fishing pole to "fish" objects out of a barrel. Typically, bombardment is followed by activities designed to stimulate production of the treatment target, although in principle it might also be provided without such a component. The most typical clinical situation in which a clinician might consider providing bombardment without a production component is as part of a stimulation program for clients in Stages 1 or 2 who are temporarily "stalled" in articulation and phonological development.

B. Stage 3 (Selected) and Stage 4

With more cognitively advanced clients in Stage 3 and clients in Stage 4, bombardment typically is used to introduce and later to prompt for treatment targets. The stimuli for bombardment activities often are specially designed stories or favorite stories containing frequent occurrences of the treatment target. A client, for example, might be instructed to "listen to a story in which the sound we're going to work on occurs lots of times." The client might also be instructed to ring a bell or raise his or her hand every time the sound occurs.

Metalinguistic Awareness

Metalinguistic awareness is the ability that allows persons to reflect on language. Techniques to facilitate metalinguistic awareness increase the client's awareness of short-term goals and treatment targets. If, for example, the treatment target is [s], the clinician might label it "the long sound" to draw attention to a perceptual property (length) and place a paper in front of the client's mouth while saying [s] to draw attention to a production property (central air emission). Many activities traditionally called discrimination and perceptual training, although probably not "teaching" discrimination or perception, serve as valuable tools to facilitate metalinguistic awareness (Bleile & Hand, 1995). Techniques particularly well-suited to facilitating metalinguistic awareness include metaphors, descriptions and demonstrations, touch cues, and word pairs.

III. METAPHORS, DESCRIPTIONS AND DEMONSTRATIONS, AND TOUCH CUES

Treatment generally proceeds more rapidly if the client is aware of the sounds and syllables that are the focus of remediation. The major techniques used to achieve this purpose are metaphors, descriptions and demonstrations, and touch cues, all of which are extremely useful when introducing new treatment targets, prompting, and promoting self-monitoring skills. Metaphors, descriptions and demonstrations, and touch cues for individual sounds are provided in Appendix 7A.

A. Metaphors

Metaphors compare some aspect of speech to something with which the client is familiar. A metaphor for [s] is "the snake sound," and a metaphor for a fricative is "the long sound." Possible metaphors for sound classes, syllables, and characteristics of words are listed in Tables 7–1, 7–2, and 7–3 (Blodgett & Miller, 1989; Flowers, 1990).

B. Descriptions and Demonstrations

Descriptions and demonstrations provide a simple means to heighten a client's awareness of selected characteristics of speech. A possible description of [p], for example, draws the client's attention to the closing lips, the build-up of air behind the lips, and the sudden release of air. A demonstration accompanying the description might involve placing a piece of paper in front of the client's lips to show the sudden release of air or gently pressing the client's lips together to show lip closure.

Table 7–1. Possible metaphors for places of production.

Place of Production	Metaphors
Bilabial	Lip sounds
Labiodental	Biting lip sounds or biting sounds
Interdental	Tongue tip sounds
Alveolar	Bump sounds, hill sounds
Postalveolar	Back of the hill sounds
Palatal	Middle sound
Velar	Back sounds
Glottal	Throat sound

Table 7–2. Possible metaphors for manners of production.

Manner of Production	Metaphors
Fricatives	Long sounds, hissing sounds
Glides and liquids (approximants)	Flowing sounds
Lateral	Side sound
Affricates	Engine chugging sounds
Nasals	Nose sounds
Stops	Short sounds, dripping sounds, and popping sounds
Voiced	Motor on, voice on, buzzing sound, hand buzzer sound, buzzing voice box, and voice box on
Voiceless	Motor off, voice off, not a buzzing sound, not a hand buzzer sound, no buzzing voice box, and voice box off

Table 7–3. Possible metaphors for consonant clusters, syllables, and words.

Sound Units	Metaphors
End of word	End sound
Multisyllabic words	Words with parts
Single syllable words	Words with one part
Initial consonants	Starting sounds
Consonant clusters	Sound friends

Source: Adapted from: Easy Does It for Phonology by E. Blodgett and V. Miller, 1989, East Moline, IL: LinguiSystems.

C. Touch Cues

Touch cues draw the client's attention to production characteristics of sounds (typically, the place of production). A client, for example, might be instructed to touch the lips for bilabial oral stops, to touch above the upper lip for alveolar stops, and to touch under the back of the chin for velar stops (Bleile & Hand, 1995). Originally designed for clients with oral-motor dysfunction, touch cues are now finding their way into wider clinical use. Commonly used touch cues are listed in Table 7–4.

D. Stage 1

These techniques are not applicable with clients in Stage 1.

Table 7–4. Possible touch cues for place and manner of production.

Sound Class	Example	Touch Cue
Nasals	[m]	Fingers and thumb hold lips together, ask client to feel vibration on neck
	[n]	Lay finger over front of cheek bone
Oral Stops	[p] [b]	Lay finger in front of lips
	[t] [d]	Lay finger above top lip
	[k] [g]	Lay finger at uppermost part of neck
Fricatives	[f] [v]	Lay finger below bottom lip
	[θ] [ð]	Place finger in front of lips and remind client to protrude tongue
	[s]	Point to the corner of the mouth (to indicate spread) and remind client of the teeth being together
	[ʃ]	Lay finger in front of lips and use the metaphor "quiet sound"
Liquid	[l]	Lay tip of finger on middle of upper lip
Diphthongs	[oʊ]	Trace with finger around lips and use the metaphor "blowing sound"
	[eɪ]	Lay fingers on corners of mouth and use the metaphor "smiling sound"

E. Stage 2

Metaphors, descriptions, and demonstrations are generally not effective with clients in Stage 2. Interestingly, however, some clients in Stage 2 respond well to touch cues even though they may lack the cognitive maturation required to identify places of production. Perhaps touch cues are effective with these clients because they prompt the client to produce a sound in a way that the clinician praises rather than because the cues help the client focus on a particular place of production (Bleile & Hand, 1995).

F. Stage 3

Touch cues are effective with almost all clients in Stage 3. Metaphors are effective with most clients, and descriptions and demonstrations are effective with more cognitively advanced clients.

As with clients in Stage 2, touch cues are introduced early in treatment. Metaphors for treatment targets are also introduced early in the course of treatment, preferably through negotiation with the client (Dean, Howell, Hill, and Waters, 1990). After the metaphor is established, practice is provided to help the client associate the metaphor with the treatment target. If, for example, the treatment target is [s], the clinician might ask the client, "Raise your hand when I say our snake sound. Is it [ʃ]? Is it [f]? Is it [s]?" If the client experiences difficulty associating the metaphor with the treatment target the number of features distinguishing the treatment target from the other sounds is increased. For example, if the client in the above example raised his or her hand for [f], the clinician might then contrast [s] with [l] or with vowels. Metaphors also provide a valuable means to prompt productions and to facilitate self-monitoring skills during the course of treatment. For example, if the client says [t] for [s], the client might be asked, "Was that the snake sound?"

Trial use of descriptions and demonstrations should be attempted early in treatment with more developmentally advanced clients. If the client appears unable to comprehend or benefit from this facilitative technique, the clinician should place greater reliance on touch cues and metaphors.

G. Stage 4

Metaphors, descriptions and demonstrations, and touch cues are effective with clients in Stage 4. Touch cues and metaphors may be used with less advanced clients in this stage, although care is needed to ensure that the client does not feel he or she is being treated "like a baby." Descriptions and demonstrations are valuable with clients in Stage 4 who have sufficient cognitive and attention abilities to comprehend the instructions used in these tasks. Clients with limited cognitive and attention skills who find descriptions and demonstrations confusing may benefit from treatment that makes greater use of metaphors.

Special Words

In treatment all words are not equal. Words that the client considers important to pronounce often provide the best focus for treatment activities. Treatment, for example, might focus on names of favorite objects and persons that contain the treatment target or specific words that are pronounced in such a way as to provoke teasing. Treatment with more advanced clients in Stage 4 might focus on multisyllabic words that appear in school or work assignments.

IV. WORD PAIRS

Languages use sound to distinguish the meaning of words. The difference in meaning between *cup* and *pup*, for example, is that the former begins with [k] and the latter with [p]. The contrastive nature of sound is used to facilitate perception and production through word pairs (also called minimal and maximal pairs) that differ by a single sound (Elbert, Rockman & Saltzman, 1982; Tyler, Edwards, & Saxman, 1987; Weiner, 1981). The words *bee-pea*, for example, are a word pair in which the words differ from each other by one sound, [b] and [p]. The words *bee* and *pea* are a minimal pair, because they differ by a single distinctive feature (voicing) in most distinctive feature systems. Word pairs can also differ by more than one distinctive feature (called maximal pairs), as in *pea-me*, which differ in voicing ([p] is voiceless and [m] is voiced) and nasality ([p] is an oral consonant and [m] is a nasal consonant).

Some evidence suggests that use of maximal pairs is more effective with clients in the early stages of articulation and phonological development, and that minimal pairs may be more appropriate for clients in later stages of articulation and phonological development (Gierut, 1989). Word pairs may also differ in the presence or absence of a sound, such as in *bee-beet* and *slow-low*. Lists of word pairs for word-initial consonants, word-initial consonant cluster reduction, word-final consonants, and word-final consonant deletion are provided in Appendix 7B (Walsh, 1994).

A. Stages 1 Through 3

Word pairs are not applicable for use with clients in Stage 1 and Stage 2. Nor are they useful with less cognitively advanced clients in Stage 3.

B. Stage 3 (Selected) and Stage 4

The greatest utility of word pairs is with more cognitively advanced clients in Stage 3 and clients in Stage 4.

1. Perception. Word pairs are used in contrast therapy activities to facilitate perception of newly introduced treatment targets (Elbert, Rockman, & Saltzman, 1980; Weiner, 1981). Typically, words containing the treatment target are contrasted with words containing the client's error. For example, a client whose treatment target was [p] and who pronounced [p] as [b] word-initially might be shown a picture of a pea and a bee, and be instructed, "I am going to show you two pictures. You point to the one I say. Bee. Good. Now point to pea. Good." Most commonly, 5 to 10 word pairs are presented in this manner with the clinician alternating whether the treatment target is the first or second member of the pair.

If the client experiences difficulty with the above task, real objects might be used in place of pictures, or the treatment target might be contrasted with a nonerror sound (e.g., *bee-see* for the client in the example). Reminding the client of a metaphor for the treatment target may also assist in this task. If the client is somewhat older, a list of words might be used instead of pictures or objects. In this situation, the client would be instructed, "I'm going to say two words. You tell me if the words sound the same or different. Ready? Pea-bee. Are they the same or different?"

2. Production. Word pairs are also used in contrast therapy activities as a preferred means to facilitate speech production (Elbert, Rockman, & Saltzman, 1980; Weiner, 1981). As was the case in facilitating perception, the client is presented with word pairs contrasting the treatment target with the client's error. The client discussed above, for example, might be presented a picture of a pea and a bee and be asked, "Tell me which one grows in the ground." If the client says [bi], he or she is given the picture of the bee, and the clinician explains, "But you said bee." As above, 5 to 10 word pairs are typically presented in this manner and the clinician occasionally presents word pairs the client can produce correctly, so he or she will not become discouraged. If the client experiences difficulty with this task, real objects may be used in place of pictures. Reminding the client of a metaphor for the treatment target often proves helpful, as does a description or demonstration of the treatment target.

V. BUILDING SYLLABLES AND WORDS

Most facilitative techniques target sounds rather than syllables and words. The metaphors described in Table 7–1 and 7–2, for example, describe sound classes, whereas the metaphors, descriptions and demonstrations, and touch cues appearing in Appendix 7A focus on individual sounds. The information provided in Table 7–3 represents a step in the development of a vocabulary with which to talk to clients directly about syllables and words. Bernhardt (in press) has pioneered efforts to develop techniques to facilitate syllable and word development. Three specific techniques focus on final consonants, consonant clusters, and retention of syllables.

Beyond the Isolated Word

Many of the elicitation activities described in Chapter 4 help a client move from isolated words to phrases, sentences, and spontaneous speech. Other activities include:

Read a story whose main characters and actions contain the treatment target. Then ask the client to tell you the story.

(continued)

Play a game in which the client tells a story containing characters whose names contain the treatment target. For younger clients, it sometimes helps to let the client hold a puppet that tells the story.

Take turns with the client telling a story in which the names of characters and actions contain the treatment target. The length of turns in the game can be determined by phrases, sentences or episodes.

Play a barrier game in which the names of the objects contain the treatment target.

For more mature clients, ask the client to make up phrases, sentences or short stories containing the treatment target.

A. Final Consonants

Many clients experience difficulty in using consonants to close syllables and words. A client, for example, might pronounce *beet* as [bi] through Final Consonant Deletion. Bernhardt recommends using a rhyming word task to remediate this error pattern (Bernhardt, in press). In this task, a client is first presented a story containing rhyming words ending in vowels. Once the client appears to grasp the concept of rhymes, rhyming words ending in consonants are introduced. The first story, for example, might involve *Pooh, Roo,* and cows that go *moo,* while the second story (or continuation of the first story) might involve a girl named *June* who sings a *tune* to the *moon* while standing on a *dune.*

B. Consonant Clusters

The acquisition of consonant clusters often presents a significant difficulty to clients. A client, for example, might pronounce *ski* as [ki] through Cluster Reduction. The remediation principle used to facilitate consonant cluster development is the same one that causes speakers to typically pronounce *is* as *tis* in phrases such as *It is* (Bleile, 1991b). In such phrases, the final consonant ([t] in this case) tends to migrate to the following syllable if that syllable begins with a vowel. Similarly, a consonant cluster can be introduced into word-initial position through phrases such as *ask a*, which, if said quickly, is likely to be pronounced as *a ska* (Bernhardt, in press).

C. Retention of Syllables

Even after a client is able to produce most sounds, he or she may still experience difficulty retaining unstressed syllables in longer words, words with unusual stress patterns, and word compounds. A client, for example, might be able to say *in*, but may delete the same syllable when it occurs in a word such as *serendipity* through a developmentally advanced form of Syllable Deletion.

Remediation to retain syllables is accomplished in three steps. First, the client practices multisyllabic words, producing them with equal syllable intensities and durations. Next, the client is provided practice in alternating loud-soft and short-long syllables. Third, the client is taught to use key words and rhythm cues. The STRONG-weak-STRONG stress pattern, for example, might be called "the elephant's beat," and the weak-STRONG-weak stress pattern might be called "Aladdin's beat." (Capital letters indicate primary stress.) A possible variation on this procedure is to use visual and tactile cues to illustrate the number of syllables in a word. A clinician, for example, might have the client place a bead on a string for every syllable in the word. A Hawaiian variation on this activity is to let the beads represent flowers on a lei (Imanaka-Inouye, 1994, personal communication).

D. Stages 1 and 2

Clients in Stages 1 and 2 lack the prerequisite cognitive abilities to perform these treatment tasks.

E. Stage 3 (Selected) and Stage 4

These tasks are appropriate for clients in Stage 3 who have more cognitively advanced abilities and for clients in Stage 4 without major intellectual disabilities, cognitive impairments, or limitations in attention. The word pairs for Consonant Final Deletion (Appendix 7B) can serve as a source of rhyming words, which can then be presented as a list or, more interestingly, in a story format. To help facilitate perception, the client might be asked to ring a bell or raise his or her hand whenever a rhyme is heard. For example, the client might be instructed: "Raise your hand every time you hear a word that rhymes with Pooh." To facilitate production, the client might be taught to recite an entertaining short story containing the rhyming words.

Activities for consonant clusters might include "talking over" games. A client for example, might be instructed to "say this over and over again: *ask a*." The client would then say, *askaaskaaska*, until *a ska* results. The client would then be instructed to throw away or drop the initial *a*, resulting in *ska*. The syllable *ska* might then be used as the basis from which to generalize [sk] clusters to word-initial environments. The same general technique might also be used to help facilitate word-initial consonants in clients whose speech contains Initial Consonant Deletion.

Any number of activities might be developed to facilitate retention of syllables, ranging from drills to elaborate games and stories. For example, a game could be made of saying all difficult multisyllabic words on a homework assignment with equal stress. Next, a game could be made of saying the words with exaggerated stress patterns, saying the unstressed syllables very slowly and the stressed syllables very loudly. An additional tactile cue is to play a game in which the client claps his or her hands on the stressed syllables (or slaps his or her desktop). Alternately, if the client experiences difficulty producing the most heavily stressed syllable in the word, hand clapping might be reserved for that syllable. Finally, key words are often crucial to treatment success in facilitating stress patterns. The best words for this purpose are those of well-liked animals (e.g., elephant and buffalo for STRONG-weak-strong stress patterns), cartoon characters, and, for older clients, words likely to arise in the course of school assignments.

VI. FACILITATIVE TALK

Facilitative talk is a body of techniques for talking with clients who have articulation and phonological disorders and language disorders. For some clients, facilitative talk is an adjunct to more direct instruction; for others, it is the primary means of intervention. The principle options for facilitative talk include motherese, repetitions, strategic errors, modeling, parallel talk, and requests for confirmation or clarification. Motherese is used with clients in Stage 1, and the other types of facilitative talk are used with clients in later stages. Many of the assessment activities described in Chapter 4 provide excellent venues for facilitative talk.

The Comfort Zone

Infants tend to vocalize most when they are in the comfort zone—an emotional state in which they feel secure, safe, and contented. Rapport and knowledge of an infant's likes and daily routines are far more likely to stimulate infant vocalizations than reliance on any particular facilitative technique or elicitation activity. This is why parents are more likely to facilitate their children's vocalizations than clinicians. When a parent is not available or is unable to perform this task, however, the clinician can perform it successfully—if the infant likes the clinician and the clinician knows the infant well.

A. Motherese

Motherese is a combination of facilitative talk techniques that serve to capture and keep an infant's attention (Dore, 1986; Snow, 1984). Motherese speech modifications include:

- Higher than usual pitch
- Talking about shared perceptions
- Exaggerated intonation
- Use of repetitions
- Calling attention to objects

Imitation games can be used in conjunction with motherese. Infants as young as 1 month of age are occasionally able to imitate vocalizations they already produce, and near 8 months of age most infants will occasionally imitate new types of vocalizations.

B. Expansions

Expansions "fill in the incorrect or missing speech parts." The client, for example, might say [pi] for *bee*, and the clinician might repeat the word, changing [p] to [b]. Alternately, if the client deleted [t] in *beet* the clinician might repeat the word, expanding [bi] to [bit].

C. Strategic Errors

Strategic errors are clinician-produced speech errors that mimic aspects of the clients articulation and phonological disorder. If, for example, the client pronounced word-initial [t] as [d], during the course of play the clinician might point to a doll's toe and say, *Doe*. The hoped-for response is for the client to look confused or laugh and then attempt to say the word with an initial [t].

D. Modeling

Modeling involves the use of the clinician, another person, or a favored toy as a speech example. In a modeling game, for example, the clinician might introduce a puppet as the teacher and the client and clinician as the students. The puppet teacher instructs the students to repeat what she says, which are words that contain the treatment target.

E. Parallel Talk

In parallel talk the clinician talks about the client's actions and the objects to which he or she is attending. For example, with a client who has [b] as a treatment target, the clinician might fill the clinic room with objects containing this sound. When the client looks at a ball, the clinician might say *ball*, and as the client rolls the ball across the floor, the clinician might say, "Ball rolling" or "Here comes the ball."

F. Requests for Confirmation or Clarification

Requests for confirmation or clarification are techniques designed to focus the client's attention on the communicative adequacy of his or her speech. During play, for example, a client whose treatment target was [k] might say *key* as *tea*. The clinician might ask, "Did you say tea?" or "What did you say you wanted?" or "Did you say you wanted some tea?" or "I thought I heard you say tea. Is that what you meant to say?" The hoped-for response is that the client will repeat, *key* or say something like, "I said key."

Baby Talk

Families frequently ask clinicians whether or not to use "baby talk" with young children. Family members should talk to their children in ways that are fun for the children and enjoyable and natural for the caregiver (Bleile, 1991a; Silverman, McGowan, Bleile, Fus, & Barnas, 1993). A child who has fun communicating is more likely to want to do it again. Caregivers might be counseled to keep the following questions in mind when interacting with a young child: Does the child appear interested? Is the child paying attention? Caregivers should speak in whatever way maximizes the chance that they can answer "yes" to both of these questions. For most children, "yes" answers are achieved most often if adults use simple language. Simplifying language means using short sentences and single words, talking about the "here and now," and talking about what appears to interest the child. For example, if the child appears interested in a stuffed animal, a caregiver might say, "Teddy Bear." Next, the caregiver might pet the stuffed animal, saying, "Soft," and then give the bear to the child to pet.

G. Stage 1

The primary facilitative talk technique used with clients in Stage 1 is motherese. Many investigators believe that routines provide the predictability in words and actions that facilitate the acquisition of speech and language (Bruner, 1983; Snow & Goldfield, 1983). For this reason, intervention with clients in Stage 1 typically begins with establishing routines between the client and the clinician (or caregiver). Possible routines include daily activities involving mealtime, diaper changing, and dressing, or "my turn—your turn" games such as "peek-a-boo" and "so big." Stimulation of vocal development then proceeds in the context of these shared routines.

Some clients in Stage 1 can be encouraged to vocalize through reciprocal communication games based on imitation. For example, the client says [bi] during play, and the clinician says [bi] in response, and the client then imitates the clinician. A more adult-centered variation of this game is for the clinician to introduce the vocalization that serves as the basis of the reciprocal communication. For example, the clinician says [di di] for the client to imitate. Reciprocal communication games are also used to stimulate more developmentally advanced types of vocalizations. For example, the client says [di di] (reduplicated babbling), and the clinician then says [di bi] (nonreduplicated babbling) for the client to imitate.

The Silent Infant

Vocal development can proceed even if an infant is temporarily unable to vocalize due to medical or physical reasons. In such situations, the infant can still learn about the perceptual and communicative value of sound from interacting with others. The infant's contribution to such dialogues may include eye widening, smiling, movement of the extremities, or imitative oral motor movements. Even if a child will not ever have the ability to vocalize, engaging in reciprocal communication is still valuable in promoting social and language development.

H. Stage 2

The primary facilitative talk techniques used with clients in Stage 2 are expansions, requests for confirmation or clarification, modeling, and parallel talk. Expansions are useful in helping the client perceive the contrast between the client's and the clinician's speech, as well as in providing an example for the client to reproduce. Requests for confirmation or clarification (e.g., asking "What did you say" or "I don't understand") help the client focus on the adequacy of his or her speech as a means of communication.

Modeling and parallel talk, in addition to offering the client perceptual information about the use of sounds in words, may also facilitate production as the client repeats the words spoken by the clinician. Most often, the speech model is the clinician or a family member, although some clients can also play simple versions of modeling games in which the model is a favorite stuffed animal or doll. In addition to the above techniques, a few clients in Stage 2 also respond appropriately to strategic errors, although most simply look confused and continue what they are doing.

I. Stage 3

All of the facilitative talk techniques used with clients in Stage 2 are also ideally suited to the interests and cognitive development of clients in Stage 3.

1. Expansions and Parallel Talk. As with clients in Stage 2, expansions and parallel talk expose the client to opportunities to perceive and produce speech.

2. Strategic Errors. Strategic errors are useful as a technique to help the client both identify his or her articulation and phonological errors and produce treatment targets.

3. Modeling. Modeling is a particularly useful technique to facilitate the production of treatment targets. For example, the client's speech might contain a Prevocalic Voicing pattern, and the treatment target might be [t] in the word-initial position. In one activity, a puppet might recite a list of its favorite words, sometimes pronouncing word-initial [t] as [d] and other times pronouncing it correctly. The client's role is to tell the puppet when it says the word correctly. In an alternate modeling activity, the puppet might be the teacher and the client's role is to repeat what the teacher says, thus facilitating speech production.

4. Requests for Confirmation or Clarification. Requests for confirmation or clarification are useful in facilitating the client's identification and production of treatment targets. During a game, for example, the client described above might pronounce *team* as *deem*. The clinician might then ask, "I didn't understand you—what did you say?" or "Did you say you want to play on the deem?"

J. Stage 4

Although treatment with clients in Stage 4 typically involves direct instruction, treatment can also use modified versions of strategic errors, modeling, and requests for confirmation or clarification. To illustrate, suppose a client's treatment target is word-initial [s]. When providing strategic errors, the clinician might read a story, sometimes pronouncing word-initial [s] with a frontal lisp and other times pronouncing it correctly. The client's role is to identify when an error is produced. The same activity can be altered into a speech production activity by having the client identify and correct any instances in which [s] is pronounced as a frontal lisp.

A possible modeling activity for clients in Stage 4 is to have the clinician read a word or sentence containing the treatment target and have the client say the same utterance exactly as the clinician did. A possible request for confirmation or clarification activity is to instruct the client to speak on a topic of interest. The clinician then stops the client and asks for confirmation or clarification each time a treatment target is pronounced incorrectly.

VII. DIRECT INSTRUCTION: PHONETIC PLACEMENT AND SHAPING TECHNIQUES

Phonetic placement and shaping techniques were the stock-and-trade of speech-language clinicians for much of the 20th century (Fairbanks, 1960; Nemoy & Davis, 1954). The use and knowledge of these techniques has declined in recent years, because client populations have shifted downward in age and increased in severity of involvement. Still, many clients benefit from careful use of phonetic placement and shaping techniques, especially with more cognitively advanced clients in Stage 3 and most clients in Stage 4.

Imitation

Imitation is used as a direct instruction technique with some clients in Stage 2, most clients in Stage 3, and almost all clients in Stage 4. A clinician, for example, might ask a client to imitate a treatment target when introducing a new treatment target and periodically during treatment "to remind" the client of the correct production.

A. Phonetic Placement

Phonetic placement techniques teach the tongue and lip positions used in speech production. Phonetic placement techniques to teach [t], for example, ask the client to raise the tongue tip, touch the tongue tip to the alveolar ridge, and to quickly draw the tongue tip down again. Phonetic placement techniques for American English consonants and [ɚ] are provided in Appendix 7C.

B. Shaping

Shaping techniques use a sound the client can already produce (either a speech error or another sound) to learn a new sound. Shaping techniques, for example, provide a series of steps through which a client who says [w] is taught to say [r]. Shaping techniques for American English consonants and [ɚ] are provided in Appendix 7C.

C. Stages 1 Through 3

Direct instruction techniques are not applicable for use with clients in Stages 1 and 2 or with most clients in Stage 3.

D. Stage 3 (Selected) and Stage 4

Phonetic placement and shaping techniques are sometimes useful with more cognitively advanced clients in Stage 3 and with attentive clients in Stage 4.

Phonetic placement and shaping techniques are guidelines rather than rigid procedures. The clinician should pick and choose among treatment techniques, keeping what works, discarding what does not, and (most often) modifying a technique to better suit the clinician's style and the client's needs. The activities used to teach phonetic placement and shaping techniques are limited only by the clinician's imagination. Place of production for alveolar stops, for example, might be indicated using peanut butter or by instructing the client to use his or her tongue tip to "touch the hill on the top of your mouth." Similarly, the release of air occurring during release of a stop might be indicated by placing a hand, a piece of paper, or a paper flower in front of the client's mouth.

APPENDIX 7A

Metaphors, Descriptions and Demonstr and Touch Cues

A. INTRODUCTION

Options for metaphors, descriptions and demonstrations, and touch cues for consonants and [ɝ] are listed in this appendix. Rather than list a voiced and voiceless demonstration for each pair of obstruents, ideas for demonstrating this contrast are listed in Table 7–5.

Table 7–5. Five possible methods to demonstrate voicing.

Methods	Instructions
1.	Instruct the client to listen to and identify the difference between a voiceless and voiced [ɑ].
2.	Place the client's hands over the ears and instruct him or her to hum, which heightens the sensation of vocal cord vibration.
3.	If the client is able to produce a voiced and voiceless fricative, ask him or her to cover the ears and make these sounds. Alternatively, ask the client to make [h] and [ɑ].
4.	You and the client place one hand on your throat and the other on the client's throat while making voiced and voiceless sounds together. Tell each other when the voicing goes on and off.
5.	If the client is able to produce a voiced and voiceless oral stop, attach a small piece of paper or a paper flower to the end of a tongue depressor or pencil and ask the client to "make the paper (or flower) move." The paper is more likely to move when a voiceless consonant is produced than when a voiced consonant is produced. (Be careful in providing instructions to the client, however, because a strongly articulated voiced oral stop will also move the flower.)

[p] and [b]

DESCRIPTION: Draw attention to closing the two lips, the build-up of pressure behind the lips, and the sudden release of air through the mouth. For [b], also draw attention to the buzzing voice box.

METAPHORS: [p] is the popping sound and the sound beginning *pop*, *pie*, and *pig*. [b] is the bubble sound and the sound beginning *bye*, *bee*, and *bed*. [p] and [b] are also short sounds (stops) and lip sounds (bilabials). Additionally, [b] is made with the motor on (voiced).

TOUCH CUE: Place the client's finger in front of his or her lips.

DEMONSTRATIONS:

Place (Bilabial)

First Method: Lightly touch the client's upper and lower lips with a tongue depressor, then ask the client to bring the lips together to touch the spot you touched.

Second Method: Ask the client to make kissing noises.

Manner (Oral Stop)

First Method: Use a strip of paper, a feather, or a hand held in front of the client's mouth while you produce a series of stops to demonstrate the explosive release of stops. Alternately, tape a small paper flower on the end of a pencil and encourage the client to move the flower with puffs of air.

Second Method: Place your or the client's palms together and then suddenly separate them to demonstrate the sudden release of stops.

[m]

DESCRIPTION: Draw attention to closing the lips, the build-up of pressure behind the lips, the buzzing in the throat, and the outward flow of air through the nose.

METAPHORS: The humming sound and the sound beginning *mom*, *moo*, and *me*. [m] is also a motor-on sound (voiced), a nose sound (nasal), and a lip sound (bilabial).

TOUCH CUE: Use the client's fingers and thumb to hold his or her lips together.

DEMONSTRATIONS:

Place (Bilabial)

First Method: Lightly touch the client's upper and lower lips with a tongue depressor, then ask the client to bring the lips together to touch the spot you touched.

Second Method: Ask the client to make kissing noises.

Manner (Nasal Stop)

First Method: Contrast breathing through the nose onto a mirror or piece of paper with breathing through the mouth onto a mirror or piece of paper.

Second Method: Instruct the client to take a deep breath, hold it, and let air out through the nose to produce a voiceless nasal sound.

Third Method: To demonstrate nasality with voicing, instruct the client to take a deep breath, hold it, and say "ah" with the mouth closed so air comes out the nose. Telling the client to open his or her mouth will help teach release of a nasal consonant.

[w]

DESCRIPTION: The round lip sound or the wow sound (wow!) and the sound that begins *wow*, *we*, and *why*. [w] is also a lip sound (bilabial), a back sound (velar), and a buzzing sound (voiced).

TOUCH CUES: None.

DEMONSTRATIONS:

Place (Bilabial)

First Method: Lightly touch the client's upper and lower lips with a tongue depressor, then ask the client to bring the lips together to touch the spot you touched.

Second Method: Ask the client to make kissing noises.

Manner (Approximant)

First Method: Use a strip of paper, a feather, or a hand held in front of the client's mouth while you produce several glides or liquids to draw attention to the "flowing" quality and continuous nature of the sounds. Alternately, tape a small paper flower on the end of a pencil and encourage the client to move the flower in the wind.

Second Method: Run your or the client's finger down the client's arm while making several long glides or liquids to demonstrate the "flowing" quality and length of these sounds.

[f] and [v]

DESCRIPTION: Draw attention to the lower lip touching the upper teeth and the outward flowing of air from the mouth. For [v], also draw attention to the motor being on.

METAPHORS: [f] is the angry cat sound ("ffff") and the sound beginning *feet*, *fun*, or *fish*. [v] is the jet sound, the sound beginning *very*, *volcano*, and *vanilla*. [f] and [v] are also long sounds (fricatives) and tooth sounds (labiodental). [v] is made with the motor on (voiced).

TOUCH CUE: Lay the client's finger below his or her bottom lip.

DEMONSTRATIONS:

Place (Labiodental)

First Method: Lightly touch the client's lower lip and the bottom of the upper front teeth with a tongue depressor, then ask the client to bring the upper teeth and lower lip together to touch where you touched.

Second Method: Ask the client to bite his or her lower lip gently with his upper teeth.

Manner (Fricative)

First Method: Use a strip of paper, a feather, or a hand held in front of the client's mouth while you produce several long voiceless fricatives to draw attention to the "hissing" quality and continuous nature of the sounds. An alternate method is to tape a small paper flower on the end of a pencil and encourage the client to move the flower in the wind.

Second Method: Run your or the client's finger down the client's arm while making several long voiceless fricatives to demonstrate the "hissing" quality and length of fricatives.

[θ] and [ð]

DESCRIPTION: Draw attention to the tongue tip between the upper and lower front teeth. For [ð], also draw attention to the buzzing voice box.

METAPHORS: [θ] is the leaking tire sound. [ð] is the motor-on sound. [θ] and [ð] are also long sounds (fricative) and tongue-teeth sounds (interdental). [ð] is also made with the voice on (voiced).

TOUCH CUE: Place the client's finger in front of his or her lips and remind the client to extrude his or her tongue.

DEMONSTRATIONS:

Place (Interdental)

First Method: Ask the client to stick the tongue out and then gently close his or her mouth (if the tongue is sticking out too far, push it back with a tongue depressor).

Second Method: Place a tongue depressor or piece of food in front of the client's mouth, ask the client to touch it with the tongue, and then to close the mouth gently.

Manner (Fricative)

First Method: Use a strip of paper, a feather, or a hand held in front of the mouth while you produce several long voiceless fricatives to draw attention to the "hissing" quality and continuous nature of the sounds. An alternate method is to tape a small paper flower on the end of a pencil and encourage the client to move the flower in the wind.

Second Method: Run your or the client's finger down the client's arm while making several long voiceless fricatives to demonstrate the "hissing" quality and length of fricatives.

[t] and [d]

DESCRIPTION: Draw attention to the tongue tip touching the bump behind the upper front teeth. For [d], also draw attention to the motor being on.

METAPHORS: [t] is the tick-tock sound and the sound that begins *toe*, *tummy*, and *Tommy*. [d] is the *do* sound ("I can do it") or the Homer Simpson sound (Doh!), and the sound that begins *dinner*, *doll*, and *done*. [t] and [d] are also tongue tip sounds (alveolar) and short sounds (stop). [d] is made with the voice on (voiced).

TOUCH CUE: Lay the client's finger above his or her upper lip.

DEMONSTRATIONS:

Place (Alveolar)

First Method: Ask the client to feel the bump on the roof of his or her mouth just behind the two front teeth.

Second Method: Place a little peanut butter or a favored food on a Q-tip, touch the Q-tip to the alveolar ridge, and ask the client to remove the food with the tongue tip.

Manner (Oral Stop)

First Method: Use a strip of paper, a feather, or a hand held in front of the client's mouth while you produce a series of stops to demonstrate the explosive release of stops. Alternately, tape a small paper flower on the end of a pencil and encourage the client to move the flower with puffs of air.

Second Method: Place your or the client's palms together and then suddenly separate them to demonstrate the sudden release of stops.

[n]

DESCRIPTION: Draw attention to the tongue tip touching the bump behind the upper front teeth, the buzzing in the voice box, and the air coming out through the nose.

METAPHORS: The siren sound and the first sound in *no*, *knee*, and *night*. [n] is also a nose sound (nasal) and a tongue tip sound (alveolar).

TOUCH CUE: Lay the client's finger over the front of his or her cheek bone.

DEMONSTRATIONS:

Place (Alveolar)

First Method: Ask the client to feel the bump on the roof of his or her mouth just behind the two front teeth.

Second Method: Place a little peanut butter or a favored food on a Q-tip, touch the Q-tip to the alveolar ridge, and ask the client to remove the food with the tongue tip.

Manner (Nasal Stop)

First Method: Contrast breathing through the nose onto a mirror or piece of paper with breathing through the mouth onto a mirror or piece of paper.

Second Method: Instruct the client to take a deep breath, hold it, and let air out through the nose to produce a voiceless nasal sound.

Third Method: To demonstrate nasality with voicing, instruct the client to take a deep breath, hold it, and say "ah" with the mouth closed so that air comes out the nose. Telling the client to open the mouth will help teach release of a nasal consonant.

[s] and [z]

DESCRIPTION: Draw attention to the hissing sound and the position of the tongue tip (behind the front upper or lower teeth). For [z], also draw attention to the buzzing voice box.

METAPHORS: [s] is the snake sound or the hissing sound and the sound that begins, *sun*, *sit*, and *Santa*. [z] is the bee sound and the sound that begins *zoo*, *zero*, and *zebra*. [s] and [z] are also long sounds (fricative) and tongue tip sounds (alveolar). [z] is made with the voice on (voiced).

TOUCH CUE: None. These sounds are usually acquired too late in development for the touch cue technique to be appropriate.

DEMONSTRATIONS:

Place (Alveolar)

First Method: Ask the client to feel the bump on the roof of his or her mouth just behind the two front teeth.

Second Method: Place a little peanut butter or a favored food on a Q-tip, touch the Q-tip to the alveolar ridge, and ask the client to remove the food with the tongue tip.

Manner (Fricative)

First Method: Use a strip of paper, a feather, or a hand held in front of the client's mouth while you produce several long voiceless fricatives to draw attention to the "hissing" quality and continuous nature of the sounds. Alternately, tape a small paper flower on the end of a pencil and encourage the client to move the flower in the wind.

Second Method: Run your or the client's finger down the client's arm while making several long voiceless fricatives to demonstrate the "hissing" quality and length of fricatives.

[l]

DESCRIPTION: Draw attention to the tongue tip raised to the mouth roof, the air flowing over the sides of the tongue, and the buzzing of the voice box.

METAPHORS: The singing sound (la-la-la) or the pointy sound (i.e., the tongue is pointing at the alveolar ridge), and the sound that begins *like*, *Lee*, and *low*. [l] is also a buzzing sound (voiced), a tongue tip sound (alveolar), and a flowing sound (liquid and glides).

TOUCH CUE: Lay the client's fingertip on the middle of his or her top lip.

DEMONSTRATIONS:

Place (Alveolar)

First Method: Ask the client to feel the bump on the roof of his or her mouth just behind the two front teeth.

Second Method: Place a little peanut butter or a favored food on a Q-tip, touch the Q-tip to the alveolar ridge, and ask the client to remove the food with the tongue tip.

Manner (Approximant)

First Method: Use a strip of paper, a feather, or a hand held in front of the client's mouth while you produce several glides or liquids to draw attention to the "flowing" quality and continuous nature of the sounds. Alternately, tape a small paper flower on the end of a pencil and encourage the client to move the flower in the wind.

Second Method: Run your or the client's finger down the client's arm while making several long glides or liquids to demonstrate the "flowing" quality and length of this sound.

Air Flow (Lateral)

First Method: Place a straw on the groove of the tongue and blow out to demonstrate central emission of air. Place one straw at each corner of the mouth to demonstrate lateral emission of air.

Second Method: Ask the client to breathe in with the tongue as for [s]. Cool air is felt at the central groove. Alternately, perform the straw technique above, remove the straw, and ask the client to breathe in. For lateral sounds, ask the client to breathe in with the tongue in position for [l]. Cool air should be felt on the sides of the tongue over which the air was emitted. An alternate method is to perform the straw technique above, remove the straws, and ask the client to breathe in.

[ɚ]

DESCRIPTION: For retroflex [ɚ], draw attention to the tongue tip raised and curled slightly back and the slight raising of the tongue toward the roof of the mouth. For humped [ɚ], draw attention to the tongue tip being down and the sides of the tongue touching the insides of the back teeth.

Two Types of [r] and [ɚ]

[r] and [ɚ] can be produced in two-ways—retroflex or humped. Some clinicians prefer to facilitate retroflex [ɚ] and [r], others prefer humped [ɚ] and [r].

METAPHORS: The mad dog sound (grrr), the growling tiger sound (grr), or the arm wrestling sound (errr). The sound that ends *hear*, *purr*, and *car*. [ɚ] is also a buzzing sound (voiced) and a tongue tip sound.

TOUCH CUE: None. [ɚ] is usually acquired too late in development for touch cue techniques to be appropriate.

DEMONSTRATIONS:

Same as for [r].

[r]

DESCRIPTION: For retroflex [r], draw attention to the tongue tip curled slightly back and raised toward the bump behind the front teeth. The sides of the tongue are against the sides of the teeth, and the voice box is buzzing. For humped [r], draw attention to the tongue tip being down, the back of the tongue humped up (arched) toward the soft palate, the sides of the tongue lying against the sides of the teeth, and the voice box buzzing.

METAPHORS: The starting race car sound (ruh) and the sound that begins *run*, *read*, and *red*. [r] is also a buzzing sound (voiced), a tongue tip sound (alveolar), and a flowing sound (liquid).

TOUCH CUE: None. [r] is usually acquired too late in development for the touch cue techniques to be appropriate.

DEMONSTRATIONS:

Place (Alveolar)

First Method: Have the client cup his or her hand to indicate that the tongue tip is raised and slightly curled back.

Second Method: Ask the client to feel the bump on the roof of his or her mouth just behind the two front teeth.

Third Method: Place a little peanut butter or a favored food on a Q-tip, touch the Q-tip to the alveolar ridge, and ask the client to remove the food with the tongue tip.

Manner (Approximant)

First Method: Use a strip of paper, a feather, or a hand held in front of the client's mouth while you produce several glides or liquids to draw attention to the "flowing" quality and continuous nature of the sound. Alternately, tape a small paper flower on the end of a pencil and encourage the client to move the flower in the wind.

Second Method: Run your or the client's finger down the client's arm while making several long glides or liquids to demonstrate the "flowing" quality and length of this sound.

[tʃ] and [dʒ]

DESCRIPTION: Draw attention to the contact between the tongue blade and roof of the mouth just behind the bumpy ridge behind the upper front teeth and the way the sound ends in [ʃ]. Additionally, the voice is on for [dʒ], and the sound ends in [ʒ].

METAPHORS: [tʃ] is the choo-choo sound or the sneezing sound (choo!) and the sound that begins *choo-choo train, chocolate chips,* and *cheese.* [dʒ] is the motor boat sound and the sound that begins *jump, joke,* and *Joe.* Both sounds are back-of-the-hill sounds (postalveolar) and engine chugging sounds (affricate). [dʒ] is made with the voice on (voiced).

DEMONSTRATIONS:

Place (Postalveolar)

First Method: Ask the client to run his or her tongue to where the bump on the roof of the mouth just begins to go down toward the back of the mouth (an analogy of a "hill and valley" can be used).

Second Method: Place a little peanut butter or a favored food on a Q-tip, touch the Q-tip to the postalveolar region, and ask the client to remove the food with his or her tongue blade.

Manner (Affricate)

First Method: Have the client hold his or her hands together tightly and then separate them quickly to indicate the stop onset and fricative release of affricates.

Second Method: Hold the client's hands together and then release them suddenly to indicate the stop onset and fricative release of affricates.

[ʃ] and [ʒ]

DESCRIPTION: Draw attention to the friction noise and the place where the tongue blade touches the roof of the mouth just behind the bumpy ridge in back of the upper front teeth. For [ʒ], the voice is on.

METAPHORS: The hushing sound (shh!) or the quiet sound, and the sound that begins *shoe*, *sheep*, and *show*. [ʒ] is the motor sound (zzzz) and the sound in *measure*, *beige*, and *pleasure*. Both [ʃ] and [ʒ] are also back-of-the hill sounds (postalveolar) and long sounds (fricative). The voice is on (voiced) for [ʒ].

TOUCH CUE: Lay the client's finger in front of his or her lips.

DEMONSTRATIONS:

Place (Postalveolar)

First Method: Ask the client to run the tongue to where the bump on the mouth roof just begins to go down toward the back of the mouth (an analogy of a "hill and valley" can be used).

Second Method: Place a little peanut butter or a favored food on a Q-tip, touch the Q-tip to the postalveolar region, and ask the client to remove the food with the tongue blade.

Manner (Fricative)

First Method: Use a strip of paper, a feather, or a hand held in front of the client's mouth while you produce several long voiceless fricatives to draw attention to the "hissing" quality and continuous nature of the sounds. Alternately, tape a small paper flower on the end of a pencil and encourage the client to move the flower in the wind.

Second Method: Run your or the client's finger down the client's arm while making several long voiceless fricatives to demonstrate the "hissing" quality and length of fricatives.

[j]

DESCRIPTION: Draw attention to the flowing air and the slight rise of the middle of the tongue toward the roof of the mouth. The voice is on.

METAPHORS: The *yes* sound and the sound that begins *yes*, *you*, and *year*. [j] is also a flowing sound (glides and liquids), a middle sound (palatal), and the voice is on (voiced).

TOUCH CUES: None.

DEMONSTRATIONS:

Place (Palatal)

First Method: Ask the client to run his or her tongue backward from the bump to the highest point on the roof of the mouth.

Second Method: Place a little peanut butter or a favored food on a Q-tip, and touch the Q-tip to the arch of the hard palate. Ask the client to remove the food with his or her tongue blade.

Third Method: Touch the middle of the tongue lightly with a tongue depressor and ask the client to hump up that part of the tongue toward the roof of the mouth.

Manner (Approximant)

First Method: Use a strip of paper, a feather, or a hand held in front of the client's mouth while you produce several glides or liquids to draw attention to the "flowing" quality and continuous nature of the sounds. Alternately, tape a small paper flower on the end of a pencil and encourage the client to move the flower in the wind.

Second Method: Run your or the client's finger down the client's arm while making several long glides or liquids to demonstrate the "flowing" quality and length of this sound.

[k] and [g]

DESCRIPTION: Draw attention to the back of the tongue touching the rear of the roof of the mouth, the quick separation of the articulators, and the air flowing out the mouth. [k] is made with the voice off, and [g] is made with the voice on.

METAPHORS: [k] is the coughing sound and the sound that begins *cold, king,* and *kite.* [g] is the water pouring sound (glug, glug, glug) or the *greaat!* (Tony the Tiger) sound, and the sound that begins *go, goat,* and *gate.* Both [k] and [g] are also quick sounds (stops) and tongue-back sounds (velar). (k] is a voice-off sound (voiceless), and [g] is a voice-on sound (voiced).

TOUCH CUE: Lay the client's finger at the uppermost part of his or her neck.

DEMONSTRATIONS:

Place (Velar)

First Method: Place the client's hand in contact with the underside of your mouth and repeat [k] several times while drawing attention to the muscle movements.

Second Method: Open your mouth and allow the client to observe while you say [k] several times.

Manner (Oral Stop)

First Method: Use a strip of paper, a feather, or a hand held in front of the client's mouth while you produce a series of stops to demonstrate the explosive release of stops. Alternately, tape a small paper flower on the end of a pencil and encourage the client to move the flower with puffs of air.

Second Method: Place your or the client's palms together and then suddenly separate them to demonstrate the sudden release of stops.

[ŋ]

DESCRIPTION: Draw attention to the back of the tongue touching the rear of the roof of the mouth, the air flowing through the nose, and the voice being on.

METAPHORS: The gong sound and the sound that ends *sing*, *wing*, and *ring*. [ŋ] is also a back tongue sound (velar), a voice-on sound (voiced), and a nose sound (nasal).

TOUCH CUE: Lay the client's finger at the uppermost part of his or her neck.

DEMONSTRATIONS:

Place (Velar)

First Method: Place the client's hand in contact with the underside of your mouth and repeat [ŋ] several times while drawing attention to the muscle movements.

Second Method: Open your mouth and allow the client to observe while you say [ŋ] several times.

Manner (Nasal Stop)

First Method: Contrast breathing through the nose onto a mirror or a piece of paper with breathing through the mouth onto a mirror or piece of paper.

Second Method: Instruct the client to take a deep breath, hold it, and let air out through the nose to produce a voiceless nasal sound.

Third Method: To demonstrate nasality with voicing, instruct the client to take a deep breath, hold it, and say "ah" with the mouth closed so that air comes out the nose. Telling the client to open his or her mouth will help teach release of a nasal consonant.

[h]

DESCRIPTION: Draw attention to the hissing sound in the throat.

METAPHORS: The panting dog sound and the sound that begins *hug*, *happy*, and *ho*. (Santa Claus' ho-ho-ho). [h] is also a long sound (fricative) and a voice-off sound (voiceless).

TOUCH CUES: None.

DEMONSTRATIONS:

Place (Glottal)

First Method: Point to your larynx while making [h] or a vowel.

Second Method: Instruct the client to touch his or her larynx between the first finger and thumb and swallow.

Manner (Approximant)

First Method: Use a strip of paper, a feather, or a hand held in front of the client's mouth while you produce several glides or liquids to draw attention to the "flowing" quality and continuous nature of the sound. Alternately, tape a small paper flower on the end of a pencil and encourage the client to move the flower in the wind.

Second Method: Run your or the client's finger down the client's arm while making several long glides or liquids to demonstrate the "flowing" quality and length of this sound.

APPENDIX 7B
Word Pairs[a]

A. Introduction

This appendix is designed to use in contrast therapy activities like those described earlier in this chapter. A chart showing the feature differences between treatment target sounds and other possible sounds begins on the following page. The feature differences are those of place, manner, and voicing (Williams, 1993). The remainder of the appendix consists of four lists of word pairs showing:

Word pairs for word-initial consonants,

Word pairs for cluster deletion and cluster reduction in word-initial position,

Word pairs for cluster reduction in word-final position, and

Word pairs for consonant substitutions in word-final position.

The words in the lists that follow are common nouns, common verbs, letters of the alphabet, and names from popular storybooks. For certain sounds, no words were found that met the above criteria, and the list was left blank. Extra spaces are provided at the end of each list for clinicians to add their own preferred words.

---

[a] This appendix is adapted from S. Walsh (1994).

B. Chart of Feature Differences

Sound	One Feature	Two Features	Three Features
p	b t k	d g f θ s ʃ tʃ m w h	v ð z ʒ dʒ n ŋ l r j
b	p d g m w	t k v ð z ʒ dʒ n ŋ l r j	f θ s ʃ tʃ h
t	p d k s	b g f θ z ʃ tʃ n l r h	v ð ʒ dʒ m ŋ j w
d	b t g z n l r	p k v ð s ʒ dʒ m ŋ j w	f θ ʃ tʃ h
k	p t g	b d f θ s ʃ tʃ ŋ h	v ð z ʒ dʒ m n l r j w
g	b d k ŋ	p t v ð z ʒ dʒ m n l r j w	f θ s ʃ tʃ h
f	v θ s ʃ	p t k ð z ʒ tʃ h	b d g dʒ m n ŋ l r j w
v	f ð z ʒ	b d g θ s ʃ dʒ m n ŋ l r j w	p t k tʃ h
θ	f ð s ʃ	p t k v z ʒ tʃ h	b d g dʒ m n ŋ l r j w
ð	v θ z ʒ	b d g f s ʃ dʒ m n ŋ l r j w	p t k tʃ h
s	f θ z ʃ t	p d k v ð ʒ tʃ n l r h	b g dʒ m ŋ j w
z	d v ð s ʒ n l r	b t g f θ ʃ dʒ m j w ŋ	p k tʃ h
ʃ	f θ s ʒ tʃ	p t k v d z dʒ h	b d g m n ŋ l r j w
ʒ	v ð z ʃ dʒ	b d g f θ s tʃ m n ŋ l r j w	p t k h
tʃ	ʃ dʒ	p t k f θ s ʒ h	b d g v ð z m n ŋ l r j w
dʒ	ʒ tʃ	b d g v ð z ʃ m n ŋ l r j w	p t k f θ s h

(continued)

Chart of Feature Differences (*continued*)

Sound	One Feature	Two Features	Three Features
m	n ŋ b w	p d g v ð z ʒ dʒ l r j	t k f θ s ʃ tʃ h
n	d z m ŋ l r	b t g v ð s ʒ dʒ j w	p k f ʃ tʃ h θ
ŋ	m n g	b d k v ð z ʒ dʒ l r j w	p t f θ s ʃ tʃ h
l	d z n r	b t g v ð s ʒ dʒ m ŋ j w	p k f θ ʃ tʃ h
r	d n z l	b t g v ð s ʒ dʒ m ŋ j w	p k f θ ʃ tʃ h
j	w	b d g v ð z ʒ dʒ m n ŋ l r h	p t k f θ s ʃ tʃ
w	b m j	p d g v ð z ʒ dʒ n ŋ l r h	t k f θ s ʃ tʃ
h		p t k f θ s ʃ tʃ j w	b d g v ð z ʒ dʒ m n ŋ l r

C. Word-Initial Contrasts

[p]

Sound	1 Feature	2 Features	3 Features
pear	bear, tear	hair, wear	
pea	key, bee	sea	knee, z
peas	keys	cheese	knees
potato	tomato		
pie	bye, tie	high, thigh	
peach	beach, teach		reach
pig	big	wig, dig	
pan	can	fan, man	ran
pin		fin, chin, thin, win	
parrot	carrot		
pat	cat, bat	mat, sat, hat, fat	rat
pen	ten	men, hen	
pet		wet	vet, net, jet
pond		wand	
pay		day, hay, weigh	ray, neigh
pickle	tickle		nickel
*pog		dog	log
paste	taste	waist, chased	raced
poke		soak, choke	joke, yolk
pail	tail	sail, mail, whale	nail, jail, rail, veil
purse			nurse
pick	tick, kick	sick, wick, thick	lick
paw			jaw
pink		sink, wink, think	rink
pull	bull	wool	
pop	top, cop	mop, hop, chop, shop	
pearl		girl	
pave	cave	wave, shave	

(*continued*)

[p] (*continued*)

Sound	1 Feature	2 Features	3 Features
pot		hot, dot	
peel		deal, meal, seal, wheel	
path	bath	math	
pest	test	chest, west	vest, nest
pour	core	four, door	roar
park	bark	shark, dark	
post	toast	ghost	roast
pill	bill	hill	
peep	keep, beep	deep, sheep, cheap	jeep, leap
pool	tool, cool	fool	jewel
_____	_____	_____	_____
_____	_____	_____	_____

*pog: A pog is a term used to refer to milk caps, which are used to play a game in Hawaii and often are given to children as reinforcement in place of stickers.

[b]

Sound	1 Feature	2 Features	3 Features
bee	pea	knee, z, key	sea
bug	mug	rug, jug	hug
bear	pear		hair
bird	word	nerd	third, heard
bunny	money		funny, honey, sunny
bat	mat, pat	cat, rat	fat, hat, sat
bye	pie	tie	high, thigh, sigh
big	dig, pig, wig		
box		rocks	fox, socks
bed	dead	red	head
beach	peach	reach, teach	
bow	go, mow	toe, row, no	sew, hoe
bows		toes, rose, nose	hose
boat	goat	coat, note	
ball	wall	call, tall	hall, fall
bone		cone	phone
boy		toy	
bad	mad, dad		sad
bake		cake, lake	
boo	goo, moo	two, zoo, new	shoe, chew
beef		leaf	thief, chief
book		cook, look	hook
bump		jump	hump
bath	path, math		
bell			shell
belt	melt		
bite	white	night, light, kite, write	fight
bark	park, dark		shark
bill	pill		hill

(*continued*)

[b] (*continued*)

Sound	1 Feature	2 Features	3 Features
beans		jeans	
berry			cherry, hairy, fairy
bull	wool, pull		
band fanned		tanned	hand, sand,
boom		zoom, room	
beep	deep, peep	leap, jeep, keep	sheep, cheep
bun	one	run	fun, sun
_____	_____	_____	_____
_____	_____	_____	_____

[t]

Sound	1 Feature	2 Features	3 Features
tomato	potato		
ten	pen	hen	men
tickle	pickle	nickel	
toast	post	ghost, roast	
taste	paste	chased, raced	waist
tail	pail, sail	nail, rail	mail, whale, jail, veil
teach	peach	reach, beach	
toes		rose, nose, hose, bows	
tear	pear	hair, bear	
tie	pie	high, bye, thigh	
tick	kick, pick, sick	thick, lick	wick
talk		chalk, hawk	walk
top	pop, cop	hop, chop, shop	mop
tool	cool, pool	fool	jewel
tall	call	ball, fall, hall	wall
time	dime		
toy		boy	
two		chew, goo, boo, new, zoo, shoe	moo
tire		fire	
tube	cube		
tear	deer	cheer, fear, hear	year
tanned	sand	hand, band, fanned	
test		nest, chest	west, vest
toe	sew	bow, row, go, hoe, no	mow
————	————	————	————
————	————	————	————

[d]

Sound	1 Feature	2 Features	3 Features
dog	log	pog*	
dig	big	wig, pig	
dish		wish	fish
dime	time		
dad	bad	mad, sad	
dot		pot	hot
dart		cart	heart
dive			hive, five
door	roar	core, pour	four
dark	bark	park	shark
deal		peel, meal, wheel, seal	
day	neigh, ray	pay, weigh	hay
dawn	lawn	yawn	fawn
deer	tear	year, peer	hear, fear, cheer
dirt			shirt, hurt
deep	beep, leap	peep, keep, jeep	sheep, cheep, heap
dead	bed, red		head
dust	rust		
_____	_____	_____	_____
_____	_____	_____	_____

*pog: A pog is a term used to refer to milk caps, which are used to play a game in Hawaii and often are given to children as reinforcement in place of stickers.

[k]

Sound	1 Feature	2 Features	3 Features
can	pan	fan	man
carrot	parrot		
keys	peas	cheese	knees
king		sing	ring, wing
kick	tick, pick	sick, thick	wick, lick
cop	pop, top	shop, hop, chop	mop
cat	pat	bat, sat, hat, fat	rat, mat
cool	pool, tool	fool	jewel
cut			nut
coat	goat	boat	note
call	tall	fall, hall, ball	wall
key	pea	bee, sea	knee
cone		phone, bone	
cake		bake	lake
cold	gold	hold, fold	mold, rolled
cave	pave	shave	wave
cart		dart, heart	
cook		book, hook	look
camp		lamp	
kite		bite, fight	write, white, light, night
candle		handle, sandal	
cube	tube		
curled			world
corn	torn	thorn, horn	worn
core	pour	door, four	roar
card	guard	hard	yard
keep	peep	deep, beep, cheep, sheep	jeep, leap
calf		half	laugh
————	————	————	————
————	————	————	————

[g]

Sound	1 Feature	2 Features	3 Features
goat	boat, coat	note	
girl		pearl	
gold	cold	mold, rolled	fold, hold
goo	boo	two, zoo, new, moo	chew, shoe
ghost		toast, post, roast	
gum			thumb
gasoline		Vaseline	
guard	card	yard	hard
go	bow	toe, row, mow, no	sew, hoe
gun	bun	run, one	sun, fun
_____	_____	_____	_____
_____	_____	_____	_____

[f]

Sound	1 Feature	2 Features	3 Features
fan		pan, can	man
fin	thin	pin, chin	win
fat	sat	cat, pat, hat	bat, mat, rat
fox	socks		box, rocks
fish			dish, wish
fun	sun		run, one, gun
feather			leather
fool		tool, pool, cool	jewel
fall		tall, call, hall	ball, wall
phone		cone	bone
fold		cold, hold	mold, rolled, gold
five		hive	dive
funny	sunny	honey	money, bunny
fell	shell		bell
four		core, pour	door, roar
fight		kite	white, night, write, bite, light
fire		tire	
fourth			north
fawn			lawn, yawn, dawn
fear		tear, cheer, hear	near, deer
fanned	sand	tanned, hand	band
fairy		cherry, hairy	berry
face		chase	race, lace

[v]

Sound	1 Feature	2 Features	3 Features
vest		nest, west	test, chest, pest
vine		shine, nine, sign, line	
Vaseline		gasoline	
veil		rail, mail, sail, whale, nail	pail, hail, tail
vet		wet, net, jet	pet
vein		mane, rain	
_____	_____	_____	_____
_____	_____	_____	_____

[θ]

Sound	1 Feature	2 Features	3 Features
thin		chin, pin	
thick	sick	pick, tick, kick	wick, lick
think	sink	pink	wink, rink
thief		chief	beef, leaf
thumb			gum
thigh		tie, pie, high	bye
thunder			wonder
thorn		corn, torn, horn	worn
thong	song		long
third		heard	word, bird, nerd
_____	_____	_____	_____
_____	_____	_____	_____

[ð]

Sound	1 Feature	2 Features	3 Features
No words selected			

[s]

Sound	1 Feature	2 Features	3 Features
sat	fat	pat, rat, cat, hat	mat, bat
sail	tail	pail, nail, veil, rail	whale, mail, jail
socks	fox	rocks	box
soap		rope	
sew	toe	row, hoe, no	bow, mow, go
sun	fun	run	one, bun, gun
sick	tick, thick	kick, pick, lick	wick
sink	think	pink, rink	wink
sea		pea, knee, key	bee
sad		dad	bad, mad
six		chicks	mix
seal		peel, deal	wheel, meal
sunny	funny	honey	money, bunny
sand	fanned, tanned	hand	band
Sam*		ham, lamb	jam
sign	shine	vine, nine, line	
sandal		handle, candle	
song	thong	long	
soak		poke, choke	yolk, joke, woke
sew	toe	row	go, bow
sing		king, ring	wing
sip	zip, ship	lip, hip, dip, rip	whip
_____	_____	_____	_____
_____	_____	_____	_____

*Sam: Sam is a character in the Dr. Seuss book, *Green Eggs and Ham.*

[z]

Sound	1 Feature	2 Features	3 Features
zoo	new	shoe, two, moo, goo, boo	chew
zip	lip, sip, rip	whip, ship	chip, hip
zero			hero
zoom	room	boom	
z	knee, sea	bee	pea, key
_____	_____	_____	_____
_____	_____	_____	_____

[ʃ]

Sound	1 Feature	2 Features	3 Features
shirt		hurt	dirt
shoe	chew	zoo, two	goo, boo, moo, new
ship	chip, sip	hip, zip	whip, rip, lip
shark		park	bark, dark
shine	sign	vine	nine, line
shell	fell		bell
shop	chop	pop, top, cop, hop	mop
shave		pave, cave	wave
sheep	cheep	keep, peep, jeep	deep, leap
_____	_____	_____	_____
_____	_____	_____	_____

[tʃ]

Sound	1 Feature	2 Features	3 Features
chased		paste, taste	raced, waist
chase		face	race, lace
chin		pin, thin	
cheese		peas, keys	knees
chip	ship	hip, sip	rip, lip, whip, zip, dip
chunk	junk		
chop	shop	cop, pop, top, hop	mop
chew	shoe	two	moo, goo, boo, zoo
chief		thief	beef, leaf
chicks		six	mix
chest		pest, test	vest, nest, west
cherry		fairy, hairy	berry
chalk		talk, hawk	walk
cheer		fear, hear, tear	deer, year, near
cheep	sheep, jeep		deep, leap
choke	joke	soak, poke	yolk
————	————	————	————
————	————	————	————

[dʒ]

Sound	1 Feature	2 Features	3 Features
jug		bug, mug	
jail		nail, whale, mail	pail, sail, tail
jaw			paw
junk	chunk		
jewel			fool, cool, tool, pool
Jello		yellow	
jacket		racket	
jump		bump	hump
jam		lamb	ham, Sam*
jeans		beans	
jeep	cheep	deep, sheep, leap, beep	keep, peep
germ		worm	
gym		limb	him
jet		wet, net, vet	pet
joke	choke	yolk	poke, soak

*Sam: Sam is a character in the Dr. Seuss book, *Green Eggs and Ham*.

[m]

Sound	1 Feature	2 Features	3 Features
man		pan	fan, can
mat	bat	pat, rat	fat, hat, cat, sat
mug	bug	jug, rug	hug
mail	whale, nail	pail, jail, rail, veil	sail, tail
men		pen	hen, ten
mouse			house
mice		rice	
mop		pop	shop, chop, top, cop, hop
mad	bad	dad	sad
mold		gold, rolled	hold, fold, cold
moo	new, boo	goo, zoo	chew, two, shoe
meal	wheel	peel, deal	seal
money	bunny		funny, honey, sunny
math	bath	path	
melt	belt		
mow	no	go, row	toe, hoe, sew
mix			six, chicks
mane		rain, vein	

[n]

Sound	1 Feature	2 Features	3 Features
nail	mail, rail	jail, whale, veil, sail, tail	pail
knees		peas, cheese, keys	
nose	rose	toes, bows	hose
nurse			purse
knock	rock, lock	sock	
nut			cut
note		boat, goat	coat
knee	z	sea (see), bee	pea, key
nest		vest, west, test	pest, chest
night	write, light	white, bite	fight, kite
nine	line	vine, sign	shine
neigh	day, ray	weigh	hay, pay
north			fourth
net		vet, wet, jet	pet
near	deer	year, tear	hear, fear, cheer
no	mow, row	go, sew, toe, bow	hoe
nerd		word, bird	third, heard
nickel		tickle	pickle

[l]

Sound	1 Feature	2 Features	3 Features
log	dog		pog[a]
leather			feather
lick		sick, tick, wick	pick, kick, thick
lock	rock, knock	sock	
lake		bake	cake
look		book	cook, hook
lip	zip, rip, dip	whip, sip	chip, ship, hip
lamp			camp
light	night, write	white, bite	fight, kite
line	nine	vine, sign	shine
long		song	thong
late		wait	
lawn	dawn	yawn	
leap	deep	jeep	heap, cheep, sheep, keep, peep
laugh			calf, half
limb		gym	him
life	knife	wife	
leaf			chief, thief
lamb		jam, Sam[b]	ham
lace	race		chase, face

[a] pog: A pog is a term used to refer to milk caps, which are used to play a game in Hawaii and often are given to children as reinforcement in place of stickers.

[b] Sam: Sam is a character in the Dr. Seuss book, *Green Eggs and Ham.*

[r]

Sound	1 Feature	2 Features	3 Features
rat		sat, mat, bat	pat, fat, hat, cat
rug		mug, bug, jug	hug
roast		toast	
raced		taste	chased, paste
rocks		socks, box	fox
red	dead	bed	head
reach		beach, teach	
rose	nose	toes, bows	
ring		sing, wing	king
rice		mice	
rope		soap	
row	no	bow, toe, mow, go, sew	
run		sun, bun, one, gun	fun
rink		sink, wink	think, pink
rock	lock, knock	sock	
rug		mug, bug	hug
rolled		mold, gold	fold, hold, cold
roar	door		core, four, pour
rip	zip, lip, dip	whip, sip	ship, chip, hip
racket		jacket	
write	night, light	bite, white	fight, kite
rain		vein, mane	
rust	dust		
race	lace		chase, face
room	zoom	boom	
rail	nail	whale, mail, sail, jail, veil, tail	pail
ray	day, neigh	weigh	pay, hay

[j]

Sound	1 Feature	2 Features	3 Features
yellow		Jello	
yard		guard, hard	card
yolk	woke	joke	poke, soak, choke
yawn		dawn, lawn	fawn
year		deer, hear	tear, fear, cheer
_____	_____	_____	_____
_____	_____	_____	_____

[w]

Sound	1 Feature	2 Features	3 Features
whale	mail	nail, pail, jail, rail, veil	sail, tail
wing		ring	king
one	bun	run, gun	fun, sun
wand		pond	
wick		pick, lick	kick, tick, sick, thick
wish		dish	fish
wink		pink, rink	think, sink
walk		hawk	chalk, talk
wall	ball	hall	fall, tail, call
wave		pave	shave, cave
wheel	meal	peel, heel	seal
whip		zip, rip, dip, lip, hip	chip, sip, ship
white	bite	write, night, light	fight, kite
world			curled
wonder			thunder
wet		net, vet, pet, jet	
wool	bull	pull	
worm		germ	
wand		pond	
wife		knife, life	
word	bird	nerd, heard	third
west		pest, nest, vest	chest, test
waist		raced, paced	taste, chased
wig	big	pig, dig	
weigh		ray, day, pay, neigh, hay	
wait		late	

[h]

Sound	1 Feature	2 Features	3 Features
hat		pat, cat, fat, sat	bat, rat, mat
hair		pear, wear	bear
hurt		shirt	
hen		pen, ten	men
house			mouse
hair		tear	
head			bed, dead, red
hand		tanned, sand, fanned	band
hawk		chalk, talk, walk	
hop		top, cop, chop, pop, shop	mop
hall		tall, fall, wall	mall
heard		third, word	nerd, bird
hug		tug	bug, mug, rug, jug
hold		cold, fold	mold, rolled, gold
hot		pot	dot
heart		cart	dart
hive		five	dive
honey		sunny, funny	bunny, money
hook		cook	book, look
him			gym, limb
hip		chip, ship, sip, whip	rip, lip, zip
hump			bump, jump, lump
ham			jam, lamb
hill		pill	bill
handle		candle, sandal	
hay		pay, weigh	day, neigh, lay, ray
high		thigh	
hairy		cherry, fairy	berry
horn		corn, thom	
hard		card, yard	guard

(*continued*)

[h] (*continued*)

Sound	1 Feature	2 Features	3 Features
hear		cheer, peer, fear	year, deer
hero			zero
hurt		shirt	dirt
half		calf	laugh
head			dead, red
hoe		sew, toe	row, go, mow, no
hose		toes	rose, nose, bows
_____	_____	_____	_____
_____	_____	_____	_____

D. Cluster Reduction

[l] Clusters

Sound	Word	1st Consonant	2nd or 3rd Consonant
[pl]	plane	pain	
	plants	pants	
	play	pay	lay
	please	peas	
	plate		late
	_____	_____	_____
	_____	_____	_____
[kl]	clip		lip
	club	cub	
	clock		lock
	clap	cap	lap
	cluck		luck
	cloud		loud
	clam		lamb
	claw	caw	
	climb		lime
	_____	_____	_____
	_____	_____	_____
[bl]	black	back	
	blue	boo	
	bleed	bead	lead
	block		lock
	blank	bank	
	_____	_____	_____
	_____	_____	_____

(*continued*)

[l] Clusters (*continued*)

Sound	Word	1st Consonant	2nd or 3rd Consonant
[gl]	glass	gas	
	glitter		litter
	globe		lobe (ear)
	glow		low
	glue	goo	
[fl]	floor	four	
	flight	fight	light
	flat	fat	
	flash		lash (eye)
	flip		lip
[sl]	slip	sip	lip
	slide	side	
	sleep		leap
	sleeve		leave
	sliver		liver

[r] Clusters

Sound	Word	1st Consonant	2nd or 3rd Consonant
[pr]	prize	pies	rise
	price		rice
	prince		rinse
	pray		ray
	prick	pick	
	_____	_____	_____
	_____	_____	_____
[tr]	trip		rip
	track	tack	rack
	train		rain
	tree	tea	
	tray		ray
	trap	tap	rap
	trail	tail	rail
	trash		rash
	trick	tick	
	troll		roll
	_____	_____	_____
	_____	_____	_____
[kr]	crab	cab	
	crib		rib
	crow		row
	crash	cash	rash
	croak	Coke (soda)	
	crust		rust
	_____	_____	_____
	_____	_____	_____

(*continued*)

[r] Clusters (*continued*)

Sound	Word	1st Consonant	2nd or 3rd Consonant
[br]	bread	bed	red
	broom	boom	room
	branch		ranch
	brake	bake	rake
	brain		rain
	___	___	___
	___	___	___
[dr]	drink		rink
	drive	dive	
	driver	diver	
	drill	dill	
	drawer	door	roar
	drag		rag
	drip	dip	rip
	___	___	___
	___	___	___
[gr]	grass	gas	
	grease	geese	
	great	gate	
	ground		round
	gray		ray
	grow	go	row
	___	___	___
	___	___	___
[fr]	front		runt
	fruit		root
	frog	fog	
	___	___	___
	___	___	___
[θr]	three	tree	
	throw		row
	thread		red
	___	___	___
	___	___	___

[w] Clusters

Sound	Word	1st Consonant	2nd or 3rd Consonant
[tw]	twig		wig
	twin	tin	win
	_____	_____	_____
	_____	_____	_____
[kw]	quick	kick	wick
	quack		whack
	quake	cake	wake
	_____	_____	_____
	_____	_____	_____
[sw]	see **[s] Clusters**		

[s] Clusters

Sound	Word	1st Consonant	2nd or 3rd Consonant
[sp]	spot		pot
	spout		pout
	spool		pool
	spill		pill
	spit	sit	pit
	spark		park
	spin		pin
	spade		paid
	spy		pie
	_____	_____	_____
	_____	_____	_____
[st]	stop		top
	sting	sing	
	stink	sink	
	stack	sack	tack
	stick	sick	tick
	stair		tear
	steam		team
	stool		tool
	steal	seal	
	stale	sail	tail
	stand	sand	
	stub	sub	tub
	star		tar
	stew		two
	_____	_____	_____
	_____	_____	_____

(continued)

[s] Clusters (*continued*)

Sound	Word	1st Consonant	2nd or 3rd Consonant
[sk]	school		cool
	ski	sea	key
	scale	sail	
	skunk	sunk	
	skip	sip	
[sw]	swing	sing	wing
	sweat	set	wet
	sweet	seat	
	switch		witch
[sm]	small		mall
	smell	sell	
	smile		mile
	smoke	soak	
	smack	sack	
[sn]	snack	sack	
	snail	sail	nail
	snow	sew	no
	snap		nap
	sneeze		knees
[sl]	see **[l] Clusters**		

(*continued*)

[s] **Clusters** (*continued*)

Sound	Word	1st Consonant	2nd or 3rd Consonant
[spr]	spring	sing	ring
	spray		ray, pay, pray
	Sprite (soda)		write, white
	sprinkle		wrinkle
	_____	_____	_____
	_____	_____	_____
[str]	struck	suck	truck
	strong	song	wrong
	street	seat	treat
	string	sting, sing	
	stream	steam	team
	strap		trap, rap (music)
	_____	_____	_____
	_____	_____	_____
[skr]	scream		cream
	_____	_____	_____
	_____	_____	_____
[skw]	square		wear
	squash		wash
	squeal	seal	wheel
	squeak		weak
	_____	_____	_____
	_____	_____	_____
[spl]	No words selected		

[ʃr] Clusters

Sound	Word	1st Consonant	2nd or 3rd Consonant
[ʃr]	shrub		rub
	shred		red
	shrug		rug
	_____	_____	_____
	_____	_____	_____

E. Final Consonant Deletion

Oral Stops

Sound	Word	Deletion
[p]	rope	row
	keep	key
	sheep	she
	soap	sew
	type	tie
	peep	pea
	pipe	pie
[b]	robe	row
	tube	two
	cob	caw
	rob	raw
[t]	goat	go
	date	day
	boat	bow
	beet	bee
	shoot	shoe
	seat	sea
	note	no
	plate	play
	toot	two
	boot	boo
	ate	A
	moat	mow
	bite	buy

(*continued*)

Oral Stops (*continued*)

Sound	Word	Deletion
[d]	road	row
	toad	toe
	seed	sea
	bead	bee
	dude	do
[k]	cake	K
	peek	pea
	rake	ray
	bike	buy
	beak	B
	back	baa
[g]	jog	jaw
	pog	paw
	egg	A

Fricatives

Sound	Word	Deletion
[f]	goof	goo
	roof	Roo (Winnie the Pooh)
	leaf	Ali (Alladin)
[v]	move	moo
	dive	die
	wave	weigh
	cave	K
[θ]	bath	baa
	teeth	tea
	tooth	two
[ð]	No words selected	
[s]	dice	die
	moose	moo
	ice	eye
	race	ray
	gross	grow

(*continued*)

Fricatives (*continued*)

Sound	Word	Deletion
[z]	nose	no
	rose	row
	hose	hoe
	toes	toe
	shoes	shoe
	maze	May
	crows	crow
	bows	bow
	_____	_____
	_____	_____
[ʃ]	No words selected	
	_____	_____
	_____	_____
[ʒ]	No words selected	
	_____	_____
	_____	_____

Affricates

Sound	Word	Deletion
[tʃ]	teach	tea
	peach	pea
	beach	bee
	couch	cow
	_____	_____
	_____	_____
[dʒ]	cage	K
	page	pay
	badge	baa
	_____	_____
	_____	_____

Nasal Stops

Sound	Word	Deletion
[m]	boom	boo
	time	tie
	dime	die
	home	hoe
	broom	brew
	zoom	zoo
[n]	moon	moo
	bone	bow
	cane	K
	rain	ray
	bean	bee (B)
[ŋ]	song	saw
	thong	thaw
	sing	sea
	king	key

Liquids

Sound	Word	Deletion
[l]	roll	row
	bowl	bow
	rail	ray
	tile	tie
	dial	die
	seal	sea
	hole	hoe
	pile	pie
	mole	mow
	peel	p
	cool	coo
	nail	neigh
	pail	pay
	goal	go

F. Final Consonant Substitutions

[p]

Sound	1 Feature	2 Features	3 Features
cap	cab, cat	catch, calf	can
map	mat	match, math, mad, mash	man
cup	cut		
hop	hot	hog	
rope		road	rose, roll
beep	beet, beak	beach, bead, beef	bees, bean
lip	lick		
leap	leak	leave, leaf, leash, leech	lean
————	————	————	————
————	————	————	————

[b]

Sound	1 Feature	2 Features	3 Features
cab	cap	cat, can	catch, calf
web		wet	
————	————	————	————
————	————	————	————

[t]

Sound	1 Feature	2 Features	3 Features
cut	cup		
hot	hop	hog	
cat	cap	catch, can, cab, calf	
beet	beep, beak, bead	beach, bean, bees, beef	
boat		bone	
bat	bad, back	bath	badge
mat	mad, map	math, man match	
pat	pack, pass	patch, pan	
tent		tenth	
hat		half, hatch	ham
wet		web	
_____	_____	_____	_____
_____	_____	_____	_____

[d]

Sound	1 Feature	2 Features	3 Features
bead	bees, bean, beet	beep	beef, beach
road	roll, rose	rope	
toad	toes		
mad	man, mat	map	match, math, mash
bad	bat	back, badge	bath
_____	_____	_____	_____
_____	_____	_____	_____

[k]

Sound	1 Feature	2 Features	3 Features
hawk		hall	
leak	leap	leaf, leech, leash	lean, leave
back	bat	bad, bath	badge
lick	lip		
cheek		chief	cheese
walk		wash, watch	wall
lock	log	long	lawn
rake			rain, rail
sink		sing	
beak	beep, beet	beach, bead, beef	bean, bees
————	————	————	————
————	————	————	————

[g]

Sound	1 Feature	2 Features	3 Features
hog		hot, hop	
log	lock, long	lawn	
————	————	————	————
————	————	————	————

[f]

Sound	1 Feature	2 Features	3 Features
leaf	leave, leash	leap, leak, leech	lean
beef		beep, beak, beach, beet	bean, bead, bees
half		hatch, hat	ham
chief		cheese, cheek	
calf		cat, cap, catch	cab, can
_____	_____	_____	_____
_____	_____	_____	_____

[v]

Sound	1 Feature	2 Features	3 Features
leave	leaf	leash, lean	leap, leak, leech
_____	_____	_____	_____
_____	_____	_____	_____

[θ]

Sound	1 Feature	2 Features	3 Features
bath		bat, back	badge, bad
math		mat, map, match	mad, man
tenth		tent	
path	pass	pat, pack, patch	pan
mouth	mouse		
_____	_____	_____	_____
_____	_____	_____	_____

[ð]

Sound	1 Feature	2 Features	3 Features
	No words selected		

[s]

Sound	1 Feature	2 Features	3 Features
pass	path, pat	pan, pack, patch	
mouse	mouth		

[z]

Sound	1 Feature	2 Features	3 Features
chains		change	
rose	road		rope
bees	bead, bean	beef	beep, beet, beak, beach
toes	toad		
cheese		chief	cheek
bows	bone	boat	

[ʃ]

Sound	1 Feature	2 Features	3 Features
leash	leaf, leech	leap, leak	lead, lean
wash	watch	walk	wall
mash	match		man
_____	_____	_____	_____
_____	_____	_____	_____

[ʒ]

Sound	1 Feature	2 Features	3 Features
	No words selected		
_____	_____	_____	_____
_____	_____	_____	_____

[tʃ]

Sound	1 Feature	2 Features	3 Features
patch		pat, pack, path, pass	pan
match	mash	mat, map, math	man, mad
leech	leash	leak, leaf, leave, leap	lean
beach		beep, beet, beak, beef	bean, bead, bees
hatch		hat, half	ham
watch	wash	walk	wall
catch		calf, cap, cat	can, cab
_____	_____	_____	_____
_____	_____	_____	_____

[dʒ]

Sound	1 Feature	2 Features	3 Features
change		chains	
badge		bad	bat, bath, back
————	————	————	————
————	————	————	————

[m]

Sound	1 Feature	2 Features	3 Features
swim	swing		
ham			half, hat, hatch
gum	gun		
————	————	————	————
————	————	————	————

[n]

Sound	1 Feature	2 Features	3 Features
pan		pat, pass	patch, pack, path
bone	bows	boat	
pin	pill	pit, pig	pick
lawn	long	log	lock
gun	gum		
rain	rail		rake
lean			leash, leap, leak, leaf, leave
can	cab	cat	cap, calf, catch
man	mad	mat	map, match, math, mash
bean	bead, bees	beet	beep, beak, beach, beef
————	————	————	————
————	————	————	————

[ŋ]

Sound	1 Feature	2 Features	3 Features
swing	swim		
long	lawn, log	lock	
sing		sink	
_____	_____	_____	_____
_____	_____	_____	_____

[l]

Sound	1 Feature	2 Features	3 Features
hall			hawk
roll	road, rose		rope
bowl	bone, bows	boat	
wall			wash, watch, walk
rail	rain		rake
tall			talk, top
_____	_____	_____	_____
_____	_____	_____	_____

APPENDIX 7C
Phonetic Placement and Shaping Techniques

A. Introduction

The following are phonetic placement and shaping techniques for American English consonants and [ɚ]. The instructions are "bare bones" descriptions of techniques that should be studied prior to commencing the treatment session and elaborated on in whatever way seems appropriate to the clinician. An instruction to "touch the client's lips together," for example, might be simply performed or elaborated into a complicated game, depending on the clinician's style and the client's needs.

Shaping techniques that involve common error patterns are indicated by three asterisks (***). For many sounds, more than one technique is described. When this occurs, the methods are listed in approximate order of difficulty, from least to most difficult. When cognates (pairs of sounds differing only in voicing) are presented, the instructions are for the voiceless sound. The voiced sound is facilitated by following the instructions for the voiceless sound and then asking the client to "turn on the voice" or some similar metaphor. The demonstrations of voicing listed in Table 7–5 may also be used to facilitate the production of voicing, for example, with clients with Final Consonant Devoicing, or to facilitate lack of voicing in clients with Prevocalic Voicing.

How to Avoid a Frustrating Situation

The following frustrating situation can arise when performing phonetic placement and shaping techniques. The example describes [t], but the situation can arise with any sound. The clinician carefully and successfully leads the client through all but the last step to produce [t]. Yet, when the clinician says, "Now say [t]," the client moves his or her articulators and reverts to the old pronunciation. Although there is no guaranteed way to keep this situation from arising, the chance of it occurring can be reduced if the clinician uses instructions that do not remind the client of the old pronunciation. After the client's mouth is in position for [t], for

(continued)

example, instead of saying "Now say [t]," the clinician might say, "Now let's play. Lower your tongue quickly" (or some other such instruction). After the client produces the [t]-like sound correctly approximately five times, the clinician might then say, "What you just did—that's how you say the [t] sound."

[p] and [b]

The following techniques facilitate production of [p]. To facilitate [b], follow the same steps, but also instruct the client to turn on the voice box.

PHONETIC PLACEMENT

Method:

1. Ask the client to blow out a long breath.

2. Next, instruct the client to use his or her lips to break up the breath into shorter and shorter bursts. If additional assistance is needed, manually close the client's mouth. [p] results as the client quickly opens and closes his or her lips while continuing to emit a long breath.

SHAPING

[p] from [b] (***Final Consonant Devoicing)

First Method: Instruct the client to turn off his or her "voice box," which for some clients is sufficient instruction to result in [p]. Another possible instruction is to tell the client that "We don't want the voice—we just want the air."

Second Method: Demonstrate the contrast between [b] and [p]. Alternatively, if the client is able to make a voicing contrast between other consonants (such as between [t] and [d]), draw attention to those contrasts. For some clients this is sufficient to result in [p].

[p] from [p̃]

Method: Use a mirror to demonstrate the difference between [p] and [p̃]. In more severe cases, press up the client's lower lip using a finger or a tongue depressor until the lower lip is in contact with the upper lip, which results in [p]. (*Note:* To facilitate [b], develop from [b̃]).

[p] from [ɸ]

Method: Use a mirror to demonstrate the difference between [p] and [ɸ]. In more severe cases, press the client's lips together with your fingers, which results in [p]. (*Note:* To facilitate [b], develop from [β]).

[m]

[m] is facilitated similarly to [p] and [b], except for the addition of nasality.

PHONETIC PLACEMENT

Nasality

First Method:

1. The clinician and client practice taking turns breathing out with their mouths closed, using a piece of paper or a mirror placed under their noses to draw attention to airflow.

2. Next, contrast nasal and oral airflow by placing a piece of paper or a mirror in front of the client's mouth while the client produces an oral consonant such as [b] or [d].

3. Ask the client to attempt [b] with his or her lips closed, but with the voice box vibrating and air coming out the nose. This often results in [m].

Second Method:

1. The clinician and client begin by taking a deep breath, holding it, and letting the air out through the nose. This results in a voiceless [m].

2. Next, have the client practice saying [ɑ].

3. The clinician and client alternate taking a deep breath while holding their noses and then letting air out through the nose while saying "ah" with the mouth closed, which results in [m].

SHAPING

[m] and [b]

Method: Instruct the client to produce [b] followed by a schwa with his or her mouth closed and with air coming out the nose. If needed, a mirror or piece of paper placed under the nostrils may be used to increase the client's awareness of air flowing from the nose. This often results in correct production of [m].

[w]

PHONETIC PLACEMENT

Method:

1. Ask the client to round his or her lips and to place them close together. If the lips are too close or too far apart, move them in to the correct position with a finger or a tongue depressor.

2. Next, instruct the client to raise (or hump up) the very back of his or her tongue toward the roof of the mouth. If needed, push the tongue back with a tongue depressor.

3. Instruct the client to breathe out with his or her voice box on, which often results in [wu].

SHAPING

[w] from [u]

Method:

1. Ask the client to say [u].

2. Next, while the client says [u], ask him or her to almost close the lips, resulting in [w]. (If needed, the client's lips can be moved manually to the appropriate position.)

[w] from [b]

First Method:

Instruct the client to open his or her lips and pucker them slightly while saying [bu], resulting in [wu].

Second Method:

1. Instruct the client to say [u] + [ɑ] several times as rapidly as possible, resulting in [uwɑ].

2. After [uwɑ] is established, instruct the client to "make the [u] silent," which results in [wɑ].

[f] and [v]

The following techniques facilitate [f]. To facilitate [v], follow the same steps, but also instruct the client to turn on the voice box.

PHONETIC PLACEMENT

Method: Instruct the client to touch his or her lower lip with the bottom of the upper front teeth and then to blow, which often results in [f]. In more severe cases, move the clients lip to the correct position using a finger or a tongue depressor. Alternately, instruct the client to "bite" the lower lip with the upper teeth and then to blow.

SHAPING

[f] from [v] (***Final Consonant Devoicing)

Method: Instruct the client to say [v] and then turn off the voice box. This often is sufficient to result in [f]. (*Note:* To facilitate [v], shape from [f] and instruct the client to turn on the voice box.)

[f] from [p] (***Stopping)

Method:

1. Say [f] and [p] to demonstrate the difference between bilabial and labiodental places of production.

2. Instruct the client to say [p] and then instruct him or her to retract the lower lip until the upper teeth are in contact with the lower lip.

3. Instruct the client to separate his or her teeth and lips slightly, resulting in [f]. (*Note:* To facilitate [v], develop from [b].)

[f] from [a]

Method:

1. Instruct the client to say [a].

2. Place the client's lower lip under the edge of his or her upper front teeth.

3. Next, instruct the client to blow air out between his or her lips and teeth so that friction is audible. (In more severe cases, move the client's lips to the correct position and instruct the client to blow out.)

4. Instruct the client to turn off the voice box, resulting in [f]. (*Note:* To facilitate [v], do not instruct the client to turn off the voice, since [a] and [v] are both voiced sounds.)

[θ] and [ð]

The following techniques facilitate [θ]. To facilitate [ð], follow the same steps but also instruct the client to turn on the voice box.

PHONETIC PLACEMENT

First Method:

1. Demonstrate placing the tongue between the upper and lower front teeth.

2. Place a feather or small piece of paper in front of the client's mouth, and instruct the client to blow through the teeth to make the object move, resulting in [θ].

Second Method:

1. Place a tongue depressor in front of the client's mouth, instructing the client to touch the depressor with his or her tongue tip.

2. When the client's tongue is out, gently push up the client's lower jaw so that his or her teeth and tongue come into contact.

3. Instruct the client to blow over the tongue. If the client is only able to produce an interdental [t], gently insert a Q-tip between the client's tongue tip and upper teeth to create a sufficiently broad opening to allow continuous airflow. This often results in [θ].

SHAPING

[θ] from [ð] (***Final Consonant Devoicing)

Method: Instruct the client to say [ð] and then ask him or her to turn off the voice box, resulting in [θ]. (*Note:* To facilitate [ð], instruct the client to turn on the voice while saying [θ].)

[θ] from [f]

Method:

1. Demonstrate the difference between the place of production for [f] and the place of production for [θ].

2. Next, instruct the client to say [f] while moving his or her tongue to lie between the upper and lower front teeth, resulting in [θ]. (*Note:* To facilitate [ð], develop from [v].)

[θ] **from** [s]

Method:

1. Demonstrate the difference between the place of production for [s] and the place of production for [θ].

2. Next, instruct the client to say [s] while moving his or her tongue to lie between the upper and lower front teeth, resulting in [θ]. (*Note:* To facilitate [ð], develop from [z].)

[t] and [d]

The following techniques facilitate [t]. To facilitate [d], follow the same steps but also instruct the client to turn on the voice box.

PHONETIC PLACEMENT

First Method:

1. Use a mirror as a visual aid to instruct the client to press his or her tongue tip against the bump behind the front teeth.

2. Instruct the client to lower the tongue quickly. If needed, a piece of paper or the client's hand placed in front of the mouth may help direct the client to the plosive release of the sound, which often results in a sound that approximates [t].

Second Method:

1. The clinician demonstrates by placing a tongue depressor under his or her tongue and then under the client's tongue. The tongue depressor serves as a shelf for the tongue, which is then raised to be even with the bottom of the upper teeth.

2. Next, raise the client's tongue on the shelf and ask the client to touch "the bump" rapidly with his or her tongue tip. If needed, a piece of paper or the client's hand placed in front of the mouth may help direct the client to the plosive release of the sound. This often results in a sound approximating [t]. (*Note:* To facilitate [d], instruct the client to turn on the voice.)

SHAPING

[t] from [d] (***Final Consonant Devoicing)

Method: Instruct the client to say [d] and then turn off the voice box. For some clients, this is sufficient instruction to result in [t]. (*Note:* To facilitate [d], instruct the client to turn on the voice while saying [t].)

[t] from [p]

Method:

1. Instruct the client to say [p] + schwa.

2. Ask the client to place his or her tongue tip between the lips and to say [p] + schwa again.

3. Next, ask the client to make "a sound almost like [p]" by making contact between his or her tongue tip and upper lip.

4. Instruct the client to make contact between the tongue tip and "the bump," resulting in [t]. (*Note:* To facilitate [d], develop from [b].)

[n]

[n] is facilitated similarly to [t] and [d], except for the addition of nasality.

PHONETIC PLACEMENT

Method:

1. The clinician and client take turns breathing out with their mouths closed and with the tongue in position for [d].

2. Next, place a piece of paper or a mirror under the client's nose to draw attention to air coming out the nose, then contrast this to placing a piece of paper or a mirror in front of the mouth when producing an oral consonant such as [b] or [d].

3. Ask the client to attempt [d] with his or her lips closed but with the voice box vibrating and air coming out the nose. This often results in [n].

SHAPING

[n] from [d]

Method: Instruct the client to take a deep breath, hold it with the tongue in position for [d], close the mouth, and then let the air out through his or her nose, resulting in [n].

[s] and [z]

The following techniques facilitate [s]. To facilitate [z], follow the same steps but also instruct the client to turn on the voice box.

---

[s] Up or [s] Down?

Some people produce [s] and [z] with the tongue tip up behind the upper front teeth, others say them with the tongue tip down behind the lower front teeth. Neither one is the "right way." Follow the client's lead in deciding which way to teach [s] and [z]. If the client appears to find it easier to say [s] and [z] with the tongue tip up, teach the sounds that way; if the client appears to find it easier to say [s] and [z] with the tongue tip down, teach the sounds that way.

PHONETIC PLACEMENT

First Method (tongue tip up or down):

1. Place a tongue depressor just behind the client's upper or lower front teeth and ask the client to use his or her tongue tip to hold it there.

2. Next, ask the client to keep his or her tongue still while the clinician carefully removes the tongue depressor.

3. Ask the client to breathe out, resulting in [s].

Second Method (tongue tip up or down):

1. Instruct the client to place the tip of his or her tongue behind either the upper or lower front teeth and then ask the client to pull the tongue away a little bit.

2. Close the client's teeth so the teeth are barely touching.

3. Place a finger in front of the center of the client's mouth, saying "Blow air slowly over your tongue toward my finger." The sound produced by the client when he or she blows out approximates [s].

Third Method (tongue tip up):

1. Make a shelf by placing a tongue depressor against the lower edges of the client's upper teeth.

2. Next, ask the client to place his or her tongue on the shelf. If needed, place a tongue depressor under the client's tongue tip to bring the "elevator up" so that the tongue depressor touches the lower front teeth.

3. Ask the client to breathe out through his or her mouth. The resulting sound approximates [s].

Fourth Method (tongue tip up):

1. Instruct the client to raise his or her tongue so that the sides are firmly in contact with the inner surface of the upper back teeth. An alternate method is to instruct the client to stick out his or her tongue slightly, lower the upper teeth to come into contact with the sides of the tongue, and then pull the tongue inside his or her mouth.

2. Ask the client to groove the tongue slightly along the midline. If needed, ask the client to protrude the tongue and place a clean object such as a drinking straw along the midline of the tongue. Then ask the client to raise the sides of the tongue slightly around the straw.

3. Carefully withdraw the straw.

4. Ask the client to place the tip of his or her tongue about a quarter of an inch behind the upper teeth and then ask the client to bring the teeth together.

5. Instruct the client to blow air along the groove of the tongue toward the lower teeth. If the client has difficulty directing the air along the tongue groove, insert a drinking straw into the client's mouth and instruct the client to blow through the straw, which often results in [s].

Fifth Method (tongue tip down):

1. Instruct the client to brush his or her lower gums with the tongue while attempting to say [s].

2. Ask the client to stop moving his or her tongue and to bring the upper and lower teeth close together, but not touching.

3. Instruct the client to breathe out through the mouth, resulting in [s].

SHAPING (tongue tip up or down)

[s] from [z] (***Final Consonant Devoicing)

Method: Instruct the client to say [z] and then to turn off the voice box. For some clients, this is sufficient instruction to result in [s]. (*Note:* To facilitate [z], instruct the client to turn on the voice while saying [s].)

[s] from [θ] (***Lisping)

Method:

1. Instruct the client to protrude his or her tongue between the teeth and to say [θ].

2. As client says [θ], instruct him or her to bring the tongue back into the mouth and behind the upper or lower front teeth, depending on which variety of [s] is being facilitated. An alternate method is to ask the client to scrape his or her tongue tip back along the back of the front teeth. (If needed, the tip of the client's tongue can be pushed inward with a tongue depressor.)

3. Next, ask the client to either raise or lower the tongue tip slightly, depending on which type of [s] is being taught.

4. Ask the client to blow air through the mouth, which typically results in [s]. (*Note:* To facilitate [z], develop from [ð].)

[s] from [ɪs] (***Lateralization)

First Method:

1. Demonstrate air flowing through a straw protruding from the side of the mouth when a lateral [s] is made and air flowing through a straw placed in the front of the mouth when a correct [s] is made.

2. Encourage the client to close his or her teeth and to direct the airflow through a straw placed in front of the mouth. This typically results in [s]. (*Note:* To facilitate [z], develop from lateral [z]).

Second Method:

1. Instruct the client to produce a lateral [s] [ɪs].

2. Draw imaginary circles with a Q-tip where the groove should occur in the center of the tongue to indicate to the client where the air should flow during [s].

3. Next, draw a small circle on a piece of paper and hold it in front of the client's mouth at the point where air should be emitted if the air flows over the top of the tongue.

4. Instruct the client to direct the air through the circle while saying [s]. An alternate method is to instruct the client to use his or her fingers instead of paper. If the client's fingers are used, the sensation of air is felt more keenly if the client's fingers are wet. (*Note:* To facilitate [z], develop from lateral [z].)

[s] from [t] (***Stopping)

First Method:

1. Instruct the client to say [t] in *tea* with strong aspiration. If said quickly and forcefully, [tsi] should result. As an alternative to this procedure, ask the client to say [tsi] instead of *tea*.

2. Instruct the client to say [tsi] without the vowel, resulting in [ts].

3. Ask the client to prolong the [s] portion of [ts], resulting in tsss.

4. Ask the client to make [t] silent, resulting in [s].

Second Method:

1. Ask the client to open his or her mouth and to put the tongue in position for [t].

2. Instruct the client to drop his or her tongue slightly and to send the air over the tongue. Place the client's finger in front of the mouth to feel the emission of air. The resulting sound is [s].

[s] from [ʃ]

Method:

1. Instruct the client to say [ʃ].

2. Ask the client to retract his or her lips into a smile. Often, this results in the tongue moving forward slightly into the position for [s]. If needed, however, instruct the client to move the tongue slightly forward. The resulting sound is [s]. (*Note:* To facilitate [z], develop from [ʒ], or instruct the client to turn on his or her voice box.)

[s] from [d] (***Stopping and ***Prevocalic Voicing)

Method:

1. Ask the client to place his or her tongue in position for [d].

2. Instruct the client to release the tongue a little bit and to force the air over the tongue.

3. Ask the client to tum off the voice. The sound that results when the client turns off the voice is [s]. (*Note:* To facilitate [z], develop from [d] or use [s] and instruct the client to turn on his or her voice box.)

[s] from [i]

Method:

1. Instruct the client to say [i].

2. Ask the client to turn off his or her voice and gradually close the teeth until [s] results. (*Note:* To facilitate [z], instruct the client to keep the voice box on.)

[s] from [h]

Method:

1. Instruct the client to gradually close the teeth while saying [h].

2. Ask the client to raise his or her tongue tip gradually while producing a prolonged [h] until the resulting sound is [s]. (*Note:* To facilitate [z], instruct the client to turn on the voice.)

[s] from [f]

Method:

1. Instruct the client to lift his or her tongue tip slowly while making a prolonged [f].

2. Ask the client to bring the front teeth close together but not quite touching. If needed, gently pull out the client's lower lip slightly.

3. Ask the client to smile while making the sound, resulting in [s]. (*Note:* To facilitate [z], develop from [v] or use [s] and instruct the client to turn on his or her voice box.)

[l]

PHONETIC PLACEMENT

First Method:

1. Touch the client's alveolar ridge with a tongue depressor, peanut butter, or lollipop to indicate the place of production for [l].

2. Ask the client to place his or her tongue tip in the place indicated, to relax, and to let air flow out from the sides of the tongue. The resulting sound is voiceless [l].

3. Instruct the client to turn on the voice box, resulting in [l].

Second Method:

1. Place a straw midline on the client's tongue groove to demonstrate central air emission. Ask the client to blow out onto an open hand or a piece of paper. An alternative (or additional) demonstration of central air emission is to ask the client to prepare his or her mouth to say [s] but to breathe in. Cool air is felt midline on the upper tongue surface.

2. Next, place a straw in each corner of the client's mouth. Ask the client to breathe out into his or her open hand or on a piece of paper. If an additional demonstration is needed, remove the straws and ask the client to breathe in and to feel the cool air on the sides of the tongue over which the air is emitted. To demonstrate the feel of the air more vividly, ask the client to suck on a piece of peppermint candy for a few minutes before performing the demonstration.

3. After lateral emission of air is obtained, ask the client to place his or her tongue tip in contact with the roof of the mouth behind the upper front teeth and to blow out over the sides of the tongue. If needed, place straws in the side of the clients mouth while the tongue tip is held in contact with the roof of the mouth.

4. Then instruct the client to blow air out the side straws, which results in voiceless [l].

5. Voicing is obtained by asking the client to turn on the voice box. The resulting sound is [l].

Third Method:

1. Place a tongue depressor under the client's tongue tip and raise the tongue tip behind the upper front teeth.

2. Ask the client to say [l] while maintaining contact between the tongue tip and the roof of the mouth. The resulting sound is [l].

Fourth Method ([l] in consonant clusters):

Instruct the client to place the tongue in the position for [l] before initiating the cluster, resulting in a consonant cluster containing [l].

SHAPING

[l] from [θ] or [ð]

Method:

1. Instruct the client to place the tongue tip between the teeth as for [θ].

2. Lower the client's jaw.

3. Instruct the client to slowly draw the tongue tip backward but to keep the tongue tip in contact with the back of the teeth and the ridge behind the two front teeth.

4. Next, instruct the client to say [l], being sure that contact between the tongue and the roof of the mouth is maintained.

[l] from [i] or [u]

Method:

1. Instruct the client to open his or her mouth wide as for [ɑ] but to raise the tongue as for [i].

2. Ask the client to keep the tongue up as for [i] but to say [ɑ], resulting in a light (alveolar) [l]. (*Note:* For a dark [velar] [l], follow the same steps but ask the client to say [u] instead of [i].)

[ɚ]

PHONETIC PLACEMENT

First Method (retroflex or humped):

Instruct the client to growl like a tiger ([ɚ]). Alternately, ask the client to make the "arm wrestling sound" ([ɚ]) while arm wrestling with the clinician.

Second Method (retroflex or humped):

Instruct the client to lie on his or her back, relax the mouth, and say [ɚ].

Third Method (humped):

1. Instruct the client to lower his or her tongue tip.

2. Ask the client to hump up the back of the tongue as for a silent [k].

3. Ask the client to make the sides of the back of the tongue touch the insides of the back teeth.

4. Ask the client to turn on the voice box, resulting in [ɚ].

SHAPING

[ɚ] (humped) From [w] (***Gliding)

Method:

1. Lower the client's jaw slightly.

2. Ask the client to say [w] but to "let the lips go to sleep." An alternate method is to tell the client, "No kissing frogs" to prompt an unround tip position. If needed, push the client's lips back with a tongue depressor to an unrounded position.

3. While reminding the client to keep the lips asleep, instruct him or her to make the tongue position for [d].

4. Ask the client to retract the tongue slightly while lowering the tongue tip and to say [ɚ].

[ɚ] (retroflex) from [ð]

Method:

1. Instruct the client to place his or her tongue as for [ð].

2. Ask the client to quickly draw the tongue tip back and slightly up, which typically results in [ɚ].

[ɚ] (humped) from [d]

Method: Lower the client's jaw slightly as for [d]. While the client's jaw is lowered, ask him or her to pull back the tongue slightly, to lower the tongue tip, and to say [ɚ].

[ɚ] (retroflex) from [ʃ]

Method:

1. Instruct the client to say [ʃ], but to curl the tongue tip back while keeping contact with the tongue on the insides of the back teeth.

2. Ask the client to turn on the voice box, resulting in [ɚ].

[ɚ] (retroflex) from [l]

Method:

1. Lower the client's jaw slightly and instruct the client to say [l] + [2].

2. While the client says [l] + [2], instruct him or her to curl back the tongue tip until [ɚ] results. (If needed, a tongue depressor can be used to push the tongue back.)

[ɚ] from [ɑ]

Method:

1. Instruct the client to say "ah."

2. Next, ask the client to raise his or her tongue slightly toward the roof of the mouth and say [ɑr]. (If needed, instruct the client to raise the tongue tip or to raise his or her tongue slightly and to say [ɑ] forcibly.) The resulting sound is [ɑr].

[ɚ] (retroflex) from [i]

Method:

1. Instruct the client to say [i].

2. While the client is saying [i], ask him or her to lift the tongue and curl back the tongue tip to say [ɚ].

[r]

PHONETIC PLACEMENT

First Method:

Instruct the client to make a sound like a motor starting up ([rɚ]).

Second Method:

1. Ask the client to place his or her tongue tip behind the upper front teeth. (If needed, place the client's tongue tip on a shelf made with a tongue depressor.)

2. Next, ask the client to curl the tongue backward without touching the roof of the mouth until it cannot go back farther.

3. Lower the client's jaw slightly and instruct the client to say [ru].

Facilitation of [r]

With some clients, correct production of [ɚ] generalizes to [r] without the need for treatment.

SHAPING

[r] from [ɚ]

Method:

1. Ask the client to say [ɚ].

2. Next, ask the client to say [ɚ] followed by [i] or some other vowel.

3. Instruct the client to say [ɚi] several times as quickly as possible, resulting in [ɚri]. After [ri] is established, instruct the client to say [ɚ] silently, resulting in [ri].

[tʃ] and [dʒ]

The following techniques facilitate [tʃ]. To facilitate [dʒ], follow the same steps, but also instruct the client to turn on the voice box.

PHONETIC PLACEMENT

Method:

1. Ask the client to pucker the lips slightly.

2. Ask the client to make the tongue tip touch "the bump" behind the two upper front teeth.

3. Next, instruct the client to make the sneezing sound (choo!) while keeping the lips slightly puckered and the tongue tip on the alveolar ridge. If [ts] results, instruct the client to move the tongue tip back slightly while maintaining contact with the roof of the mouth, resulting in [tʃ].

SHAPING

[tʃ] from [ʃ]

Method: Instruct the client to say a quick [ʃ] with the tongue tip touching "the bump," resulting in [tʃ]. (*Note:* To facilitate [dʒ], develop from [ʒ].)

[tʃ] from [t] or [ʃ]

Method:

1. Explain that [tʃ] is [t] and [ʃ] said together very quickly.

2. Next, ask the client to say [ʃ].

3. Instruct the client to say [t] and then to draw the tongue tip back a little and say [t] again.

4. With the client's tongue tip in the position for the "back" [t], instruct the client to quickly say [t] followed by [ʃ], resulting in [tʃ]. (*Note:* To facilitate [dʒ], develop from [d] and [ʒ].)

[ʃ] and [ʒ]

The following techniques facilitate [ʃ]. To facilitate [ʒ], follow the same steps but also instruct the client to turn on the voice box.

PHONETIC PLACEMENT

Method:

1. Ask the client to part his or her teeth and lips.

2. Touch the client's tongue just behind the tip with a tongue depressor. Instruct the client to move the place just touched to the roof of the mouth behind the "bumpy part." (If needed, a tongue depressor may be used to push the tongue back from the upper front teeth.)

3. Next, instruct the client to lower the tongue slightly. (If needed, direct the tongue down slightly with a tongue depressor.)

4. Ask the client to hold this position, pucker his or her lips slightly, and breathe out through the mouth, which results in [ʃ].

SHAPING

[ʃ] from [ʒ] (***Final Consonant Devoicing)

Method: Instruct the client to say [ʒ] and then turn off the voice, resulting in [ʃ]. (*Note:* To facilitate [ʒ], instruct the client to turn on the voice while saying [ʃ].)

[ʃ] from [s] (***Fronting)

Method: Ask the client to say [s]. While the client is saying [s], instruct him or her to pucker the lips slightly and to draw the tongue back a little until [ʃ] results.

[ʃ] from [i] or [ɑ]

Method:

1. Instruct the client to say [i] or [ɑ], first with the voice on and then with the voice off.

2. Next, ask the client to pucker the lips slightly.

3. Raise the client's lower jaw slightly.

4. Ask the client to breathe out silently while raising the tongue, resulting in [ʃ].

[j]

PHONETIC PLACEMENT

Method:

1. Instruct the client to place the tongue flat in the mouth. (If needed, gently press down the tongue with a tongue depressor.)

2. Open the client's mouth and gently tap the middle portion of the tongue, asking the client to slightly raise the place you touched.

3. Ask the client to breathe out with the voice on, resulting in [j].

SHAPING

[j] from [ʒ]

Method: Instruct the client to say [ʒ] several times quickly. Often, this results in [j]. An additional cue is to ask the client to lower the tongue slightly.

[k] and [g]

The following techniques facilitate [k]. To facilitate [g], follow the same steps but also instruct the client to turn on the voice box.

PHONETIC PLACEMENT

First Method:

1. Instruct the client to place a hand in contact with the underside of your mouth.
2. While holding the client's chin stationary, direct the client's attention to the muscle movements that occur as you repeat [k] several times.
3. Ask the client to imitate you, resulting in [k].

Second Method:

Ask the client to drop his or her head back and say [ku], which sometimes is sufficient to result in [k].

Third Method:

Ask the client to pretend to cough up a fish bone from the throat. Alternately, ask the client to imitate you while you pretend to shoot a gun, resulting in [ku ku ku].

Fourth Method:

1. Press your hand underneath the client's chin near the juncture of the jaw and neck where [k] is produced.
2. Instruct the client to whisper [ku] as you release the pressure, resulting in a soft [k].

Fifth Method:

1. Ask the client to place the tongue tip behind the lower front teeth. (If needed, a tongue depressor may be used to keep the tongue in place.)
2. Ask the client to hump the back of the tongue and say [ku].

Shaping

[k] from [t] (***Fronting)

Method:

1. Ask the client to place the tongue tip behind the two lower front teeth while making [t]. (If needed, the tongue tip may be held down with a tongue depressor.)

2. Next, ask the client to hump up the back of the tongue and say [k]. (*Note:* For [g], shape from [d].)

[k] from [g] (***Final Consonant Devoicing)

Method: Instruct the client to say [g] and then to turn off the voice box. For some clients, this is sufficient instruction to result in [k]. (*Note:* To facilitate [g], instruct the client to turn on the voice while saying [k].)

[k] from [i]

Method:

1. Instruct the client to say [i].

2. Next, ask the client to say a long [i] but to raise up the back of the tongue as the vowel ends, resulting in [k]. If needed, instruct the client to turn off the voice. (*Note:* To facilitate [g], do not ask the client to turn off the voice.)

[ŋ]

[ŋ] is facilitated similarly to [k] and [g] except for the addition of nasality.

PHONETIC PLACEMENT

Method:

1. Ask the client to breathe out with his or her mouth closed.

2. Next, place a piece of paper or a mirror under the client's nose, drawing attention to air coming out the nose. Contrast this with placing a piece of paper or a mirror in front of the client's mouth while producing an oral consonant such as [b] or [d].

3. Ask the client to attempt [g] with the lips closed, voice box vibrating, and air coming out the nose, resulting in [ŋ].

SHAPING

None recommended.

[h]

PHONETIC PLACEMENT

First Method: Instruct the client to practice blowing out a candle, resulting in [h].

Second Method: To produce [h] in conjunction with a vowel, ask the client to say a vowel and then to blow out the vowel that follows [h], resulting in [h] + vowel.

SHAPING
None typically is required.

CHAPTER

8

Options in Assessment and Treatment

The following topics are discussed in this chapter:

I. OVERVIEW

This chapter summarizes many of the major care options presented in previous chapters. Case studies of clients are presented to illustrate similarities and differences in providing care at four stages in articulation and phonological development. Each client is a composite of several real clients seen either by the author or his colleagues.

II. MAJOR CARE OPTIONS FOR CLIENTS IN STAGE 1

A. The Client: Bill

Bill was born with Down syndrome, a genetic disorder occurring in approximately 1 in 700 births. Children with Down syndrome typically are moderately retarded and suffer from heart conditions, weak muscle tone, and respiratory problems. In his first months at home Bill developed slowly but steadily, although he was a difficult child to feed. Bill underwent heart surgery at 6 months of age to correct a faulty heart valve, and during that time in the hospital he appeared to regress in some of his earlier developmental gains. Bill was referred to a speech-language clinician when he was 10 months of age.

B. Legal Basis of Care (Chapter 2)

Bill was eligible to be considered for articulation and phonological care under the Individuals with Disabilities Education Act (IDEA). Importantly, even if Bill was not delayed in development, he is eligible to receive developmental services, because the law recognizes that Down syndrome is a genetic disorder which places Bill at high risk for future developmental delays.

C. Screening and Assessment (Chapter 4)

The assessment consisted of three steps: an initial observation, collection of a sample of vocalizations, and hypothesis testing. The assessment began by talking with Bill's caregivers and observing Bill at rest in his mother's arms. To obtain a sample of vocalizations, the clinician's options were either to elicit vocalizations or to ask one of Bill's caregivers to perform this function. In almost all cases, a caregiver elicits vocalizations more easily from an infant than someone less familiar with the client's habits and likes, so the clinician chose to have Bill's parents act as the elicitors. Hypotheses raised during the initial evaluation session were addressed during subsequent treatment sessions.

1. **Sample Size.** The clinician obtained 10 vocalizations during the initial assessment and 14 more during the elicitation portion of subsequent treatment sessions. Although not a large sample, it was deemed sufficient to begin treatment.

2. **Transcription System.** The clinician's options were to transcribe and record Bill's vocalizations or to utilize a check mark system such as that presented in Appendix 5J. The clinician elected to use the check mark system.

3. **Types of Speech Samples.** The clinician's options were spontaneous speech, elicited speech, or a combination of both. Bill's level of development precluded all but spontaneous speech.

4. **Elicitation Activities.** The following objects were available to elicit vocalizations: a mirror, bubbles, pop-up toys, manipulable toys, a toy drum, and several toy cars.

5. **Options for Published Assessment Instruments.** None.

6. **Related Assessments.** In addition to the articulation and phonological assessment, the clinician performed a parent interview, a hearing screening, a complete language evaluation, and an oral-mechanism evaluation.

D. Analysis (Chapter 5)

The following options were considered (the order of assessments reflects their presentation in Chapter 5 and does not reflect the order in which they were performed):

Severity

Age norms

Better abilities

Related analyses

1. **Severity.** The principle clinical options were calculation of percentage of development and severity rating scales such as those presented in Chapter 5. The clinician selected a severity rating scale. The results indicated that Bill was severely delayed in vocal development compared to both his language reception abilities and chronological age.

2. **Age Norms.** The clinical option was analysis of prespeech vocalizations. Results of the assessment indicated that Bill's vocalizations approximated those of an infant near 1 to 2 months of age. The

clinician also noted that one instance of cooing (a back vowel) was observed.

3. Better Abilities. The clinical option was stimulability. Results of this analysis indicated that Bill was unstimulable for any type of vocalization.

4. Related Analyses. The clinical options were adjusted age and developmental age. Because Bill was not born prematurely, adjusted age was not calculated. Results of the language evaluation indicated that Bill's language reception and play abilities approximated those of an infant near 6 months of age.

E. Treatment (Chapter 6)

Bill was accepted into treatment as an outpatient in a hospital-based early intervention program.

1. Purpose. Articulation and phonological care focused on facilitating the acquisition of vocal skills that underlie later speech development.

2. Long-term Goals. The long-term treatment goal for Bill was for his articulation and phonological development to be commensurate to his developmental age. A second long-term treatment goal was to facilitate parent education and training.

3. Short-term Goals. The options for short-term goals were to: (1) increase Bill's opportunities to vocalize, (2) acquire developmentally advanced vocalizations, (3) teach functional, high-frequency words in familiar contexts, and (4) facilitate conversational turn-taking. The first goal might have been selected if Bill was hospitalized or suffering from neglect, because in those situations providing regular opportunities to play and vocalize sometimes is sufficient to result in impressive developmental changes. However, because Bill was delayed in vocal development despite many opportunities to vocalize, the clinician chose the second option.

4. Selecting Treatment Targets. The clinician considered behaviors in advance of Bill's present level of vocal development. Syllables containing back consonants and vowels were given the highest consideration, because during the evaluation Bill produced one instance of cooing, showing that the behavior—although infrequent—was within Bill's vocal capacities.

5. **Most and Least Knowledge Methods.** The options were to select treatment targets slightly or substantially in advance of Bill's present vocal abilities. In the vast majority of cases infants progress by small steps in vocal development, and so, perforce, the most knowledge method was selected.

6. **Number of Treatment Targets.** The treatment options were to train wide or deep. Training wide was selected because this choice seemed better suited to Bill's cognitive and developmental abilities.

7. **Changing Treatment Targets.** The clinician's options were flexibility, time, and percentage. A flexible approach was selected because it seemed better suited to Bill's level of cognitive development. The clinician, for example, arrived at each treatment session prepared to facilitate a variety of back consonants and back vowels; the exact choice of the session's treatment target was based on the sounds that Bill was willing to attempt.

8. **Linguistic Level to Introduce Treatment Targets.** This option was not pertinent to Bill's care.

F. Administrative Decisions (Chapter 6)

The administrative options involved session length, group or individual care, length of individual treatment activities, and types of activities. The clinician elected to facilitate vocal development in a group that met four times a week for 30 minute sessions. Ten minutes was devoted primarily to stimulating vocal and language development. All of the activities involved play, and individual vocal stimulation activities lasted from a few seconds to a few minutes. Bill's parents were encouraged to participate in group activities. Additional counseling of parents regarding vocal development was provided in individual weekly meetings.

G. Facilitative Techniques (Chapter 7)

The clinician's primary options for facilitative techniques were motherese and, occasionally, imitation. Language was stimulated simultaneously with vocal development.

Throughout the session, the clinician and Bill engaged in routines that had been found to encourage Bill to vocalize. While playing, the clinician occasionally produced vocalizations for Bill to imitate. If Bill imitated the vocalization, that utterance became the treatment target for the next few minutes as the clinician and Bill engaged in reciprocal vocalizations. If, however, Bill produced a different vocalization, that became the treatment target for the next few minutes. The clinician praised and looked excited when Bill produced any type of vocalization; when Bill cooed, the clinician praised him even more.

H. Assessing Clinical Progress (Chapter 6)

The clinician's primary options were pre- and post-tests, ongoing information gathering, and parent questionnaires. The clinician assessed treatment progress using the vocal development check-list (Appendix 5J) and a severity scale as pre- and post-tests. A parent interview designed to ascertain both the family's knowledge of vocal development and their degree of satisfaction with Bill's therapeutic progress was also undertaken. Results of the post-tests indicated good clinical progress; Bill's family demonstrated increased knowledge of vocal development in response to questions asked by the clinician and they expressed satisfaction with their son's clinical progress.

III. MAJOR CARE OPTIONS FOR CLIENTS IN STAGE 2

A. The Client: Mary

Mary was born 2 months prematurely, but she did not experience overt medical complications resulting from her prematurity and was discharged from the hospital shortly after her original due date, small but healthy. It was explained to Mary's family, however, that she was at risk for future developmental problems due to possible damage to her immature neurological system. Mary was referred to a speech-language clinician at 23 months of age.

B. Legal Basis of Care (Chapter 2)

Like Bill, Mary was eligible to receive articulation and phonological care under IDEA. It should be noted that, even if Mary was not delayed in development, she would have been eligible to receive developmental services because the law recognizes that prematurity places children at risk for future developmental delays.

C. Assessment (Chapter 4)

The assessment consisted of three steps: initial observation, collection of the speech sample, and hypothesis testing. The assessment began by observing Mary while she and her mother played. The clinical options for collecting the speech sample were for the clinician or Mary's mother to act as the elicitor. The clinician chose the latter option because in almost all cases a caregiver elicits speech from a toddler more easily than someone unfamiliar with the child's likes and dislikes. Hypotheses raised about Mary's speech during the initial evaluation were pursued during subsequent treatment sessions. Gradually, the clinician became the elicitor as the clinician and Mary grew more comfortable with each other.

1. **Sample Size.** A speech sample of 50 to 100 utterances, which is often obtained with older children, is seldom feasible with most toddlers, especially those under 18 months of age. The clinician obtained a total of 13 different renditions of 10 different words on the first day of evaluation, and an additional 9 different renditions of 4 additional words were obtained over subsequent evaluations undertaken concurrent with the onset of treatment.

2. **Transcription System.** The clinician transcribed whole words using the International Phonetic Alphabet (IPA). The non-English symbols and diacritics expected to be used in the transcription included labiodental stops, bilabial fricatives, unaspirated voiceless stops, wet sounds, and glottal stops. Additional symbols and diacritics were included as needed (see Chapter 2 for recommended extensions of the International Phonetic Alphabet).

3. **Types of Speech Samples.** The clinician's options were to sample spontaneous speech, elicited speech, or a combination of both. Mary's level of development precluded all but spontaneous speech and occasional use of speech imitations (elicited speech).

4. **Elicitation Activities.** The following objects were available to help elicit speech: several simple picture books, a play telephone, a wagon and a toy tricycle, a Mr. Potato head, a doll, blocks, and several big-piece puzzles.

5. Options for Standardized Assessment Instruments. None.

6. Related Assessments. In addition to the articulation and phonological assessment, the clinician performed a parent interview, a hearing screening, a complete language evaluation, and an oral-mechanism evaluation.

D. Analysis (Chapter 5)

The following options were considered (the order of assessments reflects their presentation in Chapter 5 and does not reflect the order in which they were performed):

Severity or intelligibility

Age Norms

Better abilities

Related analyses

1. Severity or Intelligibility. The major clinical options were calculation of percentage of development and clinical judgment scales. The clinician selected a clinical judgment scale. The results indicated that Mary was mildly delayed in articulation and phonological development compared to her adjusted chronological age (21 months).

2. Age Norms. The major clinical options were analysis of phonetic inventories, error patterns, and consonants.

   a. Phonetic Inventories. The clinical options were to use age norms based on either intelligible words or both intelligible and unintelligible words. The former option was selected because Mary's speech appeared largely intelligible. The number and types of consonants in Mary's phonetic inventory approximated those of a child near 16 months of age.

   b. Error Patterns. The most pervasive error patterns in Mary's speech were Fronting, Stopping, Cluster Reduction, Final Consonant Deletion, Weak Syllable Deletion, and Prevocalic Voicing. Cluster Reduction, Final Cluster Deletion, and Weak Syllable Deletion occurred on nearly 100% of all possible occasions. Fronting, Stopping, and Prevocalic Voicing occurred on 60% of all possible occasions.

    c. Consonants. Mary's speech contained two established consonants ([b] and [d]) and three emerging consonants ([f], [p], and [k]). [f], [b], [p], and [d] occurred word-initially and [k] occurred word-finally.

3. Better Abilities. The clinical options were stimulability, key environments, and key words. Mary was stimulable for [f]. No key environments or key words were found.

4. Related Analyses. The clinical options were developmental age, adjusted age, dialect, and acquisition strategies. Mary's developmental age approximated a child of 20–24 months of age. Mary's adjusted age was 21 months. No clinically relevant dialect characteristics were noted in Mary's or her family's speech. The options for acquisition strategies that the clinician considered included regressions, favorite sounds, selectivity, word recipes, homonyms, word-based learning, and gestalt learning. No prominent acquisition strategies were noted.

E. Treatment (Chapter 6)

Mary was accepted into treatment in an early intervention program.

1. Purpose. Articulation and phonological care focused on facilitating the acquisition of sounds in specific words.

2. Long-term Goals. The long-term goal of treatment for Mary was for articulation and phonological development to be commensurate with her adjusted chronological age. A second long-term treatment goal was to facilitate parent education and training.

3. Short-term Goals. The clinical options were: (1) stimulate expressive vocabulary development, (2) encourage speech for communication, (3) reduce homonyms, (4) reduce variability, and (5) maximize established speech skills. Mary's speech did not contain a lot of homonyms or variability, so goals directed to remediating those areas were not considered further. Mary also did not appear stalled in development according to parental report, only somewhat slower compared to other children of her age, so maximization of established speech abilities was not considered as a possible short-term treatment goal. The remaining option, elimination of errors affecting sound classes, was selected as Mary's short-term goal. An error pattern approach was selected. Prevocalic Voicing, Stopping, and Fronting were selected as the first foci of treatment because Mary had demonstrated some ability to produce sounds affected by these errors.

4. **Selecting Treatment Targets.** The clinical options were to select treatment targets that occurred in key words or were emerging, stimulable, or both. When considering the latter two options (emerging and stimulable), the clinician gave greatest priority to potential treatment targets that were both emerging and stimulable but did not exclude potential treatment targets that met one of the other criterion.

5. **Most and Least Knowledge Methods.** The options the clinician considered were to select treatment targets most like the client's existing sound (a traditional most knowledge method) or treatment targets least like the client's existing sounds (least knowledge method). The clinician selected the latter option, hoping this would improve the likelihood that Mary would generalize treatment success to untreated sounds. For this reason [k] was considered a preferred treatment target compared to [p], because [k] differed from Mary's established consonants in both place and voicing, whereas [p] differed from Mary's established consonants only in voicing. Similarly, [f] was considered a preferred treatment target compared to both [k] and [p], because [f] differed from Mary's established consonants in place, manner, and voicing.

6. **Number of Treatment Targets.** The clinical options were to train wide or train deep. The clinician selected training wide (three or more treatment targets) to maximize Mary's opportunities to generalize treatment success to untreated sounds.

7. **Changing Treatment Targets.** The clinician's options were flexibility, time, and percentage. The clinician selected time because it appeared best-suited to Mary's level of cognitive development. If, however, Mary had appeared to have attention difficulties or more substantive cognitive limitations, the clinician would likely have selected flexibility.

8. **Linguistic Level to Introduce Treatment Targets.** The clinical options are isolated sounds, nonsense syllables, words, and phrases. Mary's level of development precluded all but words from consideration.

F. Administrative Decisions (Chapter 6)

The administrative decisions involved session length, group or individual care, length of individual treatment activities, and types of activities. The clinician elected to provide treatment as part of an early intervention program three times a week. Group sessions typically lasted approximately 45 minutes, 15 minutes of which were devoted primarily to speech and language development. The length of specific activities in treatment sessions was approximately 5 minutes. Activities were presented in a therapeutic play format.

G. Facilitative Techniques (Chapter 6)

The clinician's options for facilitative techniques were bombardment, parallel talk, expansions, touch cues, modeling, and requests for confirmation or clarification.

Treatment was organized in cycles. The first cycle provided treatment for Fronting, Prevocalic Voicing, and Stopping. In principle, up to one half of the sounds in an error pattern received treatment. In practice, the requirements of stimulability or emerging sounds restricted the treatment targets to far fewer sounds. The first cycle continued until all treatment targets had received remediation. Error patterns were treated in subsequent cycles until Mary's production of sounds within the error pattern was commensurate with that of children of her adjusted chronological age. Additional error patterns were added to treatment as ongoing evaluation indicated additional sounds in the error patterns became either stimulable or emerging.

Prior to beginning treatment on an error pattern, the clinician and Mary's parents identified the words that were to receive special attention during treatment and at home. Treatment for [k], for example, began with bombardment using approximately 10 words beginning with [k]. Included among these words were three words that were also to be facilitated at home. The words referred to objects that the clinician named as they were drawn out of a "magic box." Production activities involved therapeutic play during which the primary facilitative technique was expansion, supplemented by parallel talk, modeling, and requests for confirmation or clarification. Touch cues for treatment sounds were also introduced. The session concluded with a bombardment activity similar to the one at the beginning of the session.

H. Assessing Clinical Progress (Chapter 6)

The clinician's primary options were pre- and post-tests, ongoing information gathering, and parent questionnaires. The clinician elected to use a clinical judgment of severity and the word lists presented during treatment as pre- and post-tests. A parent interview designed to ascertain both the family's knowledge of speech development and their degree of satisfaction with Mary's progress in speech development was also undertaken. Results of post-testing indicated fair clinical progress; Mary's family demonstrated increased knowledge of speech development in response to questions asked by the clinician and they expressed satisfaction with their daughter's clinical progress.

IV. MAJOR CARE OPTIONS FOR CLIENTS IN STAGE 3

A. The Client: Robert

Robert was born after an unremarkable pregnancy and delivery. Robert's medical and developmental history were similarly unremarkable; however Robert's mother noted that "Kids have trouble understanding his speech, although I usually know what he means." Robert was referred to a speech-language clinician when he entered preschool at 4 years of age.

B. Legal Basis of Care (Chapter 2)

Robert was eligible to be considered for intervention under IDEA, which mandates free and appropriate education to all children with handicaps from ages 3 through 21 years. Appropriate education includes a thorough assessment to determine the nature and degree of disability, education tailored to the individual needs of children, placement in the least restrictive environment, and the provision of supplementary services to help ensure success for each child.

C. Assessment (Chapter 4)

The assessment consisted of three steps: initial observation, collection of the speech sample, and hypothesis testing. The initial observation occurred during the parent interview while the clinician spoke with Robert's mother. For the elicitation portion of the assessment, the clinician presented Robert with pictures from a published assessment instrument and transcribed Robert's speech during naming activities while playing. The hypothesis testing occurred during the initial assessment and the beginning of one subsequent treatment session. The clinician concentrated on Robert's most prevalent error patterns using the error probes presented in Appendix 4C. Due to time limitations, error patterns that appeared relatively minor (e.g., deletion of [d] in *window*) were set aside for later consideration.

1. **Sample Size.** The clinician's option was to collect between 50 to 100 utterances either in the form of sentences, single words, or a combination of both.

2. **Transcription System.** The clinician transcribed whole words using the International Phonetic Alphabet (IPA). The non-English symbols and diacritics expected to be used in the transcription of Robert's speech included labiodental stops, unaspirated voiceless stops, wet sounds, glottal stops, [w] coloring of [r], lisping, lateralization, and bladed productions of [s] and [z]. Additional symbols and diacritics were included as needed (see Appendix 3A for recommended extensions of the International Phonetic Alphabet).

3. **Types of Speech Samples.** The clinician's options were to obtain samples of spontaneous speech, elicited speech, or a combination of both. During the initial observation, the clinician noted errors occurring in Robert's spontaneous speech. The major portion of the speech sample, however, was derived from single words.

4. **Elicitation Activities.** The clinician selected elicitation activities from those listed in Chapter 4.

5. **Options for Standardized Assessment Instruments.** The following published instruments offered options to assess error patterns:

   The Assessment of Phonological Processes—Revised

   Bankson-Bernthal Test of Phonology

   Compton-Hutton Phonological Assessment

   The Khan-Lewis Phonological Analysis

   Natural Process Analysis

   Phonological Process Analysis

   Smit-Hand Articulation and Phonology Evaluation (SHAPE)

The clinician elected to use pictures from the *Bankson-Bernthal Test of Phonology* to assist in the collection of the speech sample. Nonstandardized techniques were used to analyze the speech sample.

6. **Related Assessments.** In addition to the articulation and phonological assessment, the clinician performed a parent interview, a hearing screening, a complete language evaluation, and an oral-mechanism evaluation.

D. Analysis (Chapter 5)

The following assessment options were considered (the order of assessments reflects their presentation in Chapter 5 and does not reflect the order in which they were performed):

Severity or intelligibility

Age norms

Better abilities

Related analyses

1. **Severity or Intelligibility.** The major clinical options were percentage of consonants correct, calculation of percentage of development, and clinical judgment scales of severity and intelligibility. The clinician selected a clinical judgment scale of severity. The clinicians judgment was that Robert was moderately delayed in articulation and phonological development compared to his chronological age.

2. **Age Norms.** The major clinical options were phonetic inventories, error patterns, and consonant and consonant clusters.

   a. **Phonetic Inventories.** This analysis was not performed because Robert's articulation and phonological development proved more advanced than that of clients who typically benefit from analysis of phonetic inventories.

   b. **Error Patterns.** The results of the error probes indicated the following error patterns: Fronting, Cluster Reduction, Final Consonant Deletion, and Stopping. Robert's speech was largely restricted to syllables that were V, CV, and VCV. Robert's consonants were mainly stops and glides. The analysis of the error probes indicated that Fronting occurred on 3 out of 10 words

(30%), Cluster Reduction occurred on 9 out of 10 words (90%), and Final Consonant Devoicing and Stopping occurred on 4 out of 10 words (40%).

c. Consonants and Consonant Clusters. The consonants and consonant clusters that Robert produced correctly were similar to those of a child near 3 years of age.

3. **Better Abilities.** The clinical options were stimulability, key environments, and key words. The clinical options for stimulability testing were sound probes (Appendx 4B), error probes (Appendix 4C), or stimulability probes (Appendix 5O). The clinician selected the error probes, because these probes had already been used with Robert and, thus, were readily available. Robert was found to be stimulable for [k], [f], [s], and word-final [d]. The analysis revealed no key environments and several key words.

4. **Related Analyses.** The clinical options were acquisition strategies, developmental age, and dialect. The acquisition strategies and developmental age analyses were not performed because Robert's articulation and phonological development was beyond that of clients who benefit most from acquisition strategy analyses, and results of the language assessment indicated age-appropriate abilities in language comprehension. Robert's family spoke Hawaiian Creole. The dialect assessment (see Appendix 5S) indicated pronunciation of [t] and [d] for interdental fricatives. This was not considered evidence of an articulation and phonological disorder.

E. Treatment (Chapter 6)

Robert was accepted into treatment in a community speech-language program. Because the clinical options for clients in Stages 2 and 3 are generally similar, this section is more abbreviated than previous sections.

1. **Purpose.** Articulation and phonological care focused on eliminating errors affecting classes of sounds.

2. **Long-term Goals.** The long-term treatment goal for Robert was for articulation and phonological development to be commensurate with his chronological age. A second long-term treatment goal was to facilitate parent education and training.

3. **Short-term Goals.** If Robert had been either a younger preschooler or a child with a more severe articulation and phonological disability, the treatment options would have been the same as for Mary. For clients of Robert's age and general level of disability the options for short-term goals were: (1) reduce or eliminate errors affecting classes of speech elements, (2) facilitate speech in phrases and sentences, and (3) encourage use of speech in settings outside the home. The clinician selected to reduce or eliminate errors affecting classes of speech elements. Within this option, the clinical choices were to utilize either a distinctive feature or error pattern approach. The clinician selected an error pattern approach. The first error patterns selected for treatment were Fronting, Final Consonant Devoicing, and Stopping. Consonant Cluster Reduction was not selected as an early short-term treatment goal because Robert displayed limited success producing sounds affected by that error.

4. **Selecting Treatment Targets.** The clinical options were to select treatment targets that were in key words or that were emerging, stimulable, or both. The clinician elected to treat key words and treatment targets that were both emerging and stimulable, but did not exclude potential treatment targets that met one or the other criteria.

5. **Most and Least Knowledge Methods.** The options that the clinician considered were to select treatment targets most like the client's existing sounds (most knowledge method) or treatment targets least like the client's existing sounds (least knowledge method). The clinician selected the latter option, hoping this would improve the likelihood that Robert would generalize treatment success to untreated sounds.

6. **Number of Treatment Targets.** The clinical options were to train wide or train deep. The clinician selected training wide (three or more treatment targets) to maximize Robert's opportunities to generalize treatment success to untreated sounds.

7. **Changing Treatment Targets.** The clinician's options were flexibility, time, and percentage. Time is an appropriate criterion for changing targets with the vast majority of clients in Stage 3. Those who lack the cognitive and attention abilities needed for a time criterion might be provided treatment using the flexible approach described for Bill and Mary. More advanced clients in Stage 3 with good attention skills may be provided treatment using a percentage criteria. The clinician selected a time criterion for Robert.

8. Linguistic Level to Introduce Treatment Targets. The clinical options are isolated sounds, nonsense syllables, words, and phrases. The clinician selected the word level to help facilitate generalization to other settings and persons.

F. Administrative Decisions (Chapter 6)

The administrative decisions involved session length, group or individual care, length of individual treatment activities, and types of activities. Robert received 30-minute individual sessions three times a week. Individual activities in treatment sessions lasted approximately 10 minutes. The types of activities used during treatment were structured play and drill play.

G. Facilitative Techniques (Chapter 7)

A wide range of clinical options were available, including bombardment, metaphors, descriptions and demonstrations, touch cues, word pairs, techniques to facilitate syllables and words, and facilitative talk (parallel talk, expansions, modeling, and requests for confirmation or clarification).

Treatment was organized in cycles. The error patterns treated in the first cycle were Fronting, Final Consonant Devoicing, and Stopping. From two sounds up to one half of the sounds in an error pattern received treatment in each cycle. When a new treatment target was introduced (e.g., [f]), the client and clinician negotiated to find a metaphor and a touch cue for [f]. Simple descriptions and demonstrations of [f] were also provided.

At the beginning of each session Robert was bombarded with words containing the treatment target. During the session Robert and the clinician engaged in structured play and drill play using word pairs, "talk over" games, and key words to focus on perceptual and production aspects of the treatment target. The clinician used facilitative talk techniques during both perceptual and production activities and during the "play break." The session concluded with auditory bombardment and a review of "what we have learned about our sound today." A home program for Robert's family was included as part of treatment to facilitate generalization to the home and other persons.

H. Assessing Clinical Progress (Chapter 6)

The clinician's primary options were pre- and post-tests, ongoing information gathering, and parent questionnaires. The clinician elected to use a clinical judgment of severity and the probes of error patterns (Appendix 4C) as pre- and post-tests. A parent interview designed to ascertain both the family's knowledge of speech development and their degree of satisfaction with Robert's progress in speech development was also undertaken. Results of the post-tests indicated excellent clinical progress. Like Mary's family, Robert's family demonstrated increased knowledge of speech development in response to questions asked by the clinician and they expressed satisfaction with their child's clinical progress.

V. MAJOR CARE OPTIONS FOR CLIENTS IN STAGE 4

A. The Client: James

James' medical history was remarkable for frequent illnesses during the first year of life. One of these resulted in a hospitalization for failure to thrive. James' developmental history was remarkable for the presence of speech and language delays during preschool and early grade school years. Intervention was provided, and James' language problem appeared to be remediated by the end of the 1st grade. In 3rd grade, when James' class began reading for comprehension, it was discovered that James experienced a learning disability. James was referred by his regular teacher for a re-evaluation of speech when he was 9 years of age. The reason for the referral was described as, "James has trouble with some sounds. He gets some teasing when he says things like *wabbit* for *rabbit*.

B. Legal Basis of Care (Chapter 2)

Like Robert, James was eligible to be considered for intervention under IDEA, which mandates free and appropriate education to all children with handicaps from ages 3 through 21 years. Appropriate education includes a thorough assessment to determine the nature and degree of disability, education tailored to the individual needs of each child, placement in the least restrictive environment, and the provision of supplementary services to help ensure success.

Differential Diagnosis

Would treatment improve if clinicians could make clear differential diagnoses between articulation and phonological disorders? Should a client with an articulation disorder, for example, receive a treatment specifically designed to remediate problems in the speech motor component, and should a client with a phonological disorder receive a different treatment program designed specifically to remediate the phonological component of a language disorder? Or are articulation and phonology so closely interrelated that treatment for both disorders would be the same no matter what the source of the client's problem? Clearly, the conceptual difference between language (phonology) and speech motor control (articulation) is significant, but whether this distinction will lead to differences in treatment remains to be determined.

C. Assessment (Chapter 4)

The assessment consisted of three steps: initial observation, collection of the speech sample, and hypothesis testing. The initial observation occurred during the first minutes after James entered the treatment room while he and the clinician spoke together about James' classes, favorite subjects, and favorite activities. For the elicitation portion of the assessment, the clinician asked James to name pictures from a published assessment instrument. For the hypothesis testing portion of the assessment the clinician asked James to name words that contained sounds James had produced in error during the initial observation and elicitation. Stimulability testing and brief trials using phonetic placement and shaping techniques were also attempted. The word lists used during hypothesis testing are contained in Appendix 4B, and the phonetic placement and shaping techniques are described in Chapter 7.

1. **Sample Size.** The clinician's option was to collect 50 to 100 utterances in the form of sentences, single words, or a combination of both. The major portion of the speech sample was single words.

2. **Transcription System.** The clinician began by transcribing the entire word but changed to simply transcribing sounds in error after

it became clear that James' errors involved late-acquired consonants and consonant clusters. The clinician transcribed using the International Phonetic Alphabet (IPA). The non-English symbols and diacritics expected to be used in the transcription of James' speech included [w]-coloring of [r] and lisped, lateralized, and bladed production of [s] and [z]. Additional symbols and diacritics were included as needed. (See Appendix 3A for recommended extensions of the International Phonetic Alphabet.)

3. **Types of Speech Samples.** The clinician's options for speech samples were spontaneous speech, elicited speech, or a combination of both. During the initial observation the clinician noted errors occurring in James' spontaneous speech; the major portion of the speech sample, however, consisted of single words.

4. **Elicitation Activities.** The clinician selected elicitation activities from those listed in Chapter 4.

5. **Options for Standardized Assessment Instruments.** The following published instruments offer options to assess individual consonants and consonant clusters:

Arizona Articulation Proficiency Scale

Clinical Probes of Articulation Consistency

A Deep Test of Articulation

Edinburgh Articulation Test

Fisher-Logemann Test of Articulation Competence

Goldman-Fristoe Test of Articulation

Lindamood Phoneme Sequencing Program for Reading, Spelling, and Speech (LIPS)

Phonological Awareness Test

Photo Articulation Test

Smit-Hand Articulation and Phonology Evaluation (SHAPE)

The Templin-Darley Tests of Articulation

Test of Minimal Articulation Competence

Test of Phonological Awareness

Weiss Comprehensive Articulation Test

Yopp-Singer Test of Phonemic Segmentation (Yopp-Singer)

The clinician elected to use the *Smit-Hand Articulation and Phonology Evaluation (SHAPE)* for the collection of the speech sample. Nonstandardized techniques were used to analyze the speech sample.

6. **Related Assessments.** In addition to the articulation and phonological assessment, the clinician performed a parent interview, a hearing screening, a complete language evaluation, and an oral-mechanism evaluation.

D. Analysis (Chapter 5)

The following assessment options were considered (the order of assessments reflects their presentation in Chapter 5 and not the order in which they were performed):

Severity or intelligibility

Age norms

Better abilities

Related analyses

1. **Severity or Intelligibility.** The major clinical options were calculation of percentage of development, ACI, and clinical judgment scales of severity and intelligibility. The clinician selected a clinical judgment scale of severity. The clinician's judgment was that James was mildly delayed in articulation and phonological development compared to his chronological age peers.

2. **Age Norms.** The clinical option was consonants and consonant clusters. James produced the following errors: lateral [s] for [s] and [w] for [r]. The sounds [s] and [r] are typically acquired near 3;6 by 50% of children, and [s] is acquired near 5;0 by 75% of children, and [r] is acquired near 6;0 by 75% of children.

3. **Better Abilities.** The clinical options were stimulability, key environments, key words, and phonetic placement and shaping. The clinical options for stimulability testing were the sound probes (Appendix 4B) and stimulability probes (Appendix 5O). The clinician selected

the sound probes, because these probes were already being used with James and, thus, were readily available. James was found to be stimulable for [r], but not for lateral [s]. No key environments or key words were discovered. Both [r] and lateral [s] appeared to be responsive to shaping and phonetic placement techniques.

4. **Related Analyses.** The clinical options were developmental age and dialect. James' developmental level was found to approximate a child about 8 years of age. James spoke a variety of American English that did not require special assessment.

E. Treatment (Chapter 6)

James was accepted into the speech-language treatment program in his school.

1. **Purpose.** Articulation and phonological care focused on eliminating errors affecting late-acquired consonants, consonant clusters, and unstressed syllables in more difficult multisyllabic words.

2. **Long-term Goals.** The long-term treatment goals for James were for articulation and phonological development to be commensurate with his developmental age and to eliminate speech characteristics that affected his quality of life. A concomitant long-term treatment goal was to facilitate parent education.

3. **Short-term Goals.** The options for short-term goals were: (1) facilitate mastery of late-acquired consonants and consonant clusters, (2) teach pronunciation of literary and scientific vocabulary, (3) increase phonological awareness, and (4) encourage use of speech in social and educational settings.

4. **Selecting Treatment Targets.** The clinical options were to select treatment targets in key words, or treatment targets that were emerging, stimulable, or capable of being produced using either phonetic placement or shaping techniques. The clinician selected to treat [r], both because it was stimulable and because the [w] for [r] error led to James being teased. The clinician also elected to treat lateral [s], because a quick session of trial therapy indicated that James could produce [s] through phonetic placement and shaping techniques.

5. **Most and Least Knowledge Methods.** The options the clinician considered were to select treatment targets most like the client's existing sounds (most knowledge method) or treatment targets least like the client's existing sounds (least knowledge method). Only the former option was relevant due to the small number of errors in James' speech.

6. **Number of Treatment Targets.** The clinical options were to train wide or train deep. Perforce, the clinician selected training deep (one or two treatment targets).

7. **Changing Treatment Targets.** The clinician's options were flexibility, time, and percentage. The clinician selected percentage, because James had the attention skills and other cognitive abilities to make this approach feasible.

8. **Linguistic Level to Introduce Treatment Targets.** The clinical options were isolated sounds, nonsense syllables, words, and phrases. The clinician selected the word level to facilitate generalization to other settings and persons. Isolated sounds and nonsense syllables were utilized as prompts when James experienced failure at the word level.

F. Administrative Decisions (Chapter 6)

The administrative decisions involved session length, group or individual care, length of individual treatment activities, and types of activities. Ideally, James would have received individual sessions four to five times a week. Due to caseload size, James received treatment twice a week, once in a group and the other time individually. The group sessions lasted approximately 45 minutes, and the individual session lasted approximately 30 minutes. Activities in both group and individual sessions lasted approximately 10 to 15 minutes. The format for activities was drill play.

G. Facilitative Techniques (Chapter 7)

The options included the full range of facilitative techniques discussed in Chapter 5: bombardment, metaphors, descriptions and demonstrations, touch cues, word pairs, techniques to facilitate syllables and words, facilitative talk (parallel talk, expansions, modeling, and requests for confirmation or clarification), and direct instruction techniques (phonetic placement and shaping). Touch cues and facilitative talk were not selected because the clinician judged that James would find them "immature."

Each treatment target received treatment until it was produced correctly 75% of the time in spontaneous speech, after which the next treatment target received attention until the same percentage criterion was reached. When a new treatment target was introduced (e.g., [r]), the client and clinician negotiated to find a metaphor, and James was taught basic perceptual and production characteristics of the treatment target using simple descriptions and demonstrations. Games involving word pairs and stories containing [r] were used to help James identify the occurrence of the treatment target.

At the beginning of each session, the clinician and James briefly reviewed the previous session. Next, the clinician engaged James in production activities selected from the following list: phonetic placement and shaping games, games involving word pairs, barrier games, and storytelling activities involving names and objects containing the treatment target. During treatment breaks, the clinician listened to observe James' progress in producing the treatment target in spontaneous speech. The session concluded with a brief review of the day's progress. A home program for James' family was included as part of the treatment to facilitate generalization to the home and other persons.

H. Assessing Clinical Progress (Chapter 6)

The clinician's primary options were pre- and post-tests, ongoing information gathering, and parent and client questionnaires. The clinician elected to use a clinical judgment of severity and the error lists presented during treatment as pre- and post-tests. A parent interview designed to ascertain both the family's knowledge of speech development and their degree of satisfaction with James' progress in speech development was also undertaken. Results of the post-tests indicated good clinical progress. James' family demonstrated increased knowledge of speech development in response to questions asked by the clinician and they expressed satisfaction with their son's clinical progress.

REFERENCES

Anthony, A., Bogle, D., Ingram, T., & McIsaac, M. (1971). *The Edinburgh Articulation Test.* Edinburgh, UK: Churchill Livingstone.

Bailey, C., & Chen, M. (1988). Morphological basis of short-term habilitation in *Aplysia*. *Journal of Neuroscience, 8*, 2452–2459.

Bankson, N., & Bernthal, J. (1990). *Quick Screen of Phonology.* Chicago, IL: Riverside Press.

Bankson, N., & Bernthal, J. (1990). *Bankson-Bernthal Test of Phonology.* Chicago, IL: Riverside Press.

Batshaw, M. (Ed.) (1997). *Children with Disabilities (4th Ed).* Baltimore, MD: Paul H. Brookes.

Bauman-Waengler, J. (2000). *Articulatory and Phonological Impairments: A Clinical Focus.* Boston: Allyn and Bacon.

Becker, L., Armstrong, D., & Chan, F. (1986). Dendritic atrophy in children with Down's syndrome. *Annals of Neurology, 20*, 520–526.

Benes, F. (1997). Corticolimbis circuitry and the development of psychopathology during childhood and adolescence. In N. Krasnegor, G. Lyon, & P. Golman-Rakic (Eds), *Development of the prefrontal cortex: Evolution, neurobiology, and behavior.* Baltimore, MD: Paul H. Brookes.

Bernbaum, J., & Hoffman-Williamson, M. (1991). *Primary Care of the Preterm Infant.* St. Louis: CV Mosby/Yearbook.

Bernthal, J., & Bankson, N. (1998). *Articulation and phonological disorders (4th ed.).* Boston: Allyn & Bacon.

Bernhardt, B. (1992). Developmental implications of nonlinear phonological theory. *Clinical Linguistics and Phonetics, 6*, 259–281.

Bernhardt, B., & Stemberger, J. (1998). *Handbook of Phonological Development from the Perspective of Constraint-based Nonlinear Phonology.* San Diego, CA: Academic Press.

Bickerton, D. (1990). *Language & Species.* Chicago, IL: The University of Chicago Press.

Blache, S. (1989). A distinctive feature approach. In N. Creaghead, P. Newman, W. Secord (Eds.), *Assessment and remediation of articulatory and phonological disorders* (pp. 361–382). Columbus, OH: Charles E. Merrill.

Black, J., Isaacs, K., Anderson, B., Alcantara, A., & Greenbough, W. (1990). Learning causes synaprogenesis, whereas motor activity causes angiogenesis, in cerebellar cortex in adult rats. *Proceedings of the National Academy of Sciences, 87*, 5568–5572.

Bleile, K. (1987). *Regressions in the Phonological Development of Two Children*. University of Iowa: Iowa City, Iowa.

Bleile, K. (1988). A note on vowel patterns in two normally developing children. *Clinical Linguistics and Phonetics, 3*, 203–212.

Bleile, K. (1991a). Communication disorders. In M. Batshaw, *Your child has a disability: A complete sourcebook of daily and medical care* (pp. 139–151). Boston, MA: Little, Brown.

Bleile, K. (1991b). *Child Phonology: A Book of Exercises for Students*. San Diego, CA: Singular Publishing Group.

Bleile, K. (Ed.). (1993a). *The Care of Children with Long-term Tracheostomies*. San Diego, CA: Singular Publishing Group.

Bleile, K. (1993b). Children with long-term tracheostomies. In K. Bleile (Ed.), *The care of children with long-term tracheostomies* (pp. 3–19). San Diego, CA: Singular Publishing Group.

Bleile, K. (1996). *Articulation and Phonological Disorders: A Book of Exercises for Students (2nd Ed)*. San Diego, CA: Singular Publishing Group.

Bleile, K. (1998). Speech development in the absence of babbling. In R. Paul (Ed.), *Speech/language connection, vol. 6*. Baltimore, MD: Paul H. Brookes.

Bleile, K. (2002). Evaluating articulation and phonological disorders when the clock is running. *American Journal of Speech-Language Pathology, 11*, 243–249.

Bleile, K., & Burda, A. (2003). Speech disorders in children: Birth related risk factors. In R. Kent (Ed.), *MIT Encyclopaedia of Communicative Disorders*. pp. 188–190. Boston: MIT Press.

Bleile, K., & Hand, L. (1995). Metalinguistics. *Journal of Clinical Linguistics and Phonetics, 1*, 25–28.

Bleile, K., & Miller, S. (1994). Toddlers with medical needs. In J. Bernthal & N. Bankson (Eds.), *Articulatory and phonological disorders in special populations* (pp. 81–100). New York: Thieme.

Bleile, K., Stark R., & Silverman McGowan, J. (1993). Evidence for the relationship between babbling and later speech development. *Clinical Linguistics and Phonetics, 7*, 319–337.

Bleile, K., & Tomblin, J. (1991). Regressions in the phonological development of two children. *Journal of Psycholinguistic Research, 20*, 483–499.

Bleile, K., & Trenary, B. (2002). Language intervention with infants and toddlers. In L. McCormick, D. Fromm Loeb, & R. Schiefelbusch (Ed.), *Supporting children with communication disorders in inclusive settings (2nd Ed.)*. New York, NY: Allyn & Bacon.

Bleile, K., & Wallach, H. (1992). A sociolinguistic investigation of the speech of African American preschoolers. *American Journal of Speech-Language Pathology, 1*, 54–62.

Blodgett, E., & Miller, V. (1989). *Easy Does It for Phonology*. East Moline, IL: Lingui-Systems.

Boysson-Bardies, B., & Vihman, M. (1991). Adaptation to language: evidence from babbling and first words in four languages. *Language, 67*, 297–319.

Bradley, D. (1989). A systematic multiple-phoneme approach. In. N. Creaghead, P. Newman, & W. Secord (Eds.), *Assessment and remediation of articulatory and phonological disorders* (pp. 305–322). Columbus, OH: Charles E. Merrill.

Bricker, P., Bailey, E., & Bruder, M. (1984). The efficacy of early intervention and the handicapped infant: A wise or wasted resource? In M. Wolraich & D. Routh (Eds.), *Advances in developmental and behavioral pediatrics* (pp. 373–423). Greenwich, NY: JAI Press.

Brookshire, R. (1997). *An Introduction to Neurogenic Communication Problems (5th Ed.).* St. Louis, MO: Mosby.

Brown, R. (1973). *A First Language: The Early Stages.* Cambridge, Mass: Harvard University Press.

Bruner, J. (1983). *Child's Talk: Learning to Use Language.* New York: W. W. Norton.

Buell, S., & Coleman, P. (1979). Dendritic growth in the aged human brain and failure of growth in senile dementia. *Science, 206*, 854–856.

Canfield, R., Henderson, C., Cory-Slechta, D., Cox, C., Jusko, T., & Lanphear, B. (2003). Intellectual impairment in children with blood lead concentrations below 10μm per deciliter. *New England Journal of Medicine, 348*, 1517–1526.

Capute, A., Palmer, F., Shapiro, B., Wachtel, R., Schmidt, S., & Ross A. (1986). Clinical Linguistic and Auditory Milestone Scale: Prediction of cognition in infancy. *Developmental Medicine and Child Neurology, 28,* 762–771.

Carrow, E. (1974). *Austin Spanish Articulation Test.* Austin, TX: Teaching Resources Corporation.

Casey, B., Gledd, J., & Thomas, K. (2000). Structural and functional brain development and its relation to cognitive development. *Biological Psychology, 54*, 241–257.

Center on Addiction and Substance Abuse, 1996. *Substance Abuse and the American Woman.* New York: Columbia University.

Chang, F., & Greenbough, W. (1984). Transient and enduring morphological correlates of synaptic efficacy change in rat hippocampal slice. *Brain Research, 309*, 35–46.

Chang, P., Isaacs, K., & Greenbough, W. (1991). Synapse formation occurs in association with the induction of long-term potentiation in two-year-old rat hippocampus in vitro. *Neurobiology of Aging, 12*, 517–522.

Cheng, L. (1987). *Assessing Asian Language Performance: Guidelines for Evaluating Limited-English-proficient Students.* Rockville, MD: Aspen.

Chomsky, N. (1980). *Rules and Representations.* New York: Columbia University Press.

Cole, L., & Taylor, O. (1990). Performance of working class African American children on three tests of articulation. *Language, Speech, and Hearing Services in Schools, 21*, 171–176.

Compton, A., & Hutton, S. (1978). *Compton-Hutton Phonological Assessment.* San Francisco, CA: Carousel House.

Corballis, M. (2002). *From Hand to Mouth: The Origins of Language.* Princeton: Princeton University Press.

Costello, J., & Onstein, J. (1976). The modification of multiple articulation errors based on distinctive feature theory. *Journal of Speech and Hearing Disorders, 31*, 199–215.

Coupe, C., & Hombert, J. (2002). *Language at 70,000 BP: Evidence from sea crossings.* Paper from the 4th Conference on The Evolution of Language, Harvard University.

Cragg, B. (1975). The development of synapses in kitten visual cortex during visual deprivation. *Experimental Neurology, 46*, 445–451.

Creaghead, N., Newman, P., & Secord, W. (1989). *Assessment and Remediation of Articulatory and Phonological Disorders.* Columbus, OH: Charles E. Merrill.

Curtiss, S. (1977). *Genie: A Psycholinguistic Study of a Modern-day "Wild Child."* New York: Academic Press.

Curtiss, S., & de Bode, S. (1999). Age and etiology as predictors of language outcome following hemispherectomy. *Developmental Neuroscience, 21*, 174–181.

Curtiss, S., de Bode, S., & Mathern, G.W. (2001). Spoken language outcomes after hemispherectomy: Factoring in etiology. *Brain and Language, 79*, 379–396.

Curtiss, S., Katz, W., & Tallal, P. (1992). Delay versus deviance in the language acquisition of language-impaired children. *Journal of Speech and Hearing Research, 35*, 373–383.

Dean, E., & Howell, J. (1986). Developing linguistic awareness: A theoretically based approach to phonological disorders. *British Journal of Disorders of Communication, 21*, 223–238.

Dean, E., Howell, J., Hill, A., & Waters, D. (1990). *Metaphon resource pack.* Windsor, UK: NFER-Nelson.

Dean, E., Howell, J., & Waters, D. (1993, November). *Metaphon: An approach to treating children with phonological disorder.* Paper presented to the annual conference of the American Speech-Language-Hearing Association. Anaheim, CA.

Dean, E., Howell, J., Waters, D., & Reid, J. (1995). Metaphon. A metalinguistic approach to the treatment of phonological disorder in children. *Journal of Clinical Linguistics and Phonetics.*

De Bellis, M., Keshavan, M., Clark, D., Casey, B., Giedd, J., Boring, A., Frustaci, K., & Ryan, N. (1999). Developmental traumatology part II: Brain development. *Biological Psychiatry, 45*, 1271–1284.

de Waal, F. (2001). *Tree of Origins.* Cambridge, Mass: Harvard University Press.

Diedrich, W. (1983). Stimulability and articulation disorders. In J. Locke (Ed.), *Seminars in Speech and Language, 4.*

Dodd, B., & Gillon, G. (2001). Exploring the relationship between phonological awareness, speech impairment and literacy. *Advances in Speech-Language Pathology, 3(2)*, 139–147.

Dore J. (1986). The development of conversational competence. In R. Schiefelbusch (Ed.), *Language competence: Assessment and intervention* (pp. 3–59). San Diego, CA: College-Hill Press.

Dunbar, R. (1999). *The Evolution of Culture: An Interdisciplinary View.* R. Dunbar, C. Knight, and C. Power (Eds.). New Brunswick, NJ: Rutgers University Press.

Dunn, L., & Dunn, L. (1981). *Peabody Picture Vocabulary Test—Revised.* Circle Pines, MN: American Guidance Service.

Dyson, A. (1988). Phonetic inventories of 2- and 3-year-old children. *Journal of Speech and Hearing Disorders, 53*, 89–93.

Edwards, M. (1986). *Introduction to Applied Phonetics.* San Diego, CA: College-Hill Press.

Elbert, M., & Gierut, J. (1986). *Handbook of Clinical Phonology: Approaches to Assessment and Treatment.* Austin, TX: Pro-Ed.

Elbert, M., Powell, T., & Swartzlander, R. (1991). Toward a technology of generalization: How many examples are sufficient? *Journal of Speech and Hearing Research, 34*, 81–87.

Elbert, M., Rockman, B., & Saltzman, D. (1980). *The Use of Minimal Pairs in Articulation Training.* Austin, TX: Exceptional Resource.

Elbert, M., Rockman, B., & Saltzman, D. (1982). *The Sourcebook: A Phonemic Guide to Monosyllabic English Words.* Austin, TX: Exceptfonal Resources.

Ellison, P. (2001). *On Fertile Ground: A Natural History of Human Reproduction.* Boston, MA: Harvard University Press.

Elman, J. L., Bates, E. A., Johnson, M. H., Karmiloff-Smith, A., Parisi, D., & Plunkett, K. (1997). *Rethinking Innateness: A Connectionist Perspective on Development.* Cambridge, MA: MIT Press.

Ethnologue (2002). *www.ethnologue.com*

Evans, O. B., & Hutchins, J. B. (2002). Development of the nervous system. In Duane E. Haines (Ed.), *Fundamental Neuroscience,* (pp. 71–89). New York: Churchhill Livingstone.

Fairbanks, G. (1960). *Voice and Articulation Drill Book.* New York: Harper & Row.

Fenson, L., Dale, P., Reznick, J., Thal, D., Bates, E., Hartung, J., Pethick, S., & Reilly, J. (1993). *MacArthur Communicative Development Inventories.* San Diego: Singular Publishing Group.

Ferguson, C., & Farwell, C. (1975). Words and sounds in early language acquisition: English initial consonants in the first fifty words. *Language, 51,* 419–439.

Ferguson, C., & Macken, M. (1983). The role of play in phonological development. In K. Nelson (Ed.), *Child language IV* (pp. 256–282). Hillsdale, NJ: Lawrence Erlbaum.

Fey, M. (1992). Articulation and phonology: Inextricable constructs in speech pathology. *Language, Speech, and Hearing Services in Schools, 23,* 225–232.

Fisher, H., & Logemann, J. (1971). *The Fisher-Logemann Test of Articulation Competence.* Boston, MA: Houghton Mifflin.

Flowers, A. (1990). *The Big Book of Sounds.* Austin, TX: Pro-Ed.

Fluharty, N. (1978). *Speech and Language Screening Test for Preschool Children.* Bingingham, MA: Teaching Resources.

Folkins, J., & Bleile, K. (1990). Taxonomies in biology, phonetics, phonology, and speech motor control. *Journal of Speech and Hearing Disorders, 55,* 596–611.

Fridy, J., & Lemanek, K. (1993). Developmental and behavioral issues. In K. Bleile (Ed.), *The care of children with long-term tracheostomies.* San Diego: Singular Publishing Group, pp. 141–166.

Fudala, B., & Reynolds, W. (1986). *Arizona Articulation Proficiency Scale.* Los Angeles, CA: Western Psychological Services.

Geschwind, N., & Galaburda, A. (1987). *Cerebral Lateralization: Biological Mechanisms, Associations, and Pathologies.* Cambridge Mass: MIT Press.

Gibson, K. R. (1990). New perspectives on instincts and intelligence: Brain size and the emergence of hierarchical mental constructional skills. In S. T. Parker & K. R. Gibson (Eds.) *"Language" and intelligence in monkeys and apes: Comparative developmental perspectives,* Cambridge University Press.

Gierut J. (1989). Maximal opposition approach to phonological treatment. *Journal of Speech and Hearing Disorders, 54,* 9–19.

Gierut J. (1990). Differential learning of phonological oppositions. *Journal of Speech and Hearing Research, 33,* 540–549.

Gierut J. (1992). The conditions and course of clinically induced phonological change. *Journal of Speech and Hearing Research, 35,* 1049–1063.

Godolphin, F. (1942). *The Greek Historians: The Complete and Unabridged Historical Works of Herodotus.* New York: Random House.

Goldman, R., & Fristoe, M. (1986). *Goldman-Fristoe Test of Articulation.* Circle Pines, MN: American Guidance Service.

Goldstein, B. (2000). *Cultural and Linguistic Diversity: Resource Guide for Speech-language Pathologists.* New York: Singular Thomson Learning.

Gordon-Brannan, M. (1994). Assessing intelligibility: Children's expressive phonologies. *Topics in Language Disorders, 14,* 17–25.

Gould, S. (1992). *Ever Since Darwin: Reflections in Natural History.* Norton: New York.

Graham, C., Lam, E., Lee, A., Loader, S., Tan, I., & To, T. (2003). *Pers comm.*

Grunwell, P. (1986). *Phonological Assessment of Child Speech.* Boston, MA: College-Hill Press.

Guyer, B., Strobino, D., & Ventura, S. (1995). Annual summary of vital statistics: 1994. *Pediatrics 96*: 1029–1039.

Handler, S. (1993). Surgical management of the tracheostomy. In K. Bleile (Ed.), *The care of children with long-term tracheostomies* (pp. 23–40). San Diego: Singular Publishing Group.

Hauser, M. (1996). *The evolution of communication.* Cambridge, Mass: MIT Press.

Hedrick, D., Prather, E., & Tobin, A. (1984). *Sequenced Inventory of Communication Development.* Seattle, WA: University of Washington Press.

Hewes, G. (1992). History of glottogonic theories. In J. Wind, B. Chiarelli, B. Bichakjian, & A. Jonker (Eds.), *Language origin: A multidisciplinary approach* (pp. 3–20). Dordrecht, Netherlands: Kluwer.

Highnam, C. (2002). Screening Tool for Phonological Awareness. *Pers comm.*

Highnam, C. (2003). *Pers comm.*

Hockett, C. (1960). The origin of speech. *Scientific American, 203,* 88–111.

Hodson, B. (1985). *Computer Analysis of Phonological Processes: Version 1.0.* [Computer program]. Danville, IL: Interstate Publishers and Printers.

Hodson, B. (1986a). *Assessment of Phonological Processes—Revised.* Danville, IL: Interstate Publishers and Printers.

Hodson, B. (1986b). *The Assessment of Phonological Processes—Spanish.* San Diego, CA: Los Amigos Association.

Hodson, B. (1989). Phonological remediation: A cycles approach. In N. Creaghead, P. Newman, & W. Secord (Eds.), *Assessment and remediation of articulatory and phonological disorders* (pp. 323–333). Columbus, OH: Charles E. Merrill.

Hodson, B. (1994a). Foreword. *Topics in Language Disorders, 14,* vi–viii.

Hodson, B. (1994b). Becoming intelligible, literate, and articulate. *Topics in Language Disorders, 14,* 1–16.

Hodson, B., & Paden, E. (1991). *Targeting Intelligible Speech.* Austin, TX: Pro-Ed.

Hoffman, P., Schuckers, G., & Daniloff, R. (1989). *Children's Phonetic Disorders: Theory and Treatment.* Boston: Little, Brown.

Huttenlocher, R. (1991). Dendritic and synaptic pathology in mental retardation. *Pediatric Neurology, 7,* 79–85.

Infant Health and Development Program. (1990). A multisite, randomized trial. *Journal of the American Medical Association, 263,* 3035–3042.

Ingram, D. (1975). Surface contrast in children's speech. *Journal of Child Language, 2,* 287–292.

Ingram, D. (1986). Explanation and phonological remediation. *Child Language Teaching and Therapy, 2,* 1–19.

Ingram, D. (1989). *Phonetic disability in children*. New York: American Elsevier.

Ingram, D. (1994). Articulation testing versus conversational speech sampling: A response to Morrison and Shriberg (1992). *Journal of Speech and Healing Disorders, 37*, 935–936.

International Clinical Phonetics and Linguistics Association. (1992). Recommended phonetic symbols: Extensions to the IPA. *Clinical Linguistics and Phonetics, 6*, 259–261.

International Clinical Phonetics and Linguistics Association. (1992). The international phonetic alphabet (revised to 1989). *Clinical Linguistics and Phonetics, 6*, 262.

Irwin, J., & Weston, A. (1975). The paired-stimuli monograph. *Acta Symbolica, 6*, 1–76.

Jacobs, B., Schall, M., & Scheibel, A. (1993). A quantitative dendritic analysis of Wernicke's area II. Gender, hemispheric, and environmental factors. *Journal of Comparative Neurology, 237*, 97–111.

Jay, V., Chan, F-W, & Becker, L. (1990). Dendritic arborisation in the human fetus and infant with trisomy 18 syndrome. *Developmental Brain Research, 54*, 291–294.

Judd, J. S. (1990). *Neural Network Design and the Complexity of Learning*. Cambridge, MA: MIT Press.

Jusczyk, P. (1992). Developing phonological categories from the speech signal. In C. Ferguson, L. Menn, & C. Stoel-Gammon (Eds.), *Phonological Development: Models Research, Implications*. Timonium, MD: York Press, pp. 17–64.

Kehoe, M. (1997). Stress error patterns in English-speaking children's word productions. *Clinical Lingistics and Phonetics, 11*, 389–409.

Kent, R., & Forner, L. (1980). Speech segment durations in sentence recitations by children and adults. *Journal of Phonetics, 8*, 157–168.

Kent, R., Miolo, G., & Bloedel, S. (1994). Children's Speech Intelligibility Test. *American Journal of Speech-Language Pathology, 3*, 81–95.

Kent, R., & Murray, A. (1982). Acoustic features of infant vocalic utterances at 3, 6, and 9 months. *Journal of the Acoustical Society of America, 72*, 353–365.

Khan, L., & Lewis, N. (1986). *The Khan-Lewis Phonological Analysis*. Circle Pines, MN: American Guidance Service.

Killackey, H. (1995). Evolution of the human brain: A neuroanatomical perspective. In M. Gazzaniga (Ed.), *The cognitive neurosciences*. Cambridge, Mass: The MIT Press.

Kitley, D., & Buzby-Hadden, J. (1993). Legal rights to education services. In K Bleile (Ed.), *The care of children with long-term tracheostomies* (pp. 187–202). San Diego, CA: Singular Publishing Group.

Kitto, H. D. F. (1951). *The Greeks*. London: Penguin Books.

Khoury-Ghata, V. (2003). Words. *The New Yorker*, Feb 10, p. 99.

Knutson, J., & Sullivan, P. (1983). Communicative disorders as a risk factor in abuse. *Topics in Language Disorders, 13*, 1–14.

Krasnegor, N., Reid Lyon, G., & Goldman-Rakic, P. (Eds.) (1997). *Development of the Prefrontal Cortex*. Baltomore, MD: Paul H. Brookes.

Kretschmann, H., Kammradt, G., Krauthausen, I., Sauer, B., & Wingert, F. (1986). Brain growth in man. *Bibliography of Anatomy, 28*, 1–26.

Ladefoged, P. (2001). *Vowels and Consonants*. Cambridge, Mass: Blackwell.

Lai, C., Fisher, S., Hurst, J., Vargha-Khadem, F., & Monaco, A. (2001). A forkhead-domain gene is mutated in severe speech and language disorder. *Nature, 413*, 519–523.

Leinonen-Davies, E. (1988). Assessing the functional adequacy of children's phonological systems. *Clinical Linguistics and Phonetics, 2*, 257–270.

Leonard, L. (1985). Unusual and subtle behavior in the speech of phonologically disordered children. *Journal of Speech and Hearing Disorders, 50*, 4–13.

Lepore, E., & Pylyshyn, Z. (1999). *What Is Cognitive Science?* Malden, MA: Blackwell.

Lieberman, P. (1984). *The Biology and Evolution of Language*. Cambridge, Mass: Harvard University Press.

Lieberman, P. (1999). *http://www.arts.uwa.edu.au/LingWWW/LIN102_99/Notes/origin.html*

Lindamood, P., & Lindamood, P. (1998). *Lindamood Phoneme Sequencing Program for Reading, Spelling, and Speech*. Austin, TX: Pro-Ed.

Liston, C., & Kagan, J. (2002). Memory enhancement in early childhood. *Nature, 419*, 896.

Locke, J. (1983a). Clinical phonology: The explanation and treatment of speech sound disorders. *Journal of Speech and Hearing Disorders, 48*, 339–341.

Locke, J. (1983b). *Phonological acquisition and change*. New York: Academic Press.

Locke, J., & Pearson, D. (1992). Vocal learning and the emergence of phonological capacity: A neurobiological approach. In C. Ferguson, L. Menn, & C. Stoel-Gammon (Eds.), *Phonological development: Models, research, implications* (pp. 91–130). Timonium, MD: York Press.

Long, S., & Fey, M. (1994). *Computerized Profiling* [Computer program]. Austin, TX: The Psychological Corporation.

Lowe, R. (1986). *Assessment Link Between Phonology and Articulation*. East Moline, IL: LinguiSystems.

Lowe, R. (1994). *Phonology: Assessment and Intervention Applications*. Baltimore, MD: Williams & Wilkins.

Lyons, D. (1994). *The effects of Hawaiian Creole on speech and language assessments*. Unpublished master's project, Division of Speech Pathology and Audiology, University of Hawaii, Honolulu.

Madison, C. (1979). Articulation stimulability review. *Language, Speech, and Hearing Services in Schools, 10*, 185–190.

Mantovani, J., & Powers, J. (1991). Brain injury in premature infants: Patterns on cranial ultrasound, their relationship to outcome, and the role of developmental intervention in the NICU. *Infants and Young Children, 4*, 20–32.

Marks, J. (2002). *What it means to be 98% chimpanzee*. Berkeley: University of California Press.

Marler, P. (1998). Animal communication and human language. In N. Jablonski and L. Aiello (Eds), *The Origin and diversification of language*. San Francsco, CA: California Academy of Sciences.

Mason, R., & Wickwire, N. (1978). Examining for orofacial variations. *Communique, 8*, 2–26.

Masterson, J., & Pagan, F. (1994). *The Macintosh Interactive System for Phonological Analysis* [Computer program]. San Antonio, TX: The Psychological Corporation.

Mattes, L. (1993). *Spanish Articulation Measures*. Oceanside, CA: Academic Communication Associates.

Mayr, E. (2001). *What Evolution Is*. New York: Basic Books.

McCabe, R., & Bradley, D. (1975). Systematic multiple phonemic approach to articulation therapy. *Acta Symbolica, 6*, 1–18.

McDonald, E. (1964). *Articulation Testing and Treatment: A Sensory-motor Approach*. Pittsburgh, PA: Stanwix House.

McDonald, E. (1968). *Screening Deep Test of Articulation.* Pittsburgh, PA: Stanwix House.

McDonald, E. (1964). *A Deep Test of Articulation.* Pittsburgh, PA: Stanwix House.

McLeod, S. (2003). General trends and individual differences: Perspectives on normal speech development. In S. P. Sohov (Ed.), *Advances in Psychology Research (Vol. 22,* pp. 189–202). New York: Nova Science.

McLeod, S. (2002). Part I: The plethora of available data on children's speech development. *ACQuiring Knowledge in Speech, Language and Hearing, 4,* 141–147.

McLeod, S., van Doorn, J., & Reed, V. A. (2002). Typological description of the normal acquisition of consonant clusters. In F. Windsor, L. Kelly, & N. Hewlett (Eds.), *Themes in Clinical Phonetics and Linguistics* (pp. 185–200). Hillsdale, NJ: Lawrence Erlbaum.

McLeod, S., van Doorn, J., & Reed, V. A. (2000). The challenges of discerning the link between perception and production in young children's speech. C. Lind (Ed.), *Proceedings of the National Australia Speech Pathology Conference.* Melbourne, Australia: Speech Pathology Australia.

McLeod, S., van Doorn, J., & Reed, V. A. (2001a). Normal acquisition of consonant clusters. *American Journal of Speech-Language Pathology, 10,* 99–110.

McLeod, S., van Doorn, J., & Reed, V. A. (2001b). Consonant cluster development in two-year-olds: General trends and individual difference. *Journal of Speech, Language, Hearing Research, 44,* 1144–1171.

McReynolds, L., & Bennett, S. (1972). Distinctive feature generalization in articulation training. *Journal of Speech and Hearing Disorders, 37,* 462–470.

McReynolds, L., & Engmann, D. (1975). *Distinctive Feature Analysis of Misarticulations.* Baltimore, MD: University Park Press.

McReynolds, L., & Kearns, K. (1983). *Single-subject experimental designs in communication disorders.* Baltimore, MD: University Park Press.

Menn, L. (1976). *Pattern, control and contrast in beginning speech: A case study in the development of word form and word function.* Unpublished doctoral dissertation, University of Illinois, Champagne-Urbana.

Mercader, J., Panger, M., & Boesch, C. (2002). Excavation of a chimpanzee stone tool site in the African rain forest. *Science, 296,* May 24, 1452–1455.

Metz, S. (1993). Ventilator assistance. In K. Bleile (Ed.), *The care of children with long-term tracheostomies* (pp. 41–55). San Diego, CA: Singular Publishing Group.

Miller, J. (1992). Lexical development in young children with Down syndrome. In R. Chapman (Ed.), *Processes in language acquisition and disorders* (pp. 202–216). Philadelphia, PA: Mosby Year Book.

Milner, P. M. (1999). *The Autonomous Brain: A Neural Theory of Attention and Learning.* Mahwah, NJ: Lawrence Erlbaum Associates.

Morrison, J., & Shriberg, L. (1992). Articulation testing versus conversational speech sampling. *Journal of Speech and Hearing Disorders, 35,* 259–273.

Morrison, J., & Shriberg, L. (1992). Response to Ingram letter. *Journal of Speech and Hearing Disorders, 37,* 936–937.

National Geographic. (1989, October [1889]): Did Neanderthals speak? New bone of contention.

Nemoy, E., & Davis, S. (1954). *The Correction of Defective Consonant Sounds.* Magnolia, MA: Expression.

Neville, H. (1991). Neurobiology of cognitive and language processing: effects of early experience. In K. R. Gibson & A. C. Peterson (Eds.), *Brain maturation and cognitive development*, Amsterdam: Aladine de Gruyter Press.

Office of Scientific and Health Reports (1988). *Developmental Speech and Language Disorders: Hope through Research* (NIH Publication No. Pamphlet 88-2757). Bethesda, MD: National Institute of Neurological and Communicative Disorders and Stroke.

Ojemann, J. (1991). Cortical organization of language. *Journal of Neuroscience, 11*, 2281–2287.

Oller, K. (1980). The emergence of the sounds of speech in infancy. In G. Yeni-Komshian, J. Kavanagh, & C. Ferguson (Eds.), *Child phonology: Production* (pp. 93–112). New York: Academic Press.

Oller, K. (1992). Description of infant vocalizations and young child speech: Theoretical and practical tools. *Seminars in Speech and Language, 13*, 178–192.

Oller, K., & Delgado, R. (1990). *Logical International Phonetic Programs* [Computer program]. Miami, FL: Intelligent Hearing Systems.

Parker, F. (1976). Distinctive features in speech pathology: Phonology or phonemics? *Journal of Speech and Hearing Disorders, 41*, 23–39.

Pascallis, O., de Haan, M., & Nelson, C. (2002). Is face processing species specific during the first year of life? *Science, 296*, 1321–1323.

Passingham, R. (1982). *The Human Primate*. San Francisco, CA: Freeman.

Paul, R. (1991). Profiles of toddlers with slow expressive language. *Topics in Language Disorders, 11*, 1–13.

Paul, R. (2001). *Language Disorders from Infancy Through Adolescence: Assessment and Intervention*. St. Louis, MO: Mosby.

Paul, R., & Shriberg, L. (1982). Associations between phonology and syntax in speech-delayed children. *Journal of Speech and Hearing Research, 25*, 536–547.

Pendergast, K., Dickey, S., Selmar, T., & Soder, A. (1969). *Photo Articulation Test*. Danville, IL: Interstate Publishers and Printers.

Peters, A. (1977). Language learning strategies: Does the whole equal the sum of the parts? *Language, 53*, 560–573.

Peters, A. (1983). *The Units of Language Acquisition*. New York: Cambridge University Press.

Pinker, S. (1995). *The Language Instinct: How the Mind Creates Language*. New York: HarperPerennial.

Powell, T. (1991). Planning for phonological generalization: An approach to treatment target selection. *American Journal of Speech-Language Pathology, 1*, 21–27.

Powell, T., Elbert, M., & Dinnsen, D. (1991). Stimulability as a factor in phonological generalization of misarticulating preschool children. *Journal of Speech and Hearing Research, 34*, 1318–1328.

Proctor, A. (1989). Stages of normal noncry vocal development in infancy: A protocol for assessment. *Topics in Language Disorders, 10*, 26–42.

Quartz, S., & Sejnowski, T. (1997). The neural basis of cognitive development: A constructivist manifesto. *Behavioral and Brain Sciences, 20 (4)*, 537–596.

Ramey, C., & Campbell, F. (1984). Preventive education for high-risk children: Cognitive consequences of the Caroline Abecedarian Project. *American Journal of Mental Deficiency, 88*, 515.

Ray, J. (in preparation). Phonological processes in Hindi-English bilingual children.

Robb, M., & Bleile, K. (in press). Consonant inventories of young children from 8 to 25 months. *Clinical Linguistics and Phonetics.*

Robb, M., & Bleile, K. (1994). Consonant inventories of young children from 8 to 25 months. *Clinical Linguistics and Phonetics, 8,* 295–320.

Robertson, C., & Salter, W. (1997). *The Phonological Awareness Test.* East Moline, IL: LinguiSystems.

Sander, E. (1972). When are speech sounds learned. *Journal of Speech and Hearing Disorders, 37,* 55–63.

Schade, J. P., & van Groenigen, W. B. (1961). Structural organization of the human cerebral cortex. I. Maturation of the middle frontal gyrus. *Acta Anatomica, 47,* 72–111.

Scheibel, A. B. (1993). Dendritic structure and language development. In B. de Boysson-Bardies (Ed.), *Developmental neurocognition: Speech and face processing in the first year of life,* Kluwer Academic Publishers.

Schoenborn, C., & Marano, M. (1989). *Current Estimates from the National Health Interview Survey, United States.* National Center for Health Statistics. Vital and Health Statistics, Series 10, No. 173. DHHS Pub. No. (PHS) 89-1501. Public Heath Service, Washington, DC: Government Printing Office.

Scollon, R. (1976). *Conversations with a One Year Old: A Case Study of the Developmental Foundation of Syntax.* Honolulu: The University Press of Hawaii.

Schwartz, R. (1988). Phonological factors in early lexical acquisition. In M. Smith & J. Locke (Eds.), *The emergent lexicon: The child's development of a linguistic vocabulary* (pp. 185–222). New York: Academic Press.

Schwartz, R., & Leonard, L. (1982). Do children pick and choose: An examination of phonological selection and avoidance in early lexical acquisition. *Journal of Child Language, 9,* 319–336.

Secord, W. (1981a). *Clinical Probes of Articulation Consistency.* San Antonio, TX: The Psychological Corporation.

Secord, W. (1981b). *Test of Minimal Articulation Competence.* San Antonio, TX: The Psychological Corporation.

Shanahan, 2002. *New Yorker,* October 14 & 21st, 173.

Shaywitz, B., Shaywitz, S., Pugh, K., Mencl, W., Fulbright, R., Skudlarski, P., Constable, R., Marchione, K., Fletcher, J., Lyon, G., & Gore, J. (2002). Disruption of posterior brain systems for reading in children with developmental dyslexia. *Biological Psychiatry, 52, 2,* 101–110.

Shelton, R., & McReynolds, L. (1979). Functional articulation disorders: Preliminaries to treatment. In N. Lass (Ed.), *Introduction to communication disorders* (pp. 263–310). Englewood Cliffs, NJ: Prentice-Hall.

Shewan, C. (1988).1988 omnibus survey: Adaptation and progress in times of change. *Asha, 30,* 27–30.

Shine, R. (1989). Articulatory production training: A sensory-motor approach. In N. Creaghead, P. Newman, & W. Secord (Eds.), *Assessment and remediation of articulatory and phonological disorders* (pp. 355–359). Columbus, OH: Charles E. Merrill.

Shriberg, L. (1986). *Programs to Examine Phonetic and Phonologic Evaluation Records: Version 4.0.* [Computer program]. Hillsdale, NJ: Lawrence Erlbaum.

Shriberg, L. (1993). Four new speech and prosody-voice measures for genetics research and other studies in developmental phonological disorders. *Journal of Speech and Hearing Research, 36,* 105–140.

Shriberg, L., & Kent, R. (1982). *Clinical Phonetics.* New York: John Wiley.

Shriberg, L., & Kwiatkowski, J. (1980). *Natural Process Analysis.* New York: John Wiley.

Shriberg, L., & Kwiatkowski, J. (1982). Phonological disorders III: A procedure for assessing severity of involvement. *Journal of Speech and Hearing Disorders, 47,* 256–270.

Shriberg, L., & Kwiatkowski, J. (1983). Computer-assisted natural process analysis (NPA): Recent issues and data. In J. Locke (Ed.), *Seminars in Speech and Language, 4,* 397.

Shriberg, L., & Kwiatkowski, J. (1988). A follow-up study of children with phonologic disorders of unknown origin. *Joumal of Speech and Hearing Disorders, 53,* 144–155.

Silverman McGowan, J., Bleile, K., Fus, L., & Barnas, E. (1993). Communication Disorders. In K. Bleile (Ed.), *The care of children with long-term tracheostomies* (pp. 113–140). San Diego, CA: Singular Publishing Group.

Silverman McGowan, J., Kerwin, M., & Bleile, K. (1993). Oral-motor and feeding problems. In K. Bleile (Ed.), *The care of children with long-term tracheostomies* (pp. 89–112). San Diego, CA: Singular Publishing Group.

Simonds, R. J., & Scheibel, A. B. (1989). The postnatal development of the motor speech area: A preliminary study. *Brain and Language, 37,* 42–58.

Shilovskaya, A. (2003). *Pers comm.*

Slater, S. (1992). Portrait of the professions. *Asha, 34,* 61–65.

Smit, A., Hand, L., Frelinger, J., Bernthal, J., & Byrd, A. (1990). The Iowa articulation norms project and its Nebraska replication. *Journal of Speech and Hearing Disorders, 55,* 779–798.

Smit, A., & Hand, L. (1997). *Smit-Hand Articulation and Phonology Evaluation.* Los Angeles, CA: Western Psychological Services.

Smit, A. (2003). *Articulation and Phonology Resource Guide.* New York: Thomson Delmar Learning.

Smit, A. (2003). *Articulation and Phonology Resource Guide for School-age Children and Adults.* New York: Thomson Delmar Learning.

Snow, C. (1984). Parent-child interaction and the development of communicative ability. In R. Schiefelbusch & J. Pickar (Eds.), *The acquisition of communication competence* (pp. 69–108). Baltimore, MD: University Park Press.

Snow, C., & Goldfield, B. (1983). Turn the page please: Situation-specific language acquisition. *Journal of Child Language, 10,* 551–569.

Sowell, E., Dells, D., Stiles, T., & Jernigan, J. (2001). *Journal of the International Neuropsychological Society, 7,* 312.

Stark, R. (1980). Stages of speech development in the first year of life. In G. Yeni-Komshian, J. Kavanagh, & C. Ferguson (Eds.), *Child phonology. Production* (pp. 73–92). New York: Academic Press.

Stark, R., Bleile, K., Brandt, J., Freeman, J., & Vining, E. (1995). Speech-language outcomes of hemispherectomy in children and young adults. *Brain and Language, 51,* 406–421.

Stoel-Gammon, C. (1985). Phonetic inventories, 15–24 months: A longitudinal study. *Journal of Speech and Hearing Research, 28,* 505–512.

Stoel-Gammon, C., & Dunn, C. (1985). *Normal and disordered phonology in children.* Baltimore, MD: University Park Press.

Stoel-Gammon, C. (1987). Phonological skills of 2-year-olds. *Language, Speech, and Hearing Services in Schools, 18,* 323–329.

Task Force on Health Care. (1993). Task force on health care report. *Asha, 35,* 53–54.

Taylor, O., & Peters-Johnson, C. (1986). Speech and language disorders in Blacks. In O. Taylor (Ed.), *Nature of communication disorders in culturally and linguistically diverse populations.* San Diego, CA: College-Hill Press.

Teicher, M. (2002). Scars that won't heal: The neurobiology of child abuse. *Scientific American,* ———.

Templin, M., & Darley, F. (1969a). *Templin-Darley Screening Test.* Iowa City: University of Iowa Bureau of Education Research and Service.

Templin, M., & Darley, F. (1969b). *The Templin-Darley Tests of Articulation.* Iowa City: University of Iowa Bureau of Educational Research and Service.

Tetterall, I., & Schwarz, J. (2000). *Extinct Humans.* New York: Westview Press.

Tobias, P. (1987). The brain of Homo habilus: A new level of organization in cerebral evolution. *Journal of Human Evolution, 16,* 741–761.

Topbas, S. (1997). Phonological acquisition of Turkish children: Implications for phonological disorders. *European Journal of Disorders of Communication, 32, 4,* 377–396.

Torgesen, J., & Bryant, B. (1994). *Test of Phonological Awareness.* Austin, TX: Pro-Ed.

Trevathan, W. (1987). *Human Birth: An Evolutionary Perspective.* Aldine de Gruyter.

Turner, R., & Greenbough, W. (1985). Differential rearing effect on rat visual cortex synapses. I. Synaptic and neuronal density and synapses per neuron. *Brain Research, 329,* 195–203.

Tyler, A. (1993, November). *Different goal attack strategies in phonological treatment.* Paper presented to the annual Conference of the American Speech-Language-Hearing Association, Anaheim, CA.

Tyler, A., Edwards, A., & Saxman, J. (1987). Clinical application of two phonologically based treatment procedures. *Journal of Speech and Hearing Disorders, 52,* 393–409.

Tyler, A., Tolbert, L., Miccio, A., Hoffman, P., Norris, J., Hodson, B., Scherz, J., & Bleile, K. (2002). Five views of the elephant: Perspectives on the assessment of articulation and phonology in preschoolers. *American Journal of Speech-Language Pathology, 11,* 213–249.

U.S. Department of Education. Twelfth annual report to Congress on the implementation of The Education of the Handicapped Act. Washington, DC: Government Printing Office.

U.S. Department of Education (1994). *To assure the free appropriate public education of all Americans: Sixteenth annual report to Congress on the implementation of the Individuals with Disabilities Education Act* (ED/OSERS Publication No. 065-000-00700-2). Washington, D.C.: U.S. Government Printing Office.

Vannucci, J. (1994). *Assessment of vocal behaviors during the first year of life.* Unpublished masters' project, Division of Speech Pathology and Audiology, University of Hawaii, Honolulu.

Van Riper, C. (1978). *Speech correction: Principles and methods* (6th ed.). Englewood Cliffs, NJ: Prentice-Hall.

Van Riper, C., & Erickson, J. (1968). Predictive Screening Test of Articulation. *Journal of Speech and Hearing Disorders, 34,* 214–219.

Vargha-Khadem, F., Carr, L., Isaacs, E., Brett, E., Adams, C., & Mishkin, M. (1997). Onset of speech after left hemispherectomy in a nine-year-old boy. *Brain, 120,* 159–182.

Vihman, M. (1996). *Phonological Development: The Origins of Language in the Child.* Cambridge, Mass: Blackwell.

Vihman, M., Ferguson, C., & Elbert, M. (1986). Phonological development from babbling to speech: Common tendencies and individual differences. *Applied Psycholinguistics, 7,* 3–40.

Wallace, K. (1967). *Francis Bacon on the Nature of Man; The Faculties of Man's Soul: Understanding, Reason, Imagination, Memory, Will, and Appetite.* Urbana: University of Illionois Press.

Walsh, S. (1994). *A resource for treatment of articulatory and phonological disorders: Minimally and maximally contrasting word pairs.* Unpublished masters' project. University of Hawaii, Honolulu.

Waterson, N. (1971). Child phonology: A prosodic view. *Journal of Linguistics, 7,* 179–221.

Weiner, F. (1979). *Phonological Process Analysis.* Austin, TX: Pro-Ed.

Weiner, F. (1981). Treatment of phonological disability using the method of meaningful minimal contrast: Two case studies. *Journal of Speech and Hearing Disorders, 46,* 97–103.

Weiner, F. (1986). *Process Analysis: Version 2.0* [Computer program]. State College, PA: Parrot Software.

Weiss, C. (1980). *Weiss Comprehensive Articulation Test.* Chicago, IL: Riverside.

Weiss, C. (1982). *Weiss Intelligibility Test.* Tigard, OR: C. C. Publications.

Weiss, C., Gordon, M., & Lillywhite, H. (1987). *Clinical Management of Articulatory and Phonologic Disorders.* Baltimore, MD: Williams & Wilkins.

Werker, J. & Polka, L. (1993). Developmental changes in speech perception: New challenges and new directions. *Journal of Phonetics, 21,* 83–101.

White, K., Mastrapierl, M., & Casto, G. (1984). An analysis of special education early childhood projects approved by the joint dissemination review panel. *Journal of the Division of Early Childhood, 9,* 11.

Whitmore, K. (2002). The evolution of school-based speech-language services: A half century of change and a new century of practice. *Communication Disorders Quarterly, 23,* 68–76.

Williams, A. L. (2000a). Multiple oppositions: Theoretical foundations for an alternative contrastive intervention approach. *American Journal of Speech-Language Pathology, 9,* 282–288.

Williams, A. L. (2000b). Multiple oppositions: Case studies of variables in phonological intervention. *American Journal of Speech-Language Pathology, 9,* 289–299.

Williams, A. L. (2002, November). Models of assessment and intervention: Phonology in clinical settings. Short course presented at the annual convention of the American Speech-Language-Hearing Association, Atlanta, GA.

Williams, L. (1991). Generalization patterns associated with training least phonological knowledge. *Journal of Speech and Hearing Research, 34,* 722–723.

Williams, L. (1993). Phonological reorganization: A qualitative measure of phonological improvement. *American Journal of Speech-Language Pathology, 2,* 44–51.

Williams, L. (2003). *Speech Disorders Resource Guide for Preschool Children.* New York: Thomson Delmar Learning.

Winfoeld, D. (1981). The postnatal development of synapses in the visual cortex of the rat and the effects of eyelid closure. *Brain Research, 206,* 166–171.

Winitz, H. (1984). *Treating Articulation Disorders.* Baltimore, MD: University Park Press.

Yavas, M., & Lamprecht, R. (1988). Processes and intelligibility in disordered phonology. *Clinical Linguistics and Phonetics, 2,* 329–345.

Yopp, K. (1995). A test for assessing phonemic awareness in young children. *The Reading Teacher, 49,* 20–29.

Zimmerman, I., Steiner, V., & Pond, R. (1992). *Preschool Language Scale 3.* Columbus, OH: Charles E. Merrill.

INDEX